Manual of Thoracic Endoaortic Surgery

Jacques Kpodonu

Manual of Thoracic Endoaortic Surgery

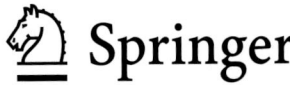 Springer

Jacques Kpodonu, MD
Division of Cardiac and Endovascular
   Surgery
Surgical Director Cardiac Hybrid
   and Endovascular Program
Hoag Heart and Vascular Institute
Hoag Memorial Hospital Presbyterian
One Hoag Drive
Newport Beach, California 92663
Jacques.Kpodonu@Hoaghospital.org

ISBN 978-1-84996-295-7   e-ISBN 978-1-84996-296-4
DOI 10.1007/978-1-84996-296-4
Springer London Dordrecht Heidelberg New York

British Library Cataloguing in Publication Data
A catalogue record for this book is available from the British Library

Library of Congress Control Number: 2010931547

Springer is part of Springer Science+Business Media (www.springer.com)

Foreword

In today's healthcare environment, the real driver is value. Maximizing outcomes and minimizing costs or providing similar outcomes with lower cost in terms of actual numbers or recovery time will dominate our healthcare delivery system. An excellent example of this evolution is in the field of cardiovascular intervention. Dr. Jacques Kpodonu's *Manual of Thoracic Endo-Aortic Surgery* is a most timely and descriptive work in this burgeoning field. It provides an excellent overview of current technology and techniques, plus the endovascular expert can drill down into the details of the devices and technologies described and significantly enhance their knowledge and perspective. Procedural detail, excellent graphics, pertinent imaging studies, and relevant instruction are the mainstays of this text.

The first chapter comprises the key overview and very comprehensively covers the platform – the hybrid OR, the tools, the accessories, and the medium – superb, state-of-the-art imaging modalities required to perform these advanced procedures. The text then moves into more technical details including options and instruction regarding access approaches and potential pitfalls of such. This is followed in ensuing chapters by dissemination of precise information, techniques, and indications for the most popular and utilized grafts including Boston Relay Stent Graft, Cook TX2 Zenith Stent Grafts, as well as the Gore and Medtronic Aortic Stent Grafts. Transitioning from the devices themselves, the ensuing chapters cover challenging clinical problems such as dissections, traumatic aorta injury, and hybrid debranching techniques as well as a chapter on fenestrated and branched graft technology for thoracoabdominal aortic pathology expertly written by an expert in the field Dr. Roselli. Points are well illustrated with case examples. A most essential final clinical chapter covers the identification, treatment, and avoidance of complications. The text is completed with a look into future technologies.

The *Manual of Thoracic Endo-Aortic Surgery* is well organized, flows efficiently, and is well written. It reflects the significant clinical experience of Dr. Kpodonu and embodies his commitment to teaching and education. It is important for any clinician in the field of cardiovascular care to be aware of the therapeutic options and imaging modalities covered in this text. Furthermore, the endo-aortic specialist will benefit most significantly by the technical details elucidated in this publication. This entire field is rapidly evolving and represents a major advance in medical therapy.

Knowledge of current therapeutic options and clinical expertise in delivering these options are essential. This text provides an important element in the foundation for that process.

Newport Beach, California   Aidan A. Raney

Preface

The development of less invasive technologies over the past decade has resulted in a changing paradigm for the management of aortic diseases. Endovascular and hybrid surgical approaches are gradually being adopted by cardiovascular surgeons which has been proven to shorten hospitalization, reduce morbidity and mortality, speed recovery, and hasten return to normal life. Clinical investigations have shown these procedures to be favorable over open surgical techniques in most situations.

Our current training programs have not been designed to easily accommodate the rapid evolution in endovascular technology, 3D imaging modalities, intravascular ultrasound technology, and advanced navigational tools. In an effort to bridge the gap which exists between our training, educational programs, and the technology explosion, it is essential that the cardiovascular surgeon of today and the future will have the fundamental knowledge and skill sets required to adequately understand and incorporate all the latest technology into the practice of aortic surgery.

Although certain limitations currently exist regarding thoracic aortic endografting techniques and their application to thoracic aortic pathologies there is every indication that most thoracic aortic pathologies will be treated with these less invasive procedures in the future. There is no substitute for learning from experience; it is my hope that the Manual of Thoracic Endoaortic Surgery will provide a useful tool for practitioners as they plan and execute treatment of patients with these various thoracic aortic pathologies as well as serve as a useful reference as this segment of the field expands.

Newport Beach, California   Jacques Kpodonu

Acknowledgments

The author would like to thank John Liu of the Division of Information Technology at Hoag Memorial Presbyterian Hospital as well as my esteemed colleagues Aidan A. Raney, Douglas Zusman, and Colin Joyo for their valuable support in putting this manual together. I also would like to acknowledge the staff of Arizona Heart Institute who were instrumental in pioneering many of the techniques described in this manual and finally to the love of my life Tiffany and our two gorgeous children Nathalie and Henri for their unwavering support in bringing this work to completion.

The author would like to acknowledge the following for his contribution to this work: Eric Roselli, MD, Department of Cardiothoracic Surgery, Cleveland Clinic, Cleveland, OH, USA.

Contents

Part XI   Future Technology

Chapter 1
The Cardiovascular Hybrid Room

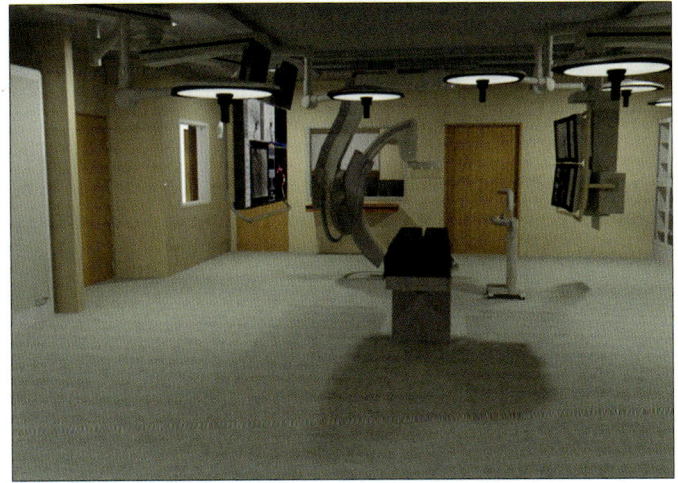

The last few years have seen a paradigm shift in the treatment of cardiovascular-related diseases from once traditional open surgical modalities to the entire cardiovascular tree being amenable to percutaneous interventions. The tremendous advances in transcatheter endovascular procedures currently been applied to the heart and the peripheral vasculature have resulted in a treatment paradigm shift in the care of the cardiovascular patient. These changing winds in the treatment of cardiovascular disease require that a new type of cardiovascular specialist code named the cardiovascular hybrid surgeon be trained to perform to provide seamless care in providing both endovascular and open surgical procedures to this increasingly complex group of patients.[1]

Patient and market forces continue to push for minimally invasive approaches over more traditional open surgical approaches with proven efficacy and long-term treatment benefit. The cardiovascular surgeon of today must be required to adapt to this new technology-driven trend. These minimal invasive procedures or hybrid procedures have resulted in markedly decreased morbidity and mortality of elderly

J. Kpodonu, *Manual of Thoracic Endoaortic Surgery*,
DOI 10.1007/978-1-84996-296-4_1, © Springer-Verlag London Limited 2010

patients who would otherwise be exposed to major operative morbidity and mortality. Currently large areas of traditional cardiac surgery as it stands are rapidly disappearing and have been substituted with less invasive percutaneous techniques. Areas of cardiovascular surgery in which transcatheter techniques are firmly established and are rapidly adapted to treat the whole spectrum of the cardiovascular tree include treatment of coronary artery disease in which coronary revascularization is increasingly being replaced by percutaneous interventions and possibly by the emerging techniques of angiogenesis and related advances in molecular genetics. Thoracic aortic aneurysms are rapidly disappearing from the surgical repertoire and are being treated with endovascular procedures. Here, a true benefit is already being observed when applying this minimally invasive, percutaneous approach in aged, polymorbid patients. Percutaneous techniques are currently used to treat atrial septal defects, patent foramen ovale, patent ductus arteriosus, and coarctation of the aorta. In the developing world, mitral and pulmonary stenosis is not being seen by surgeons: Arrhythmia surgery (Wolff–Parkinson–White syndrome, ventricular ablation, and atrial flutter) is an established domain of electrophysiologically trained interventionists who have also completely taken over the pacemaker and defibrillator implantations, previously the work of cardiac surgeons. Aortic valve stenosis is currently being treated by transfemoral and transapical valve replacement, avoiding the inherent morbidity of cardiopulmonary bypass, aortic manipulation, and prolonged intensive care unit stay with in some cases patients leaving the hospital the next day.

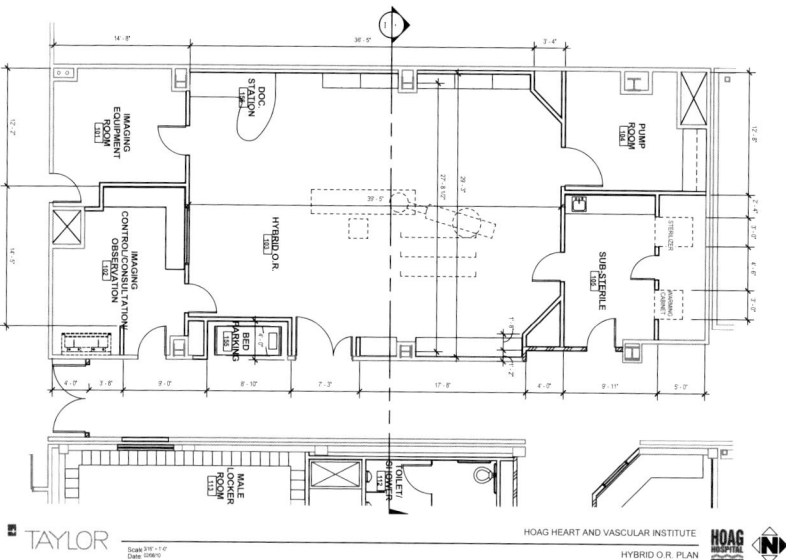

Fig. 1.1 Architectural drawing of a hybrid suite

The ability to provide such cutting-edge technology borders on the availability of a new operative environment known as the hybrid surgical suite (Fig. 1.1).

1.1 The New Operative Environment (The Hybrid Surgical Suite)

A fully integrated interventional suite combines surgical sterility[2–4] with flat-panel cardiovascular imaging, a linked workstation, post-processing, and storage facilities.[5–7] The size of the hybrid room should be of sufficient dimensions to allow anesthesiology facilities needed for full patient monitoring. Furthermore any type of supportive equipment available in the room including equipment for anesthesia, intravascular ultrasound, intra cardiac echochardiogram, transesphageal echochardiogram and rotational angiography as well as endovascular supplies must be able to fit in the room in a seamless fashion irrespective of wether the room is used for an open surgical, hybrid surgical or totally percutaneous procedure. Current peripheral suites are fitted with many interesting features to make certain procedures easier. An on-table duplex ultrasound makes puncturing easy and is a good guide during endovenous laser therapy. The possibility of storing several reference points to which the C-arm can be automatically relocated at any time during the procedure facilitates the management of even extremely complex procedures. It is obvious that routine endovascular and open surgical practice both clearly gain from performance in this dual-capability working environment. For example, classic open bypass creation is immediately controlled on-table. When improvement of inflow or outflow becomes necessary after bypass surgery, balloon dilation with or without additional stent placement can be rapidly performed without dramatically prolonging procedural time. The use of an integrated endovascular suite, however, stretches beyond hybrid procedures and opens doors to new diagnostic and treatment possibilities. Three-dimensional reconstructions generated by integrated CT or rotational angiography can make a real-time visualization of vessel morphology in any direction and improve the visibility of vessel structures. Application of 3D reconstruction during treatment of intracranial aneurysms, for instance, is a must to ensure optimal positioning of catheters, coils, balloons, and stents. An integrated setting means saving time and personnel because more procedures can be completed in the same room by the existing staff without increasing the strain on the team and without relocating equipment or personnel from another department. The hybrid suite should become the one stop shop where patients can get diagnosed and treated in one visit, for less downtime and a speedier recovery. Unique technology in the suite allows doctors across different specialties to work together on a case-by-case scenario, in the best interest of each patient. The most advanced imaging systems available provide quick and detailed information for shorter, more accurate treatment with substantially less X-ray exposure when compared to traditional devices. Complex cases are more easily treated, since the suite is designed to handle both minimally invasive percutaneous, hybrid operations and open surgical procedures.

1.2 Basic Equipment and Design of the Hybrid Endovascular Operating Room

The primary components of the hybrid suite center on intra-operative angiography and fluoroscopy as well as on carefully designed operating tables to accommodate and optimize the usefulness of the radiographic equipment. The hybrid suite imaging system provides superior image quality and higher tube heat capacity and has measurement capabilities capable of simple and complex procedures requiring high resolution. Prices range between (US $1.2 and US $5.0 million) depending on the brand, specifications, ability to provide rotational angiography, addition of a bi-planar system and with integration of various sophisticated imaging modalities like 3D echocardiography, intracardiac ultrasound, intravascular ultrasound, and electromagnetic navigation systems the cost of the room rises.

1.2.1 Size of the Hybrid Operating Room and Radiation

The operating room should ideally be between 550 and 900 square feet (Fig. 1.1), with a minimum clear area of 400–500 square feet. Floor to ceiling height should be at minimum 10 ft to accommodate floor- or ceiling-mounted C-arms capable of rotational angiography for volume rendering 3D CT-like images achieved with advanced biplanar imaging systems (Fig. 1.2). In existing operating rooms, the fixed ceiling-mounted C-arm requires some structural modifications to install the mounting plates and run electrical conduits under the floor to the components. Most states dictate that any operating room with a fixed imaging system must have lead-lined walls. Most

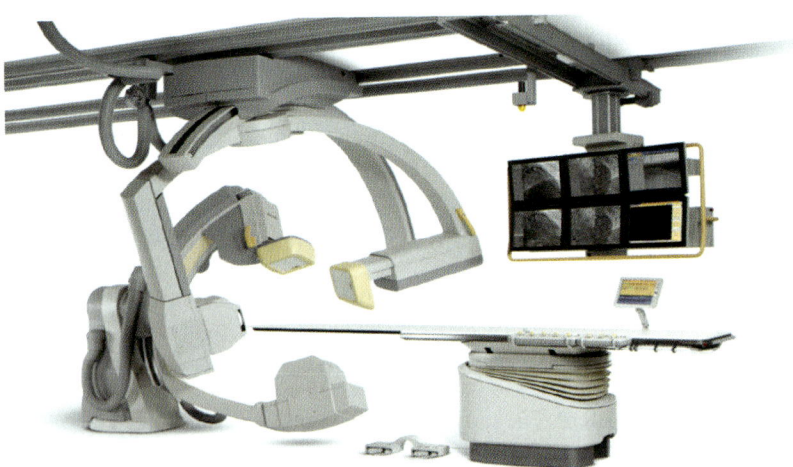

Fig. 1.2 Endovascular suite integrated in the operating room comprising a biplane digital substraction angiography unit with multipurpose surgical capabilities. The Allura Xper FD20 biplanar fixed system by Phillips

standard ORs have leaded covering 0.5 mm which is not sufficient for the radiation dose generated by a fixed unit. Lead-lined walls in the range of 2–3 mm for the fixed units may be needed and may vary from state to state (must see regulations for the state of California). The expense of these constructions/modifications can vary up to $100,000 depending on the original condition of the room, local contracting costs, architect's fees accompanies that market fixed fluoroscopic units usually provide consulting services for such alterations.

As endovascular/cardiovascular hybrid surgical procedures become more complex, the relationship of the C-arm, table, and patient's position becomes even more important. The fluoroscopic unit should be able to move in a horizontal plane from the groin along the course of the vessel with the ability to "snap images on the move." This parallel movement prevents the need for excessive contrast material and greatly expedites the procedure. When a catheter is placed in the brachial artery, the fluoroscopic unit must be capable of rapid movement over the catheter's path from the arm and through the thoracic aorta to the area of ultimate instrumentation. Obstructions from a table or a floor-mounted portable unit that hinder rapid panning over wide anatomic areas limit potential success of the procedure.

1.2.2 Carbon-Fiber Table

To optimize the usefulness of the radiographic equipment, a nonmetallic, carbon-fiber surgical table is available for the interventional techniques.[10] The preferred surgical operating table to accommodate such techniques should be preferably thin but highly stable table and should provide complete clearance beneath a panning X-ray system. The Diethrich IC 2020 Surgical Imaging Table (Fig. 1.3) is a thin carbon-fiber table supported at only one end to provide complete clearance beneath for a panning. The telescoping pedestal allows vertical travel from 28 to 48 in., 20°

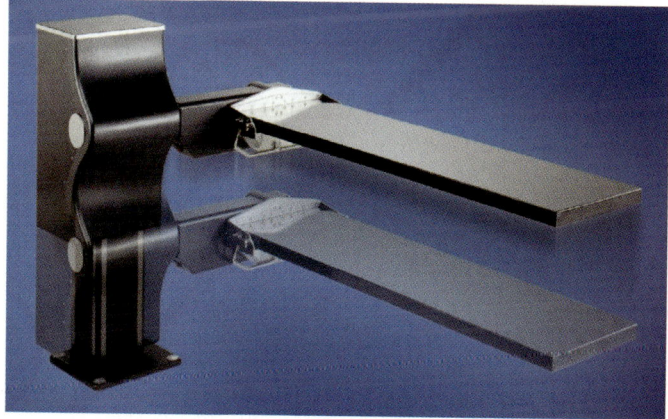

Fig. 1.3 The Diethrich IC 2020 Surgical Imaging Table

side-to-side roll, and 20° Trendelenburg tilt (reverse and standard) which makes it ideal as a surgical operating room. Complete clearance is achieved beneath for unobstructed neck to toe imaging and rapid horizontal panning is achieved with multiple position, height, tilt, and roll adjustments.

1.2.3 Flat Screens and Monitors

The surgeons, the assistants, the anesthesiologists, and the nurses should all have views of all major imaging and monitoring sources. It is therefore suggested that display of all these sources should be available in all four quadrants of an integrated room. A total of four to six ceiling-mounted flat screens as imaging tools for the procedures are necessary. Extreme care should be taken to ensure that these ceiling-mounted flat screens do not collide with operating lights. Monitors for the vital signs of the patient with provision for systemic arterial monitoring, central venous monitoring, and continuous electrocardiographic surveillance is imperative. A large 40 in. flat panel should be available as well as cameras (wall/or in-light).

1.3 Patient Monitoring

The hybrid suite must be equipped for accurate patient monitoring during the procedure; for continuous electrocardiography, surveillance is imperative. Observation of urine output is also essential for cases involving renal arteries and higher abdominal or thoracic aortic segments. Intra-arterial monitoring that includes precise measurement of pressure differentials is also important during performance of these procedures. Space for storage for the special procedure-related equipment such as stents, wires, balloons, and stent grafts, should be available.

1.4 Fluoroscopy and CT Imaging Systems

The imaging quality is dominated by the quality of the fluoroscopy unit available. Available systems can be divided roughly into two categories: portable and fixed C-arm units. Fixed C-arm units could be flooring mounted (Fig. 1.4) or ceiling mounted. There are a number of fixed fluoroscopic units available with various modifications, depending on the manufacturer (e.g., Philips, GE, OEC, Siemens, Toshiba). The image quality of fixed systems is usually superior to portable systems which can be explained by the focal spot sizes of fixed systems being significantly smaller than those of portable units.[8,9] A smaller focal spot size means higher resolution through more line pairs per millimeter. Nevertheless, the latest portable C-arm systems (Fig. 1.5) are able to reach resolutions up to 2.5–3 line pairs per millimeter, values which only could be attained by fixed systems until recently. The monitor resolution of fixed systems differs from portable systems, with the

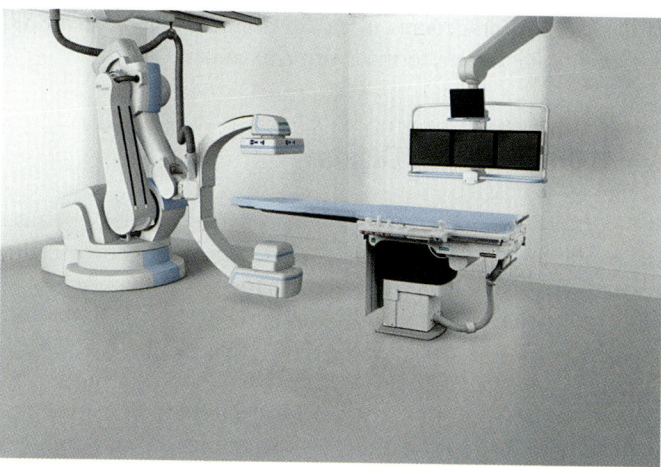

Fig. 1.4 Floor-mounted hybrid surgical system Artis zeego. Multi-axis system by Siemens

monitors of fixed systems usually having twice the lines of resolution as the monitors of portable systems. Portable systems have a smaller generator in order to keep the system "practical" while fixed systems have a large remote generator which provides more power, with better tissue penetration and improved imaging quality. Currently, portable C-arm systems are able to provide sufficient quality for the

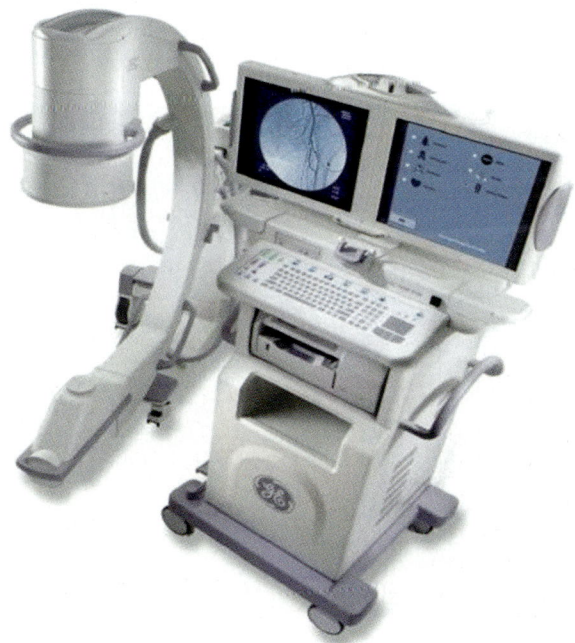

Fig. 1.5 A General Electric OC 9900 mobile fluoroscopic unit

majority of the standard procedures in cardiovascular surgery. However, the more complex procedures are best performed with a fixed unit.

1.5 Image Acquisition and Display

Traditional fluoroscopy provides real-time, high-resolution, low-contrast images in two dimensions through the use of an image intensifier. The development of a flat-panel detector to replace the image intensifier has enabled fluoroscopy to transition into three dimensions, producing a CT-like image (Fig. 1.6). The contrast resolution of CT is approximately 1 Hounsfield unit (HU), whereas the contrast resolution of a CT-like image is around 10 HU. CT fluoroscopy is not meant to replace diagnostic CT but to be used as a tool that will supplement interventional procedures. The ability to acquire data in three dimensions during an intervention has led to the fusion of 3D datasets with the 2D images displayed on typical monitors. In CT rotational angiography which the latest hybrid imaging systems have, the C-arm is used to rapidly rotate, obtaining serial images of the area in question in a radial fashion. The 3D reconstruction can be registered with subsequent real-time fluoroscopic images and projected to offer the clinician the ability to work in three dimensions. The process by which the image is registered and displayed is the subject of considerable research efforts on the part of many imaging equipment manufacturers. Data can be rendered volumetrically and overlaid on the fluoroscopic image, making the anatomy much more identifiable, a fused 2D /3D dataset can be created, or the information can be placed side by side. Further requirements of the suite's imaging system are a processing unit, a workstation, and a central image storage unit. The

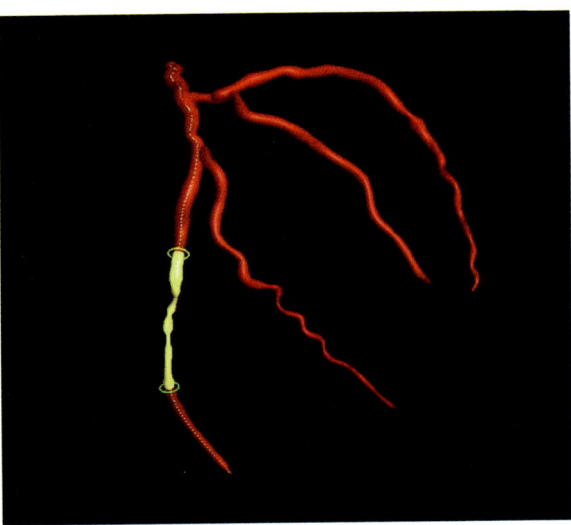

Fig. 1.6 Three-dimensional reconstruction of the left coronary artery in the projection with the least foreshortening performed with rotational angiography

potential of any C-arm equals the weakest link of each of these last three elements. While performing a procedure, smooth and fast graphic abilities are a must. Using large-size, superb-quality images from a C-arm implies that a powerful processing unit is needed. The higher the image quality, the more working memory the processing unit needs. Images from a C-arm are stored in DICOM format files, which can then be used for biometric post-processing, such as quantitative vessel analysis or 3D reconstruction. The higher the quality of the images obtained from the C-arm, the larger the size of the files that have to be processed by the workstation. Advanced imaging using Dynamic 3D Roadmap has significant clinical advantages for applications such as real-time catheter navigation and monitoring coil delivery. The image is dynamic, meaning the 3D roadmap remains displayed even if the C-arc projection, source-to-image distance, and field of view size are changed (Fig. 1.7). The 3D volume automatically follows the orientation of the C-arc in real time, so that users can choose the optimal projection view. This dynamic overlay ensures excellent positioning for catheter navigation during challenging interventions. The dynamic 3D image decreases the number of DSA acquisitions and fluoroscopy time for an examination. The user can also recall roadmap positions to reduce the need to re-mask. This reduces X-ray dose and contrast medium, which can reduce procedure costs. Dynamic 3D Roadmap provides live interventional catheter navigation.

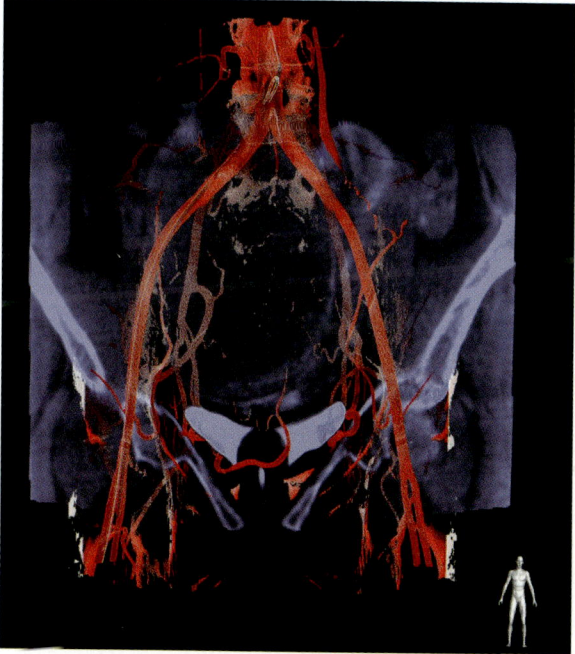

Fig. 1.7 Dynamic 3D Roadmap provides live 3D guidance through tortuous vasculature. It creates an overlay of real-time 2D fluoroscopy images and the 3D reconstruction of the vessel tree

1.6 Other Imaging Modalities

Integration of other imaging modalities like intravascular ultrasound (IVUS) (Fig. 1.8) permits more data acquisition.[11] The explosion of the endovascular revolution with particular application to the aorta has placed new demands on accurate pre-operative and intra-operative imaging to obtain accurate aortic measurements for endovascular stent grafting of the aorta.[12,13] IVUS technology requires that the user be adequately versed in the process of performing the acquisition and interpretation of the images. In patients undergoing cardiac surgery, transesophageal echocardiography and epi-aortic ultrasound have been used to characterize the severity of atherosclerosis within the ascending aorta.[14] Such information has been used to modify surgical technique, altering the location of cannula insertion, the position of aortic cross-clamps, and the placement of saphenous vein grafts, and reducing the risk of dislodging atheromatous debris.

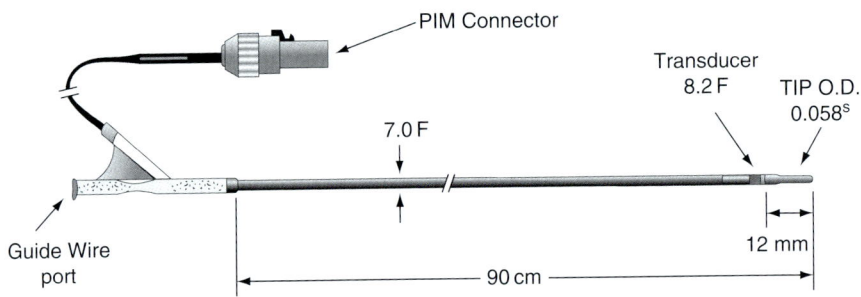

Fig. 1.8 Intravascular ultrasound 0.035 PV catheter system (PIM Connector, patient interface module connector; TIP O.D., tip outer diameter of probe)

1.7 Future Perspectives

Wireless devices would become reality in the near future and would overcome the direct limitations now present due to wire connection points. In a wireless setting, the operating table, C-arm, and other equipment can be rotated a full 360° (and beyond) at any location within the surgical/endovascular suite. Wireless equipment would also save time in case one piece of equipment needs to be repaired. A broken piece of equipment can be temporarily removed from the interventional suite and replaced by a spare. The cardiovascular surgeon or interventionist would not lose valuable operation time, and patients would not need to be put on hold. The technical team would not have to wait for spare parts or specialized tools for a certain repair because the broken piece could easily be shipped to a central repair point. Moreover, this approach would save time and costs related to the mobility of a highly specialized technical team. Integration of robotic and navigational techniques into clinical practice may lead to improved catheter accuracy, stability, and safety in comparison with conventional techniques, while minimizing radiation exposure. By maximizing the use of existing technologies while developing new approaches to treating these challenging cases, we hope that these would lead to improve overall clinical outcomes and further reduce the mortality and morbidity rates associated with managing the cardiovascular patient. It is hoped that as these new fields develop and with increasing experience with these new hybrid methods, we may well be able to maximize the applicability of minimally invasive endovascular and hybrid technology to treat a larger cohort of patients with cardiovascular disease.[15]

References

1. Zhou W, Lin PH, Bush RL, Lumsden AB. Endovascular training of vascular surgeons: have we made progress? *Semin Vasc Surg*. 2006;19:122–126.
2. Eliason JL, Guzman RJ, Passman MA, Naslund TC. Infected endovascular graft secondary to coil embolization of endoleak: a demonstration of the importance of operative sterility. *Ann Vasc Surg*. 2002;16:562–565.
3. Ducasse E, Calisti A, Speziale F, Rizzo L, Misuraca M, Fiorani P. Aortoiliac stent graft infection: current problems and management. *Ann Vasc Surg*. 2004;18:521–526.
4. Nichols RL. The operating room. In: Bennett JV, Brachman PS, Sanford JP, eds. *Hospital Infections*. 3rd ed. Boston, MA: Little, Brown; 1992:461–467.
5. Eagleton MJ, Schaffer JL. The vascular surgery operating room. Development of an up to date vascular room that would meet the up to date demands of the vascular surgery patient and the team. *Endovasc Today*. August 2007;25–30.
6. Goel VR, Ambekar A, Greenburg RK. Multimodality imaging and image-guided surgery. Advances in imaging provide physicians with the confidence to confront procedures previously thought impossible. *Endovasc Today*. March 2008;67–70.
7. Sikkink CJ, Reijnen MM, Zeebregts CJ. The creation of the optimal dedicated endovascular suite. *Eur J Vasc Endovasc Surg*. 2008;35(2):198–204.
8. Mansour MA. Endovascular and minimally invasive vascular surgery. The new operating environment. *Surg Clin North Am*. 1999;79:477–487.
9. Hodgson KJ, Mattos MA, Sumner DS. Angiography in the operating room: equipment, catheter skills and safety issues. In: Yao JST, Pearce WH, eds. *Techniques in Vascular Surgery*. Stamford, CT: Appleton & Lange; 1997:pp. 25–45.
10. Fillinger MF, Weaver JB. Imaging equipment and techniques for optimal intraoperative imaging during endovascular interventions. *Semin Vasc Surg*. 1999;12:315–326.
11. Kpodonu J, Ramaiah VG, Diethrich EB. Intravascular ultrasound imaging as applied to the aorta: a new tool for the cardiovascular surgeon. *Ann Thorac Surg*. 2008;86(4):1391–1398.
12. Garrett HE, Abdullah AH, Hodgkiss TD, et al. Intravascular ultrasound aids in the performance of endovascular repair of abdominal aortic aneurysm. *J Vasc Surg*. 2003;37:615–618.
13. van Essen JA, van der Lugt A, Gussenhoven EJ, et al. Intravascular ultrasonography allows accurate assessment of abdominal aortic aneurysm: an in vitro validation study. *J Vasc Surg*. 1998;27:347–353.
14. Davila-Roman VG, Phillips KJ, Daily BB, et al. Intraoperative transesophageal echocardiography and epiaortic ultrasound for assessment of atherosclerosis of the thoracic aorta. *J Am Coll Cardiol*. 1996;28:942–947.
15. Kpodonu J, Raney AA. The cardiovascular hybrid room a key component for multimodality for hybrid interventions and image guided surgery in the emerging specialty of cardiovascular hybrid surgery. *Interact Cardiovasc Thorac Surg*. 2009;9(4):688–692.

Part I
Accessories Used in Thoracic Endografting

Chapter 2
Balloons Used in Thoracic Aortic Endografting

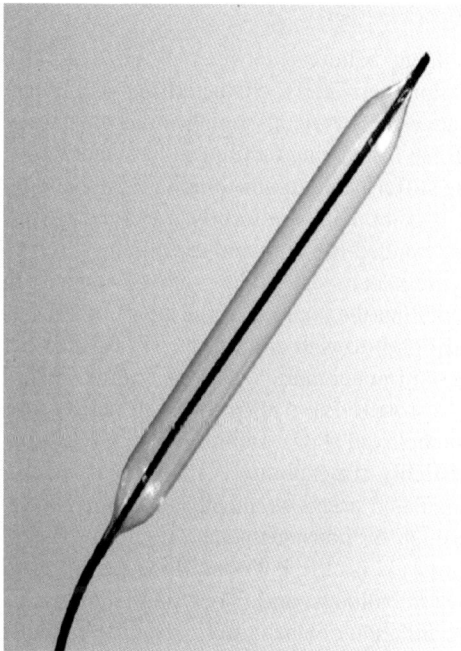

2.1 General Overview

Balloons come in different diameters and lengths and are made from diverse materials polyethylene PE, polyethylene terephthalate PET to give exact or oversized diameters, with various inflation pressures. The pressure needed to inflate the balloon to its manufactured diameter using an inflation device (Fig. 2.1) is measured in atmospheres and referred to as nominal pressure. Balloons are rated for *burst*, using a manufacturing threshold specifying that 1% of all balloons tested burst at this particular pressure. Most of the smaller balloons have a rated burst of between

J. Kpodonu, *Manual of Thoracic Endoaortic Surgery*,
DOI 10.1007/978-1-84996-296-4_2, © Springer-Verlag London Limited 2010

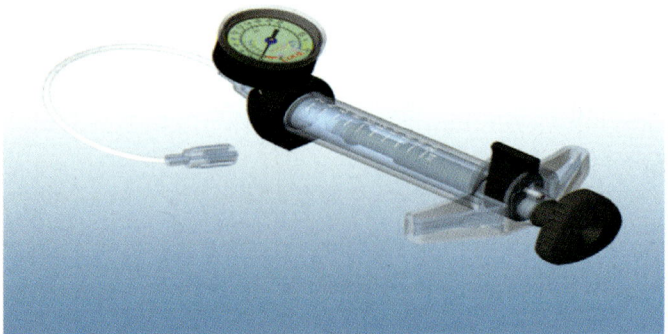

Fig. 2.1 Inflation devices used to obtain controlled inflation of balloon catheters

10 and 15 atm and large balloons between 3 and 6 atm. The degree of balloon hardness depends on the material characteristics (compliant or noncompliant). Compliant materials are usually soft and stretch or deform under pressure preventing the concentration of force from being focused at the stenosis and increase the risk of vessel dissection. The stiffer or more noncompliant the balloon material, the more dilating force it has, and the more uniformly it expands. Noncompliant balloons hold their shape despite added pressure and exert more force against a hard lesion or metal stent to increase dilatation. *Profiling* refers to a gentle inflation of the compliant balloon to smooth out the contour of the artery or gently expand a deployed stent graft and improve graft to wall apposition. Therapeutic ballooning refers to a forcible inflation of a semi-noncompliant balloon to dilate an arterial stenosis (such as an external iliac artery stenosis) to allow for graft delivery. Most balloons are of low profile in their undeployed states. Balloons are characterized by their profiles, trackability, and pushability. Trackability is the ease of advancing a balloon over a wire through an angulated artery segment. Pushability is defined as the ability to push a balloon through tortuous segments or across a lesion. There are different types of ballooning: (1) profile balloons (Fig. 2.2a), (2) therapeutic balloons (Fig. 2.2b), (3) Perfusion balloons, and (4) cutting balloons. Therapeutic ballooning refers to a forcible inflation of a semi-noncompliant balloon to dilate an arterial stenosis (such as an external iliac artery stenosis) to allow for graft delivery. A perfusion balloon has extra lumen with antegrade flow while the balloon is in inflation. A cutting balloon has micro-blades arranged lengthwise along the sides of the balloon. Once inflated, the mechanism of acute lumen gain after plain balloon angioplasty (PTCA) in calcified lesions is dissection while it is plaque compression and vessel expansion in fibrotic lesion. The balloon catheter can be advanced over a wire that passes through the lumen inside the whole length of the shaft (over-the-wire system) or only inside the distal segment (monorail system) or without an indwelling wire at all (fixed wire). In the monorail system, smaller guides can be used with better opacification and reduced fluoro time. However the wire is unable to be exchanged or reshaped without removing it, giving up position or use of a transport catheter. The over-the-wire balloon may be more trackable and the fixed-wire balloon has a

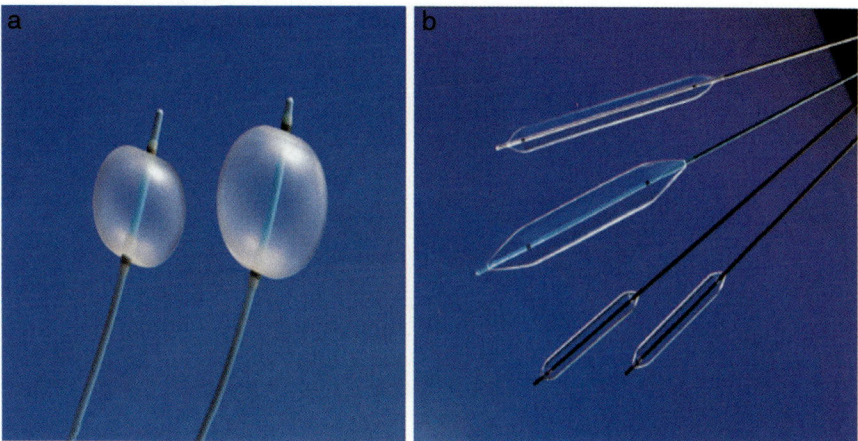

Fig. 2.2 (**a**) Medtronic Reliant profile balloon used in thoracic endografting. (**b**) Noncompliant – therapeutic ballooning

much lower profile and can be useful in tortuous arteries and extremely tight lesions. Because of the excellent result of stents to seal off dissection, the need for perfusion balloon catheters disappears, except in the case of perforation which requires prolonged inflation or in the case of poor results of initial balloon but inability to stent.

2.2 Selection of Balloon

The choice of the exact balloon and wire system is less important than the operator's overall approach to the technique of dilation, the familiarity with the system chosen, the balloon size, and the capacity to treat possible complications.[1] The ratio of the balloon:artery should be approximately 1:1. A higher balloon:artery ratio has been shown to be associated with dissection and acute closure.

2.2.1 Balloons Used for Thoracic Endografting

The **Equalizer (Boston Scientific)** can be used in thoracic aortic interventions to profile the deployed stent graft, and it comes in 20–40 mm sizes with a 7 Fr shaft and a 14 Fr sheath for introduction. It is a compliant latex balloon with radiopaque markers at its proximal and distal ends (Fig. 2.3, Table 2.1).

The **Cook Coda balloon (Cook Inc., Bloomington, IN)** (Fig. 2.4) has a 32 or 40 mm inflated diameter, a 10 Fr shaft, and a 14 Fr sheath for introduction. It is made of polyurethane and is a semi-compliant balloon with radiopaque markers that deflate very quickly, which is a benefit when temporarily occluding the thoracic aorta.

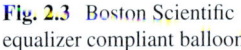 **Fig. 2.3** Boston Scientific equalizer compliant balloon

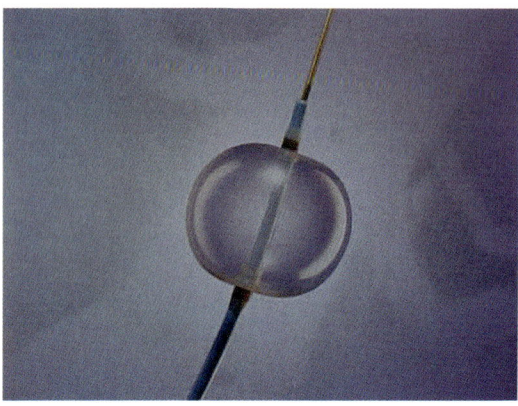

Gore Tri-lobe balloon (W.L. Gore & Associates, Flagstaff, AZ), which is probably the most advanced of the balloons described in this article, has a 26–40 mm inflated diameter, and a 105 cm working length with a 20 Fr sheath for intro-duction and radiopaque markers 5 cm apart (Fig. 2.5). Its silicone construction allows quick inflation and deflation and the tri-lobe design offers continuous flow and decreases the "wind sock" effect. This balloon is extremely useful in situa-tions in which profile ballooning is required in a tenuous landing zone to minimize the likelihood of dislodging the graft with the ballooning process secondary to wind-socking.

Medtronic Reliant Balloon (Santa Rosa) is a multi-lumen catheter non-latex compliant molding balloon which comes in a 100 cm working length. The balloon has an 8 Fr shaft and is 12 Fr sheaths compatible and a 10–46 mm inflation diameter. Usable catheter length is 100 cm with a guidewire compability of 0.038 in. or less. Maximum inflation pressure is 1 atm with the Talent Medtronic stent graft and a maximum number of inflation/deflation cycles at 20 (Fig. 2.6).

2.2.2 Adjuncts Techniques Useful in Thoracic Aortic Endografting

Advancing a balloon across tight lesion: Ensure that the guide position is coaxial to provide sufficient support for advancement of the balloon. Asking the patient to take a deep breath may help enlongate the heart and the artery making it easier for the balloon to be advanced. By applying a constant pressure on the balloon while pulling back the wire can decrease friction between wire and balloon allowing the balloon catheter to slide over the wire. The addition of a stiffer wire can help straighten out the vessel allowing the balloon catheter to track over it. If all fails changing to a lower profile balloon or use of a monorail system could help advance balloon through a tight lesion.

Table 2.1 Recommended balloons for thoracic endografting[2]

Company name	Product name	Indicated use	Material used	Maximum guidewire size/ID (in.)	Nominal/rated burst (atm)	Catheter diameter (Fr)	Catheter length (cm)	Comments
Cordis	OPTA-Pro PTA	Peripheral vessel therapeutic ballooning	Balloon-duralyn/catheter-nylon MDX-coated catheter	0.035	6 atm nominal/10 atm rated burst	5	80 cm/110 cm	Semi-compliant balloon/used for dilatation of access vessels/recommended sizes 7–10 mm diameter × 4 cm length
Abbott Vascular	Fox PTA	Peripheral vessel therapeutic ballooning	Balloon-TPX 101 nylon/catheter-polyemy SLIC-coated catheter	0.035	9 atm nominal/15 atm rated burst	5	75 cm/135 cm	Noncompliant balloon/used for dilatation of calcified access vessels/recommended sizes 7–10 mm diameter × 4 cm length
Boston Scientific	Blue-Max	Peripheral vessel therapeutic ballooning	Balloon-COEX nylon/catheter-nylon (hydrophilic-coated balloon)	0.035	20 atm rated burst	5.8	75 cm/120 cm	Extreme noncompliant balloon/used for dilatation of heavily calcified access vessels/recommended sizes 7–10 diameter × 4 cm length

Table 2.1 (continued)

Company name	Product name	Indicated use	Material used	Maximum guidewire size/ID (in.)	Nominal/rated burst (atm)	Catheter diameter (Fr)	Catheter length (cm)	Comments
Cook Inc.	CODA	Expand vascular prostheses	Polyurethane	0.035	Profile balloon up to 32 or 40 mm model	10	32 mm–100 cm/ 40 mm–120 cm	Semi-compliant balloon/used for endograft molding/14 Fr sheath compatible/ fastest inflation and deflation time of all aortic balloons
W.L. Gore & Associates	Tri-Lobe	Expand vascular prostheses	Silicon	0.035	Profile balloon up to 40 mm	16	108 cm	Compliant balloon/used for endograft molding/20 Fr sheath compatible/lobed design to allow aortic blood flow while inflated
Medtronic	Reliant	Expand vascular prostheses	Polyurethane	0.035	Profile balloon up to 46 mm	8	100 cm	Compliant balloon/used for endograft molding/12 Fr sheath compatible

Fig. 2.4 Cook Coda compliant balloon

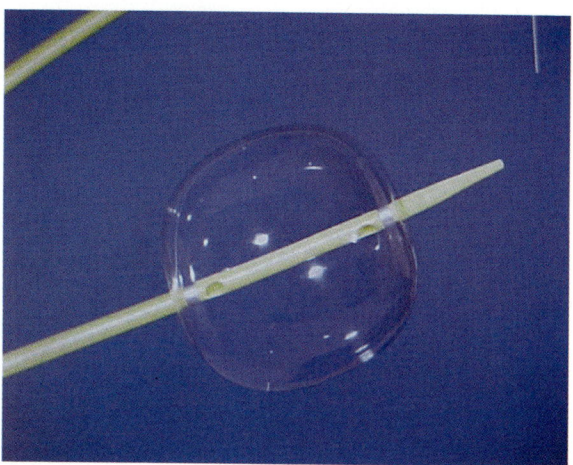

Fig. 2.5 Gore Tri-Lobe compliant balloon

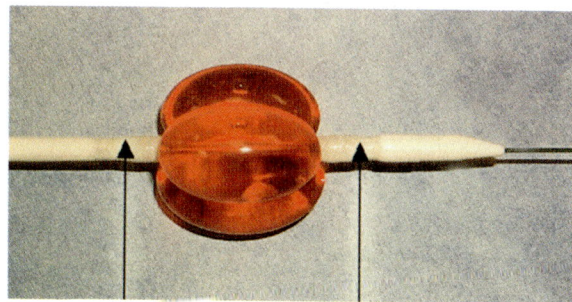

Failure to dilate a lesion: Heavily calcified lesions may prevent the full expansion of a balloon; even the balloon is inflated to near the rupture pressure. Overinflation of a balloon may be successful but may expose the patient to the risk of dissection or balloon rupture. Use of an undersized noncompliant balloon or in heavy calcified lesions the use of debulking of the plaque by rotational or orbital atherectomy or the use of a cutting balloon in undilatable fibrotic lesions with or without stent deployment may be adjunct maneuvers used to dilate complex lesions.

Failure to deflate the balloon: Inability to deflate the balloon is a rare occurrence. Possible causes are excessive twisting: more than 360° in order to cross a distal lesion [8] or entrapment in the distal portion by a tight lesion. Comparative usual maneuvers to deflate the balloon are listed below. Deflate the balloon with the inflation device. Deflate the balloon with a 50 cc syringe directly at the inflation port. Inflate the balloon to rupture it. Prepare to rupture the balloon with the back end of a wire; alternately, last option is surgical removal of balloon.

How to puncture an undeflatable balloon? Advance a small new over-the-wire balloon (OTW) immediately next to the proximal end of the entrapped and still-inflated balloon. Remove the wire of this OTW balloon, reinsert the wire back, with

Fig. 2.6 Medtronic Reliant
balloon (Santa Rosa)

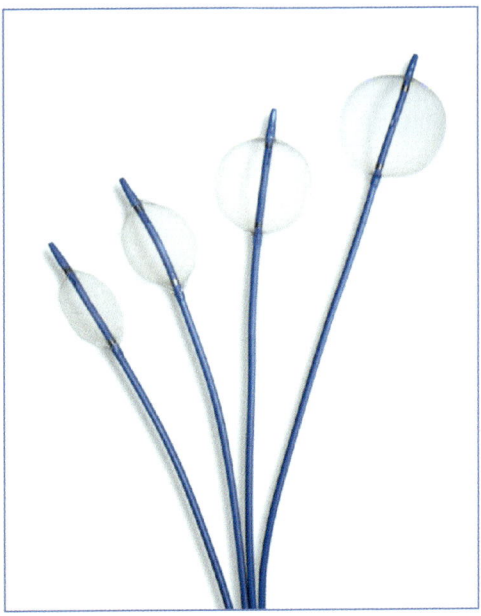

the stiff back end, and inflate the new balloon at low pressure to position the sharp
tip of the wire at the center of the vessel lumen. Try to puncture the trapped inflated
balloon with the back end of the wire which has a tapered back end. Although there
is a risk of vessel perforation, the hole would be quite small and unlikely to cause
any significant complication. In addition, vessel trauma from balloon rupture can be
much more extensive and more uncontrolled than a single pinhole puncture.

Entrapment of deflated balloon during withdrawal: Even though the incidence
of entrapment of a deflated balloon is low, once it happens it is quite traumatic to
the patient, operator, and the interventional team. The entrapment can happen in any
unpredicted way. Different options for management are listed below. There are no
best options. Different modalities of treatment can be tried on a trial-and-error basis.
Push the balloon forward and then pull it back and twist the balloon in an attempt to
rewrap the balloon before pulling back. Insert a stiffer wire alongside the entrapped
balloon before pulling the balloon back so that the artery is straighter. Advance a
second wire distally and then insert an OTW balloon alongside the entrapped balloon and inflate the new balloon at low pressure to free the entrapped balloon. If the
OTW balloon cannot be advanced, then advance a balloon on a wire alongside the
entrapped balloon and inflate it to free the entrapped balloon. Advance a commercial microsnare and tighten the loop as near to the balloon as possible, and then pull
the balloon back as you would any embolized material.

Using a commercial snare to remove a balloon: Cut the proximal end of the
balloon catheter and advance the snare using the balloon catheter as a wire. Arriving
at the entrapped balloon site, loop the snare around the balloon, tighten the loop by
advancing the transport catheter, and pull the snare and the catheter end to free the

balloon. Be prepared to unwrap the snare and pull it back alone if it is not possible to remove the trapped balloon.

Damage control for balloon rupture: Balloon rupture is seen under fluoroscope as a quick dispersion of contrast agent from the balloon, with short contrast opacification of the vessel or decrease in the inflation pressure. When this occurs, slowly withdraw the balloon proximal to the lesion and inject some contrast to detect if there is perforation. The balloon is then removed if not entrapped in the lesion. Stenting should be performed if there is dissection.

Manipulating a cutting balloon: Because of the presence of the micro-blades at its side, the cutting balloon is quite stiff and is difficult to curve around sharp bends. To overcome this problem, the cutting balloon is designed with very short length. While dilating the cutting balloon, a slow inflation strategy is used. There should be a 3–5 s interval between each atmosphere increase, to ensure that the peripheral balloon wings unfold slowly first around the blades, before inflation of the central core of the balloon. Rapid inflation could result in puncturing a hole in the balloon by the blades. The manufacturer's guidelines for balloon inflation should be adhered to (1 atm inflation every 5 s; maximum 6–8 atm). Some operators also recommend deflation of the balloon at the same gradual rate. Finally, withdrawal of the cutting balloon should not be attempted until an adequate time interval has elapsed to allow full rewrapping of the balloon.

References

1. Dotter CT, Judkins MP. Transluminal treatment of arteriosclerotic obstruction: description of a new technic and a preliminary report of its application. *Circulation*. 1964;30·654 670.
2. Wheatley GH, McNutt R, Diethrich EB Introduction to thoracic endografting: imaging, guide wires, guiding catheters and delivery sheaths. *Ann Thorac Surg*. 2007;83(1):272–278.

Chapter 3
Catheters Used in Endografting
of the Thoracic Aorta

In general, choosing the correct catheter size means picking the smallest diameter that supports the procedure. Catheters come in standard lengths that range from 65 to 110 cm in length. As with sheaths, the French scale is used to size catheters (1 Fr = 0.33 mm); however, catheters are measured at their outer diameter. Their shape is associated with function and target area. Catheters are characterized by their tractability, pushability, crossability, and steerability. Trackability describes the ability of the catheter to follow the guidewire through tortuous vessels and around corners without pulling the wire out of its intended location. Pushability refers to the amount of force at the hub of the catheter that is needed to advance the tip of the catheter. Crossability is the term that describes the ease with which a catheter follows the guidewire across a lesion or through a diseased arterial segment. Steerability refers to the responsiveness of the catheter tip to handling maneuvers performed at the hub. Catheters are made most commonly from polyurethane, polyethylene nylon and occasionally Teflon. Polyethylene catheters are pliable and have good shape memory. Polyurethane is softer and more pliable and follows guidewires more easily than polyethylene, but has a higher degree of friction. Nylon catheters (such as those by AngioDynamics) are stiff and tolerate high flow rates; nylon is actually the most common material for catheters. Teflon is sometimes used as well, but is generally reserved for use in dilators and sheaths because it is much stiffer than the other material described (Table 3.1). Almost all catheters have radiopaque tips and some flush catheters have graduated measurement markers with optimal fluoroscopic resolution for taking vessel length measurements. Among the types of catheters, there are two major types used in thoracic aortic procedures: (1) selective catheters and (2) non-selective type of catheters.

3.1 Non-selective Catheters

Non-selective catheters which include flush, diagnostic, exchange, and perfusion catheters are usually constructed of nylon and are designed to rapidly infuse large volumes of contrast agent without injuring the vessel. In order to accomplish this, the distal portion of these catheters contains multiple side holes, in addition to

J. Kpodonu, *Manual of Thoracic Endoaortic Surgery*,
DOI 10.1007/978-1-84996-296-4_3, © Springer-Verlag London Limited 2010

Table 3.1 Guidewire properties

Flexibility/ability to track guidewire to intended position				
(Greatest) 4	3	2	1	(Least)
Polyurethane	Polyethylene	Nylon	Teflon	
Coefficient of friction				
(Greatest) 4	3	2	1	(Least)
Polyurethane	Polyethylene	Nylon	Teflon	
Torqueability (turning the ex vivo portion of the catheter results in rotation of the distal tip)				
(Greatest) 4	3	2	1	(Least)
Polyurethane	Polyethylene	Nylon	Teflon	

the standard end hole. This distal portion is preformed into a shape that assists in dispersion of the contrast; e.g., Omni flush, Grollman, pigtail, straight, tennis racket, multipurpose. The following catheters are commonly used in thoracic endografting: Pigtail Marker (Angiodynamics), Pigtail/TR Flush (Boston Scientific) (Fig. 3.1), Bentson 2 (JB2) (Angiodynamics), Headhunter (Angiodynamics), straight arterial (Angiodynamics), internal mammary (Angiodynamics), and Glidecath (angled/straight) (Boston Scientific). Each of these catheters serves a unique purpose within the conduct of a thoracic endografting procedure. For example, the Bentson 2 catheter can be used to cannulate the left subclavian artery to assist with possible embolization for a type II endoleak. A summary of the catheters necessary for thoracic endografting procedures is given in Table 3.2.[1–5] Non-selective catheters are generally used only in large diameter vessels (aorta or its primary branches). Larger diameter catheters known as guiding catheters (Fig. 3.2) used to deliver endovascular devices (e.g., balloons and stents) have a braided shaft design which offers strength, flexibility, superb torque response, and maximum tactile control. Infusion catheters (Fig. 3.3) are non-selective cathers used mainly in

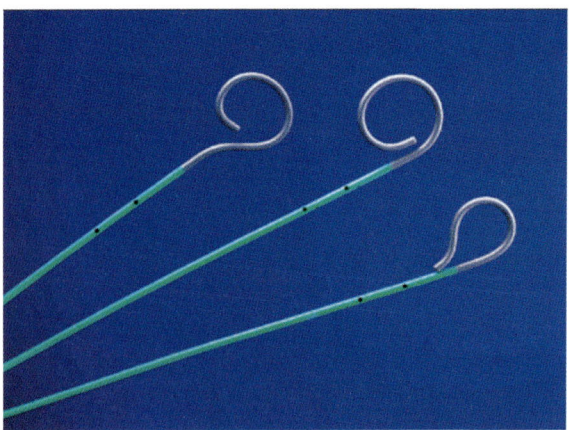

Fig. 3.1 Flush catheters

Table 3.2 Recommended commercially available ancillary catheters used in thoracic endografting

Company name	Product name	Indicated use	Material used	Maximum guidewire size/ID (in.)	Maximum flow rate/pressure limit	Catheter diameter (Fr)	Catheter length (cm)	Comments
Angiodynamics	Accu-Vu sizing pigtail	Bolus angiographic catheter	Co-extruded nylon	0.038	26 cc/1050 psi	5	100	21-Platinum heat embedded markers (measures 20 cm length)/used for aortic length measurements
Boston Scientific	Imager II TR Flush	Bolus angiographic catheter	Braided/pebax	0.038	26 cc/1050 psi	5	100	Alternative aortogram catheter
Angiodynamics	Mariner Headhunter	Shaped angiographic catheter	Duration coating/non-braided/co-extruded nylon	0.038	8 cc/272 psi	5	100	Headhunter shape is best suited for traversing tortuous aortic anatomy
Angiodynamics	Mariner Bentson 2	Shaped angiographic catheter	Duration coating/non-braided/co-extruded nylon	0.038	8 cc/272 psi	5	100	Primary catheter used to cannulate the great vessels from a CFA approach
Angiodynamics	Mariner Cobra 2	Shaped angiographic catheter	Duration coating/braided/co-extruded nylon	0.038	10 cc/254 psi	5	65	Cobra 2 catheter shape allows for easy cannulation of the celiac, SMA, or renal arteries

Table 3.2 (continued)

Company name	Product name	Indicated use	Material used	Maximum guidewire size/ID (in.)	Maximum flow rate/pressure limit	Catheter diameter (Fr)	Catheter length (cm)	Comments
Boston Scientific	Impulse IM	Shaped angiographic catheter	Braided/pebax	0.038	8 cc/1200 psi	5	100	Used for cannulating an inferior takeoff of the celiac artery. Used to assist in placing a guidewire into the descending thoracic aorta from a brachial puncture
Boston Scientific/Terumo	Radiofocus straight and angled glidecath	Wire exchange/ shaped angiographic catheter	Hydrophilic-coated nylon/ polyurethane	0.038	19 cc/1000 psi	5	100	Non-braided floppy catheter/most trackable catheter on the market
Angiodynamics	Mariner straight art	Wire exchange angiographic catheter	Duration coating/ braided/co-extruded nylon	0.038	8 cc/238 psi	5	90	Quality in expensive wire exchange catheter/used for gradient pull-through
Spectranetics	Quick-cross	Wire exchange angiographic catheter	HDP (polyethy-lene)/marker bands-nonferric platinum (10% iridium)	0.035	6.1 cc/300 psi	4.8/tapers to 3.7 Fr tip	135	Lowest profile 0.035 guidewire compatible catheter on the market/most crossable catheter behind graft or through tight access areas

Table 3.2 (continued)

Company name	Product name	Indicated use	Material used	Maximum guidewire size/ID (in.)	Maximum flow rate/pressure limit	Catheter diameter (Fr)	Catheter length (cm)	Comments
Biocardia	Morph/universal deflectable guide catheter	Guiding catheter	Braided pebax shaft/PTFE liner	0.068	50 psi	8 Fr OD/5.2 Fr ID	50/110	Deflectable tip allows for supported cannulation of any vessel/able to place 0.018 balloon-expandable stents through
Cordis	Vista Brite-tip hockey stick guide catheter	Guiding catheter	Stainless steel braided/blended nylon shaft/PTFE liner	0.088	N/A	8 Fr OD/7.2 Fr ID	100	Shape allows for supported cannulation of the great vessels; able to place most 0.035 balloon-expandable stents through
Cordis	Vista Brite-tip IM guide catheter	Guiding catheter	Stainless steel braided/blended nylon shaft/PTFE liner	0.088	N/A	8 Fr OD/7.2 Fr ID	55	Shape allows for supported cannulation of the celiac artery/able to place most 0.035 balloon-expandable stents through

CFA, common femoral artery; HDP, high-density plastic; ID, internal diameter; IM, internal mammary; OD, outer diameter; PTFE, polytetrafluoroethylene; SMA, superior mesenteric artery

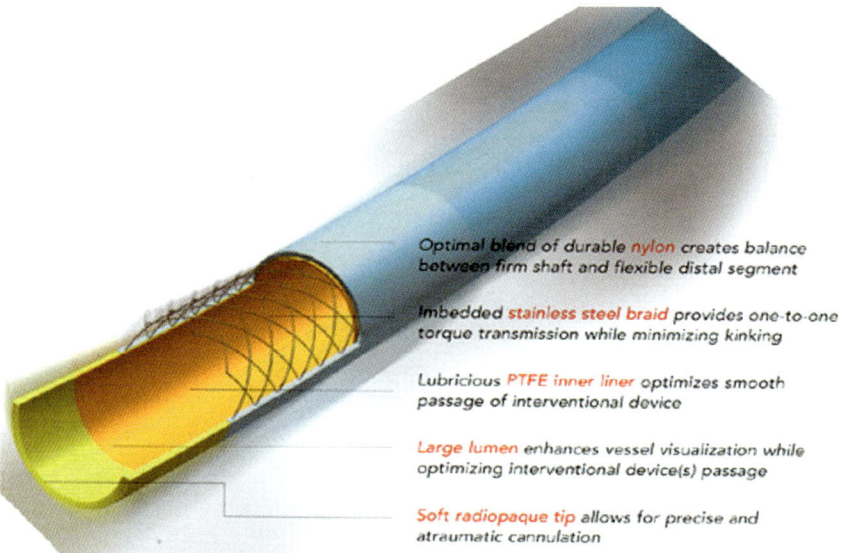

Optimal blend of durable nylon creates balance between firm shaft and flexible distal segment

Imbedded stainless steel braid provides one-to-one torque transmission while minimizing kinking

Lubricious PTFE inner liner optimizes smooth passage of interventional device

Large lumen enhances vessel visualization while optimizing interventional device(s) passage

Soft radiopaque tip allows for precise and atraumatic cannulation

Fig. 3.2 Guiding catheters

Fig. 3.3 Infusion catheters

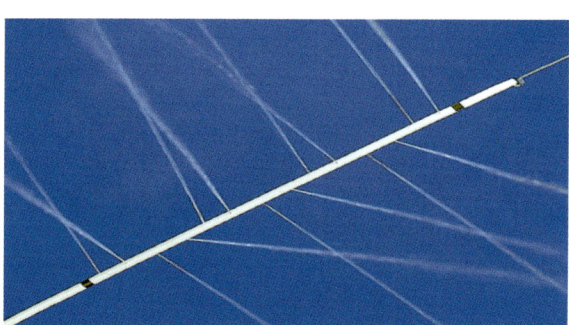

combination with thrombolytic therapy in cases of thromboembolic occlusions. Side holes allow the slow diffusion of the agent to permeate the clot, thereby speeding the process of thrombolysis.

3.2 Selective Catheters

Selective catheters, with a single end hole, are designed for the selective catheterization and contrast injection of specific branch vessels and are usually positioned at the entry of an aortic branch and a small amount of contrast is injected. An abundant selection of preformed distal ends is available to assist in the catheterization of the various anatomic branch points of the vascular system. For primary aortic access from a retrograde femoral artery approach, we prefer a Berenstein-tipped catheter (Imager II Selective BERN; Boston Scientific Corp.), which is shaped similar to a hockey stick. When it is necessary to cross-tight stenoses, an alternate angled tip hydrophilic-coated catheter may be useful (Glidecath; Terumo Medical Corp. or Slip-cath; Cook, Inc.). For selective catheterization of aortic arch branches, common catheter shapes include Berenstein or vertebral, JR4, Simmons, headhunter, and Vitek. For catheterization of renal or mesenteric arteries, popular shapes are cobra, renal double curve, Simmons, and Shepherd hook/Omni SOS. Catheter shapes commonly used for access to the contralateral iliac artery include cobra, Simmons, and pigtail. Catheters with curved distal ends are usually introduced over a guidewire with a floppy tip (e.g., Bentson), so that they may assume their preformed shape when the guidewire is withdrawn with its distal tip inside the catheter. In catheterization of branch vessels with an acute angulation from the direction of approach, a catheter with a secondary curve is helpful. These catheters, such as Simmons, Vitek, and SOS Omni, are first advanced past the target branch vessel. Then the catheter tip is made to cannulate the vessel while withdrawing the catheter back toward the access site. Catheters of this type also require manual reshaping to their preformed shape in the aorta proximal to the area of interest. To reshape, the catheter is advanced until the tip and primary curve are no longer supported by the guidewire. Then, with the tip engaged in a side branch, the main body of the catheter is either advanced or rotated, reforming the catheter into its native shape. Alternatively, a catheter may be reformed by reflection off the aortic valve or using a suture pull.

References

1. Wheatley GH 3rd, McNutt R, Diethrich EB. Introduction to thoracic endografting: imaging, guidewires, guiding catheters, and delivery sheaths. *Ann Thorac Surg.* 2007;83(1):272–278.
2. Diethrich EB, Ramaiah VG, Kpodonu J, Rodriguez JA. *Endovascular and Hybrid Management of the Thoracic Aorta. A Case Based Approach.* 1st ed. West Sussex: Wiley-Blackwell; 2008.
3. Casserly IP, Sacher R, Yadav JS, eds. *Manual of Peripheral Vascular Intervention.* Philadelphia, PA: Lippincott Williams and Wilkins; 2005.
4. Moore WS, ed. *Vascular and Endovascular Surgery: A Comprehensive Review,* 7th ed. Philadelphia, PA: Elsevier Saunders; 2006.
5. White RA, Fogarty, TJ, eds. *Peripheral Endovascular Interventions,* 2nd ed. New York, NY: Springer; 1999.

Chapter 4
Equipment Required for Thoracic Aortic Endografting

- Fluoroscope with digital angiography capabilities (C-arm or fixed unit)

  - Nonobstructive table for imaging of chest and abdomen
  - Power injector for fluoroscopic contrast studies
  - Connecting tubing for power injector
  - Digital subtraction angiography (DSA)
  - Road mapping
  - Multiplane image system

- High-resolution fluoroscopic imaging and the ability to record and recall at imaging
- Surgical suite standby in the event that emergency surgery is necessary
- Cell saver and/or auto transfuser (optional)
- Inflation device with pressure gauge
- Needles
- Radiopaque ruler with centimeter increments
- Heparinized solution
- Puncture needles 18 or 19 G
- Assorted guidewires of at least 260 cm in length, including a stiff 0.035″ wire to support the Xcelerant Delivery System
- Assorted angiographic, angioplasty, and graduated pigtail catheters
- 12 Fr introducer system to be used with the Reliant stent graft balloon catheter
- Sterile introducer sheaths of 5 or 10 Fr for vascular access to femoral arteries and to perform diagnostic imaging
- Radiopaque contrast media
- Sterile silicone lubricant or mineral oil

4.1 Supplementary Equipments

- Nitinol goose neck snare (10–15 mm)
- Angioplasty catheters 8–40 mm (depending on case)
- IVUS unit with catheters

J. Kpodonu, *Manual of Thoracic Endoaortic Surgery*,
DOI 10.1007/978-1-84996-296-4_4, © Springer-Verlag London Limited 2010

- Sterile marker
- 25–30 mm valvuloplasty balloons

4.2 Dilators

4.2.1 Percutaneous Entry Needle/Devices

Endovascular procedures require the use of a percutaneous needle. Needles come in a variety of lengths and gauges. Each needle contains two parts: the hub used when attaching the needle to the syringe and the cannula, which is the hollow shaft of the needle. The most common gauge used is the 18 G needle (Fig. 4.1). The 18 G needle will accommodate a 0.035″ guidewire. The length of needles varies between 2 and $3\frac{1}{2}$ in. Other accessories include micro-puncture sets and smart needles.

Fig. 4.1   18 G 7 cm Cook percutaneous needle

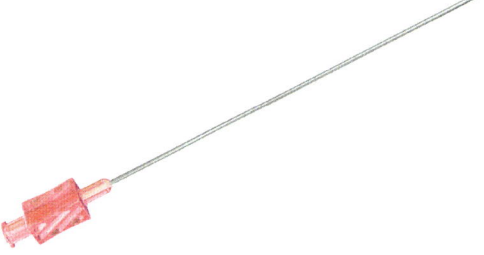

4.2.2 Vessel Dilators

These devices dilate the tract the needle has created, allowing large devices such as catheters and sheaths to be introduced into the vessel. They are placed over the guidewire that was introduced through the original puncture needle. Vessel dilators are measured in French sizes (1 Fr = 0.33 mm) and are most commonly 15–20 cm in length. "Serial dilation" can be necessary when attempting to introduce large diameter sheaths, particularly with patients that have scar tissue buildup in the CFA area. It is important not to overdilate the tract. Overdilating can allow blood to leak around your catheter or sheath not allowing you to gain hemostatic control of the vessel. Dilator sets may vary from 4 to 22 Fr × 20 cm (Fig. 4.2).

4.2.3 Guidewires

Guidewires are used to access the vessel through the percutaneous needle. In addition, they are used to help steer catheters and devices through the vascular anatomy. Guidewires are manufactured in several different ways: either they are solid steel

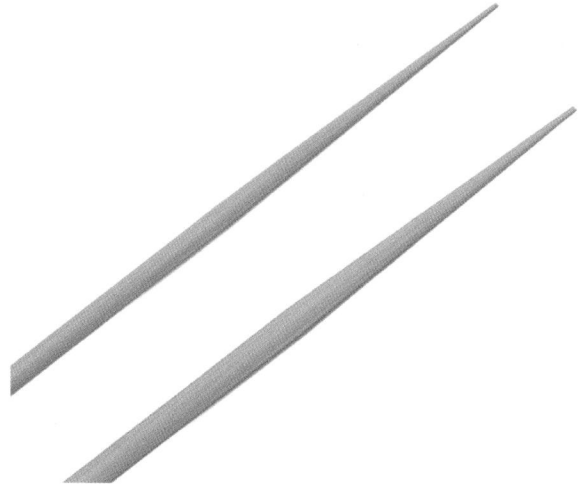

Fig. 4.2 Dilator sets

core wires, or the steel core can be wrapped in a thin steel coil. The core can also be incased in a polymer-type jacket. Recently they have started using nitinol metal for the inner core material. Guidewires usually have a floppy tip with a stiff body. The tip configuration usually includes angled tips, straight tips, J-tips, and shapable tips. The diameters of the wires are measured in thousandths of an inch, ranging from 0.014″ to 0.038″. Lengths are measured in centimeters and can range from 80 to 300 cm. However, some specialty wires can come in lengths up to 450 cm.

Some guidewires may have a hydrophilic coating making them slippery when wet. Hoag Hospital's primary work horse guidewire is the 0.035 in. Terumo-angled Glidewire. This wire has a hydrophilic coating. It is constructed with a center core of super-elastic metal alloy that tapers to a soft flexible tip. The kink-resistant core is coated with a polyurethane jacket. This jacket is bonded with a hydrophilic polymer that becomes slick when saline has been applied. There are many guidewire manufacturers (Fig. 4.3), with hundreds, possibly thousands, of wires to choose from. The wire selection is dependent on the location of the lesion, the tortuosity of the vessel, and the physician's preference.

4.2.4 Introducer Sheaths

- Sheaths are hemostatic conduits inserted into the vessel (Fig. 4.4). They allow the passage of guidewires, catheters, and interventional devices. The sheath allows these to be passed in and out of the body without damaging the vessel and reduces the blood loss. Some sheaths may have a braided wire construction to reduce kinking in acute angles. They may have a radiopaque tip for visualization under

Fig. 4.3 Ultrastiff
guidewires used in thoracic
endografting

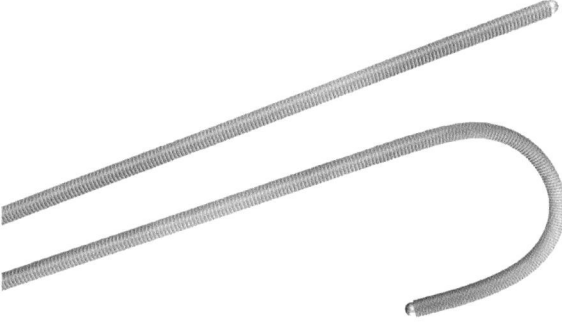

Fig. 4.4 Introducer sheaths
commonly used in
introducing balloons,
catheters, and wires for
thoracic endografting

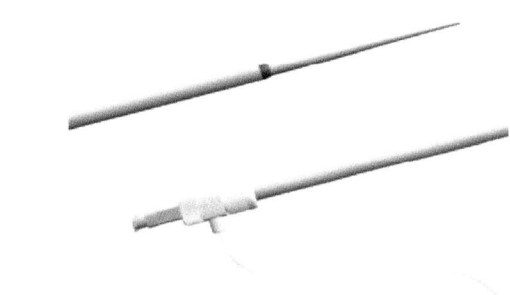

fluoroscopy. Sheaths are measured by the inner diameter in French sizes. They are universally color coated. They range in sizes from 4 to 24 Fr. Larger sized sheaths may require the surgeon to "cut down" and expose the CFA in order to repair the large arteriotomy post-procedure.

4.2.4.1 Universal Color Coating

- 4 Fr = red
- 5 Fr = grey
- 6 Fr = green
- 7 Fr = orange
- 8 Fr = blue
- 9 Fr = black
- 10 Fr = violet
- 11 Fr = yellow

4.2.5 Flush/Diagnostic/Guiding Catheters

Catheters have three primary purposes: to deliver contrast for angiographic images, to assist in directing wires through target lesions needing intervention, and to give shaped support when trying to deliver devices to these target lesions. Catheters are

Fig. 4.5 Guiding catheters
used in thoracic endografting

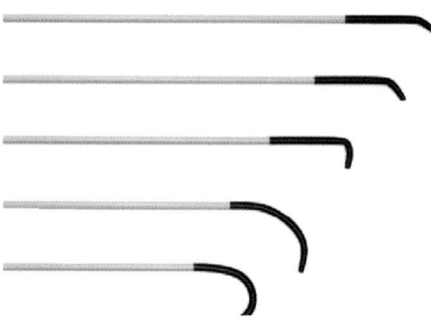

measured by the outer diameter in French sizes. The diagnostic catheters are 4–5 Fr diameters and are used to help maneuver guidewires through the vascular anatomy and to deliver contrast for angiograms (Fig. 4.5). The guide catheters are 6–12 Fr in diameter and are used to assist in the delivery of the interventional devices, such as stents and balloons. These catheters come in hundreds of shapes and lengths. They come in braided and non-braided construction. They have special features like hydrophilic coatings, radiopaque tips, and radiopaque markers used to help determine lesion lengths.

4.2.5.1 Types of Catheters

– cerebral catheters
– visceral catheters
– coronary catheters
– exchange catheters
– flush catheters
– guiding catheters

4.2.6 Angioplasty Balloons

Angioplasty balloons are used for several different reasons: they are used to assist self-expanding stent grafts with arterial wall apposition; this is called profile ballooning. They are also used to dilate lesions and for mounting stainless steel or cobalt chromium stents. These are expanded in the target lesion; this is called therapeutic ballooning. Balloons are measured in diameter (mm) and then length (mm or cm) (e.g., 5 × 10 balloon = 5 mm × 10 cm). The balloons come in many different shaft lengths and various crossing profiles. The balloons have pressure ratings called nominal and rated burst pressures. Nominal pressure is the amount of atmospheres it takes to expand the balloon to its listed diameter and length. Rated burst pressure is a conservative measurement, in which 1 out of 100 balloons tested ruptured at this atmospheric pressure. These rates and the amount of growth the balloon has when

Fig. 4.6 Compliant
Equalizer (Boston Scientific)
balloon used for profiling of
an endoluminal graft

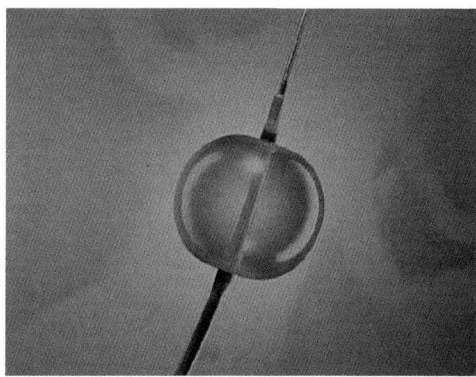

Fig. 4.7 Noncompliant
balloon used for dilating
calcified arteries

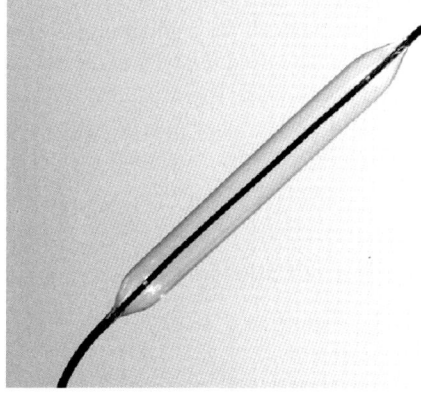

the pressure exceeds the nominal pressure determine how the balloons are classified. The classifications of the balloons are compliant (greater than 10% growth), semi-compliant (between 5 and 10% growth), and noncompliant (less than 5% growth). The more noncompliant the balloon is, the stronger the balloon is for dilating hard calcified lesions (Fig. 4.6). The more compliant the balloon is, the more suitable for profile ballooning, or pulling thrombus or an embolus out of a vessel (Fig. 4.7).

4.2.7 Stents

Stents are metallic scaffolding used to permanently dilate a lesion. There are two different types of stents: balloon-expandable and self-expanding stents. The balloon-expandable stents (Fig. 4.8) are constructed of 316L stainless steel. They have a high radial strength and are placed in ostial lesions where the vessel has low mobility, e.g., renal arteries, common iliac arteries. The stent is mounted on a balloon and placed so it straddles the lesion as the balloon is inflated prying the stent open. Self-expanding stents are constructed of nitinol (Fig. 4.9). Nitinol is a man-made metal

Fig. 4.8 Balloon-expandable
stent

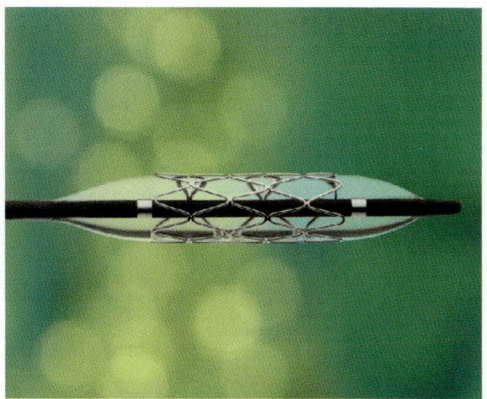

Fig. 4.9 Self-expandable
stent

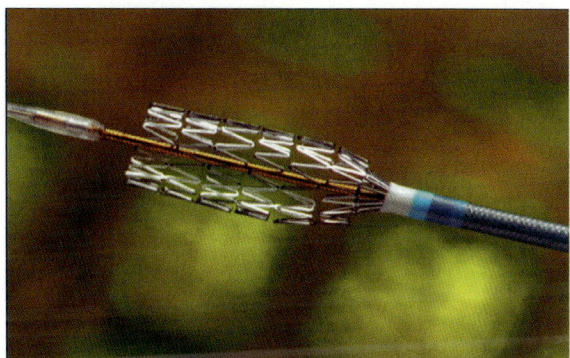

created by the navy. When nitinol is chilled the metal can be compressed so the stent
can be loaded into a delivery catheter system. This is done by the stent manufacturing company. When the stent is placed in the human body and the delivery system
is deployed, the stent expands due to body temperature. The interesting property of
nitinol is that it has memory, so it can be crushed and it will recover its manufactured specifications. Self-expanding stents are placed in lesions where the vessels
are more mobile, e.g., near joints or in limbs. Most self-expanding stents have
radiopaque markers that increase their visibility. Covered stent grafts (Fig. 4.10)
are alternatively used for arthero-occlusive disease, dissection, and rupture of
vessels.

- **ELGs (endoluminal grafts)** – ELGs are stents, primarily self-expanding, that are
  covered with PTFE material or woven Dacron. They are most commonly used in
  the aorta to exclude aneurysms. They are used in both the abdominal aorta and
  the thoracic aorta. The majority of grafts used in the abdominal aorta bifurcate
  and the limbs continue into the iliac system. Currently, there are three FDA-
  approved thoracic endoluminal graft. Most of these grafts require large sheaths
  to place into the body. FDA flexibility, conformability, ease of deployment,

Fig. 4.10 Covered stent graft

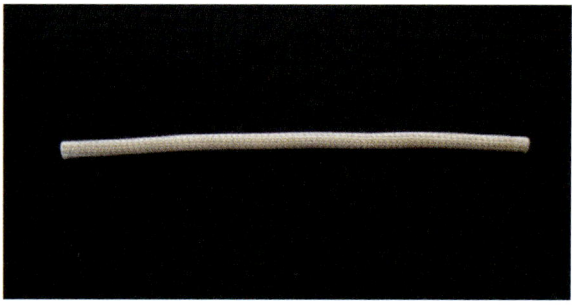

Fig. 4.11 Gore TAG thoracic
endoluminal graft

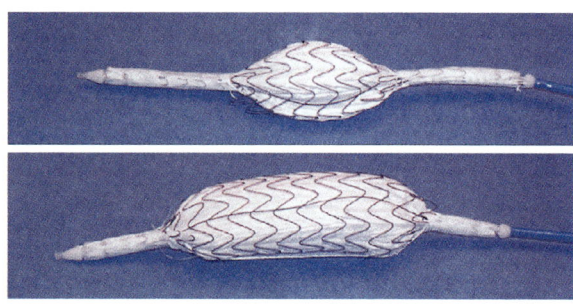

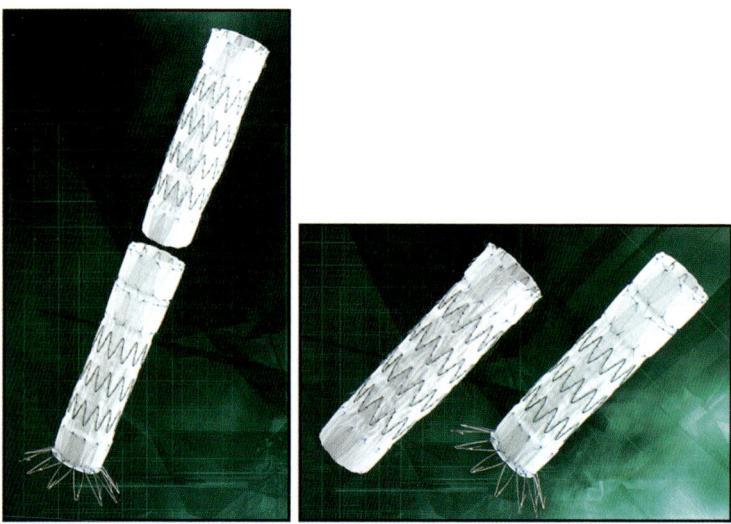

Fig. 4.12 Cook Tx2 thoracic endoluminal graft

Fig. 4.13 Medtronic Talent
thoracic endoluminal graft

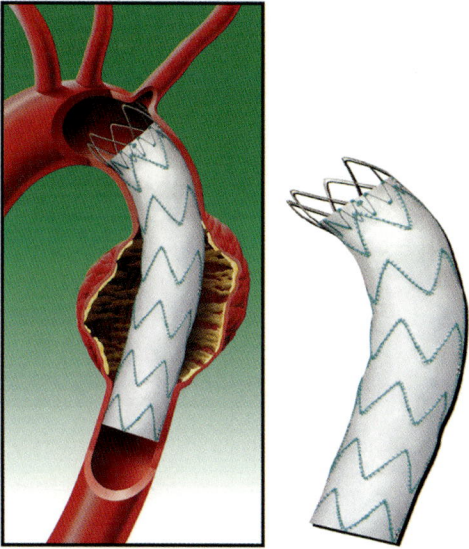

accuracy of deployment, durability, availability in a wide range of diameters and lengths, and low-profile delivery systems are desirable attributes for the ideal endograft. Several types of endograft are currently commercially available; these include the Gore TAG (W.L. Gore & Associates, Flagstaff, AZ) (Fig. 4.11), Zenith TX2 (Cook, Bloomington, IN) (Fig. 4.12), Medtronic Talent and Valiant graft (Fig. 4.13), Relay (Bolton Medical, Sunrise, FL). Evita (Jotec, Hechingen, Germany), and Endofit (Endomed Phoenix, AZ).

The technical features of the most commonly used devices are presented in Table 4.1.

4.3 Endograft Selection

The following are true about the current devices: no device is perfect. There is no good-quality scientific evidence that any one device is better than the others. The majority of devices are chosen on the basis of personal preference and experience (Table 4.1). The nitinol stent grafts are MR compatible so that the risk of irradiation can be reduced for the follow-up examinations.

In general devices are oversized by 10–20% for aneurysms and slightly less for acute dissection (e.g., 5–10%). When selecting a device diameter for use in dissections, the caliber of the aorta just proximal to the dissection should be used. This will generally be the diameter of the mid-aortic arch. In acute dissections, a device length should be chosen to cover the main entry tear.

In chronic dissection, devices should extend from just proximal to the entry tear to the diaphragm.

Table 4.1 Technical features of some commercially available devices (author's personal assessments)

Device	Introducing sheath	Introducing system size (F)	Available diameter size (mm)	Available lengths (mm)	Bare proximal portion	Delayed deployment of more proximal stent	Radial force	Flexibility	MRI compatibility (images artifacting)	Delivery system
TAG (Gore)	Y	20–24	26–40	20	N	N	+	++	Y	Pull-knob
Talent (Medtronic)	N	22–27	22–46	100	Y	N	++	+	Y	Pull-back
Valiant (Medtronic)	N	20–24	22–46	100–220 150–	Y	N	+++	++	Y	Pull-back Xcelerant System
Zenith TX2 (Cook)	Y	20–22	22–42	100–216 150–	Y	Y	++	+	N	Pull-back
Relay (Bolton)	N	22–26	22–46		Y	Y	++	+	Y	Pull-back

4.4 Accessory Tools

A variety of other tools may also be useful in thoracic aortic endografting procedures. Snares, such as the EV3 Gooseneck (EV3, Plymouth, MN) and INTER-V
Ensnare device (INTER-V, Gainesville, FL) (Fig. 4.14), are intended for use in thoracic endografting procedures to retrieve and manipulate foreign objects and are
useful when establishing brachial–femoral guidewire access to assist with delivery of the thoracic stent in cases of severely tortuous aortas. Embolization coils
(Fig. 4.15) may also be needed to treat a type II endoleak by coiling the origin of
the left subclavian artery or to deposit the coils in the sac. Peripheral vascular stents
and covered stents may be important tools when addressing iliac artery stenoses to
help with delivery of the sheath and thoracic endoprosthesis.

Fig. 4.14 INTER-V Ensnare
device

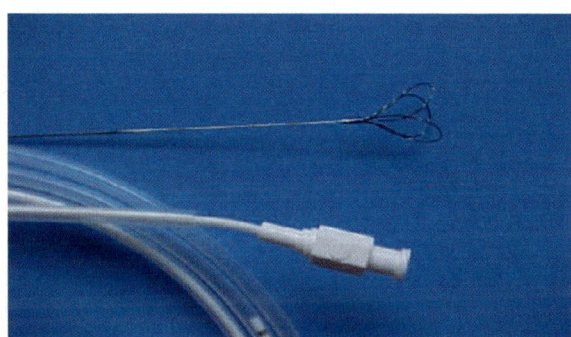

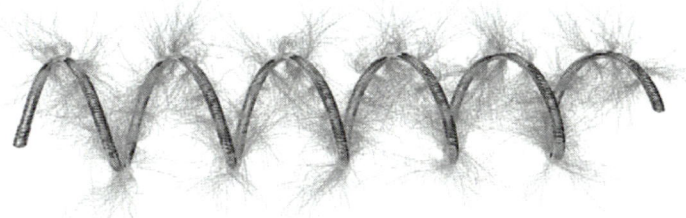

Fig. 4.15 Nestor (Cook) embolization coils used for arterial and venous embolization

Reference

1. Endovascular today 2010 Buyer's guide

Chapter 5
Guidewires Used in Thoracic Aortic Endografting

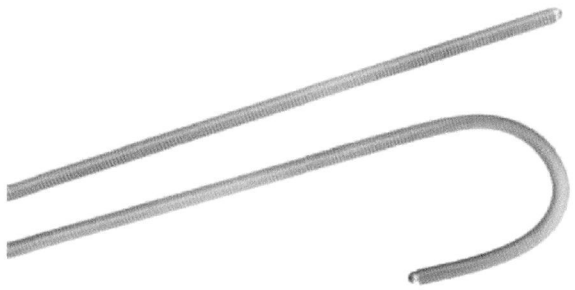

5.1 General Overview

A wire consists of two main components: (1) a central shaft of stainless steel or nitinol and (2) a distal flexible tip shaped as a spring coil made with platinum or tungsten. Wires with a nitinol core are kink resistant while those with stainless steel are more susceptible to kinking. The tip can be soft, stiff, intermediate or floppy J tipped or angled tip. Soft tip guidewires consists of an inner core end combined with tip shaping capabilities making it more aggressive in crossing tight lesions. Floppy tip has no inner core to the tip of the wire and usually comprised of a ribbon of stainless steel, nitinol, gold, or platinum which allows you to shape the wire and allows for safe traumatic selection of vessels. "J" tip allows for safe passage of wire through: irregular lesions stents (keeping wire in "true" lumen and not through struts). Angled tip is selectively used to steer wire because of tip angle. Wires can have a shaped or pre-shaped tip (Fig. 5.1). Nearly all guidewires have some form of antifriction coating, and some may have antithrombogenic/heparin coating.A tetrafluoroethylene (TFE) coating has been shown to reduce the coefficient of friction for stainless steel wires to 1/2 the uncoated value, and a silicone coating can reduce it to 1/6 the uncoated value. Many newer wires are coated with

J. Kpodonu, *Manual of Thoracic Endoaortic Surgery*,
DOI 10.1007/978-1-84996-296-4_5, © Springer-Verlag London Limited 2010

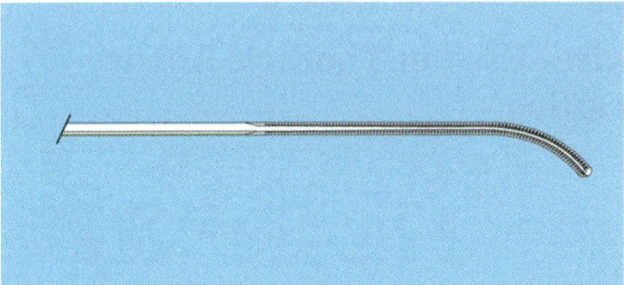

Fig. 5.1 A pre-shaped wire

a hydrophilic polymer similar to silicone; when wet, it has a slipperiness that facilitates passage through vessels and catheter exchanges (Fig. 5.2). Hydrophilic-coated wires must be meticulously cleaned and moistened in order to avoid drying out and becoming tacky.Because passage through entry needles can shear off the hydrophilic coating, these wires are not used for initial vascular access. The usual wire is the flexible tip 0.014 in. diameter lightweight wire, while the larger size wires (0.16–0.18 in.) or the much stiffer wires are used to straighten tortuous arterial segments and to provide more support for device tracking and when the support offered by a guide needs bolstering. In general, the flexible wires are less steerable and the stiffer wire offers more torque control.[1,2] However, since the wires are stiff, they can straighten the curved segment, change the vessel shape, and cause wrinkles or pseudo lesions. Disadvantages of using a stiff wire include difficulty of tracking stents because of the wire bias inducing vessel spasm, even obstruction of flow induced by vessel kinking, and wire buckling due to sharp transitions. The reason that a wire is stiff or flexible is down to its intrinsic design and material composition. A core that extends to the distal tip provides extra support and torque transmission and is therefore stiff (Fig. 5.3). The nitinol core increases wire tractability, including the ability to traverse acute artery angulations without wire prolapse. The limitations of nitinol core wire is that it tends to store, rather than transmit torque.[1] When

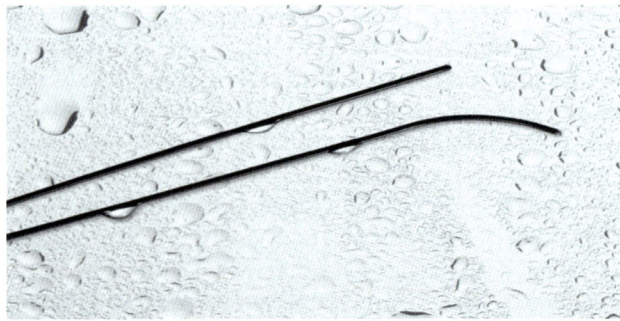

Fig. 5.2 Wire with a hydrophilic wire coating

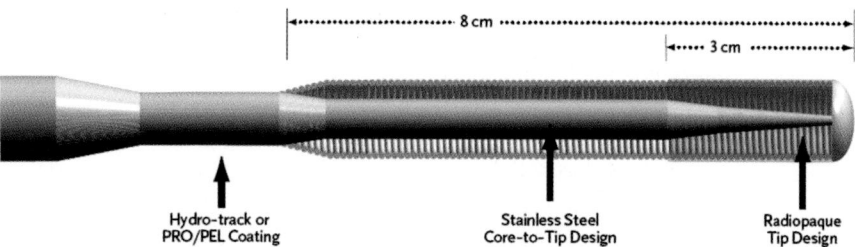

Fig. 5.3 Schematic of typical guidewire construction with a solid core component and a core taper

selection or entry to a side branch is desired, it is important to make the radius of the curve on the tip of the wire match the diameter of the main vessel proximal to the origin of that branch. A double bend can be useful if there are two different angulated segments to cross. Standard guidewire length of 145–180 cm is usually adequate for access to a specific place in a vessel, catheterization of a branch vessel, and/or crossing a lesion; however, to facilitate exchange of catheters while maintaining a lesion crossing, exchange-length guidewires (260–300 cm) are used. These longer wires will generally also have more support (i.e., are stiffer) than those used to cross lesions. The standard guidewire diameter for peripheral interventions, especially those involving large vessels, is 0.035 in. All the wires mentioned here fall into that group. However, due to improved guidewire construction, an increasing number of endovascular procedures can be performed using 0.014 or 0.018 in. wires (Table 5.1).

5.2 Technical Pearls

5.2.1 Advancing a Wire Through Severely Angulated vessel

When a wire needs to navigate a tortuous vessel, it is recommended that the tip of the wire be curved to form a large diameter curve. Once the tip enters the branch, the wire is withdrawn to prolapse the tip into the intended branch. The wire should then be rotated toward the main lumen, clockwise if the tip was pointing toward the left of the patient and counterclockwise if the tip was pointing toward the right of the patient. If there are enough stiff segments inside the side branch (not just the soft tip), then the wire will advance further, without prolapsing back (Fig. 4.1).

Crossing a stent: If a stent needs to be recrossed, the tip of the guidewire should be curved well into a wide J and the whole wire can be advanced while being rotated. This maneuver will help to avoid the inadvertent migration of the tip of the catheter under a strut, changing the direction of the whole wire to outside the stent.

Table 5.1 Commonly used guidewires for access and crossing lesions

Device	Dimensions and materials	Company	Characteristics
Benston starter	0.035″ × 180 cm stainless steel	Boston Scientific	Preferred wire for initial access, TFE-coated medium rigid wire with straight floppy tip
Safe T-J	0.035″ × 180 cm stainless steel	Cook	TFE-coated with soft J-tip
Wholey	0.035″ × 145 cm stainless steel with gold tip	Mallinckrodt	TFE-coated steerable wire with floppy tip
Glidewire	0.035″ × 180 cm nitinol core wire; polyurethane jacketwith tungsten	Terumo	Hydrophilic coated; adept at traversing difficult anatomy, dissection risk
Magic torque	0.035″ × 180 cm stainless steel	Boston Scientific	Hydrophilic-coated, calibrated wire with good support for catheters
Nitrex	0.035″ × 260 cm nitinol core wire; gold–tungsten coil with IVUS; silicone-coated	ev3	Preferred wire for reflection off aortic valve and aortic inspection
Platinum plus	0.025″ × 260 cm stainless steel withplatinum distal coil	Boston Scientific	TFE-coated with shapeable platinum floppy tip

Measure the length of a lesion with a wire: It is not easy to guess accurately the length of a lesion if some segments are foreshortened because of tortuosity. When a vessel bends in more than one plane, no single angiographic view can overcome multiple foreshortenings. Most radiolucent wires have a 20–30 mm radiopaque distal end. Position this radiopaque segment across the lesion so the length of the lesion can be estimated. Another way is to measure the lesion length with a balloon that has markers at its two ends.

Manipulating the hydrophilic wire: The hydrophilic wires such as the glidewire (Meditech/Terumo Corp, Piscataway, NJ), Choice PT phus, and Whisper wire are kink-resistant flexible wires covered with a hydrophilic polyurethane coating. The core is constructed with super elastic titanium–nickel alloy that offers extreme flexibility and kink resistance, thus optimizing pushability. A hydrophilic polymer coating results in low thrombogenicity and extreme lubricity when wet. Because it is very slippery, it has to be handled with a plastic holding device at its proximal end to avoid slippage due to its alloy core.

5.3 Guidewires Used in Thoracic Endografting

The extra-support guidewire (extra-stiff guidewire) is an essential component of thoracic endografting and is used to assist with tortuous and angled anatomy and for traversing long distances with large devices. The most common extra-stiff guidewires used in thoracic endografting include the Nitrex nitinol (ev3, Plymouth, MN), the Meier wire (Boston Scientific, Natick MA), the Amplatz (Boston Scientific), and the Lunderquist by Cook Inc. (Bloomington, IN) (Table 5.2).

5.3.1 Lunderquist Stiff Wire Guides (LES)

The Lunderquist extra-stiff guidewires (Cook Inc., Bloomington, IN) is the most commonly used extra-stiff guidewire for aortic interventional procedures because they have excellent laser-weld transition, a high degree of shaft stiffness, a Teflon coating, a stainless steel mandrel, and available in both a straight and a curved tip. The Lunderquist extra-stiff wire (Fig. 5.4) (Cook Inc., Bloomington, IN) is the preferred wire for thoracic endografting, because the floppy tip is curved and designed to sit above the aortic valve in a non-traumatic fashion and will not wander into the coronary arteries or the brachiocephalic vessels.

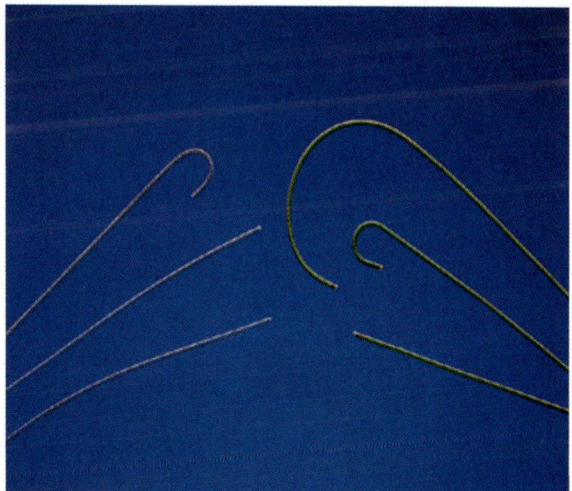

Fig. 5.4 Lunderquist stiff guidewire

5.3.2 LES3 Lunderquist Wire Guide (Curved Tip)

LES3 Lunderquist guidewire (Fig. 5.5) is a 260 cm extra-stiff wire and is used when extremely stiff exchange wire guides are required. Features include a shaped design for stability in the thoracic aorta with a curve that mimics the natural arch

Table 5.2 Recommended stiff guidewires for thoracic endografting

Company name	Product name	Material used	Guidewire size/OD (in.)	Guidewire length (cm)	Comments
Boston Scientific/Terumo	Radiofocus glidewire/angled tip/regular shaft	Hydrophilic coated/stainless steel core	0.035	260	Primary wire used for initial cannulation/used in conjunction with catheter manipulation
Boston Scientific/Terumo	Radiofocus glidewire/angled tip/stiff shaft	Hydrophilic coated/stainless steel core	0.035	260 cm	Used for extra support with catheter manipulation in tortuous aortic anatomy
Boston Scientific/Terumo	Radiofocus glidewire/angled tip/stiff shaft	Hydrophilic coated/stainless steel core	0.035	450	Used for brachiofemoral wire access/"body flossing" technique
Boston Scientific	Amplatz super stiff	Spiral wind over/stainless steel core	0.035	260	Extra-support wire for intravascular ultrasound catheter imaging procedure
Cook Inc.	Double-curved Lunderquist extra stiff (LES3)	TFE-coated stainless steel	0.035	260	Extra-support wire used to deliver the endograft
Cook Inc.	Newton LLT	TFE-coated stainless steel	0.038	145	Pusher wire for 0.038 embolization coils

OD, outer diameter; TFE, polytetrafluoroethylene

of the anatomy while offering the stiffness of a standard Lunderquist extra-stiff wire. Non-traumatic distal tip has "non-selecting" curve that will not wander into brachiocephalic vessels.

Fig. 5.5 LES3 Lunderquist guidewire

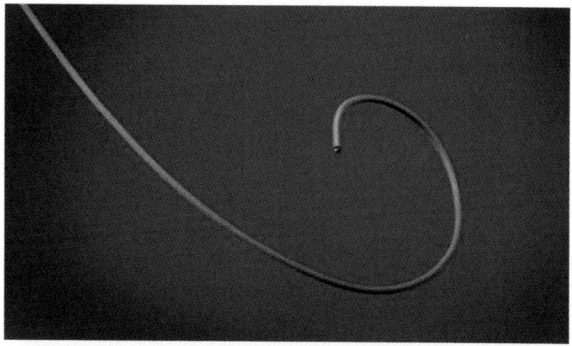

Fig. 5.6 Amplatz stiff wire

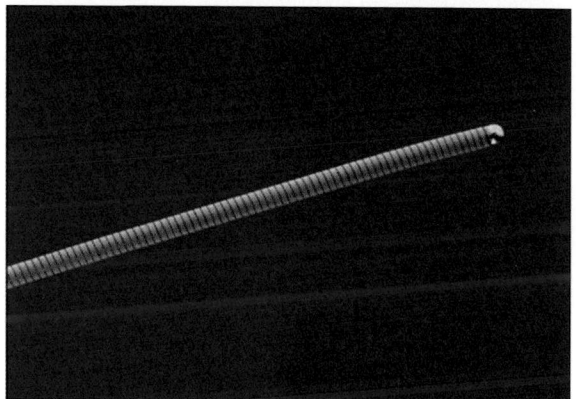

5.3.3 Amplatz Stiff Wire

Ultra-stiff wire (Fig. 5.6) guides are used for interventional cardiovascular procedures, interventional biliary drainage, abscess drainage, uroradiology procedures, and catheter exchanges.

References

1. Abbott JD, Williams DO. Coronary wire manipulation. In: King III SB, Douglas JS, eds. *Coronary Arteriography and Angioplasty*. New York, NY: McGraw-Hill; 1985:303–313.
2. Wheatley GH 3rd, McNutt R, Diethrich EB. Introduction to thoracic endografting: imaging, guidewires, guiding catheters, and delivery sheaths. *Ann Thorac Surg*. 2007; 83(1):272–278.

Chapter 6
Sheaths Used in Thoracic Aortic Endografting

Sheaths are hemostatic conduits inserted into the vessel which provide the safest method of maintaining access for an endovascular procedure. Sheaths allow passage of guidewires, catheters and interventional devices in and out of the body without damaging the vessel and reducing the blood loss.[1-3] Sheaths are essential for planned exchange of guidewires or catheters or when any large or irregular devices are to be introduced as well as all interventional procedures. Sheaths are introduced during initial vascular access over guidewire after cannulation of the artery using the Seldinger technique. Appropriately sized dilators aid the insertion of the larger sheath into the small puncture made by the initial needle. Subsequent to insertion, all exchange or introduction of guidewires, catheters, and devices will take place through the lumen of the sheath. The benefit of the sheath lies in the exclusion of the vessel puncture site from this activity. Each guidewire or catheter introduced directly into the vessel carries a risk of localized hematoma formation or vessel trauma (enlarging the puncture site, dissection of an intimal flap, tearing of vessel walls, etc.), but the sheath serves to minimize vessel trauma and extravasation of blood while maintaining vascular access. Sheaths and dilators (Fig. 6.1) are usually constructed of Teflon (tetrafluoroethylene), with the braided construction making

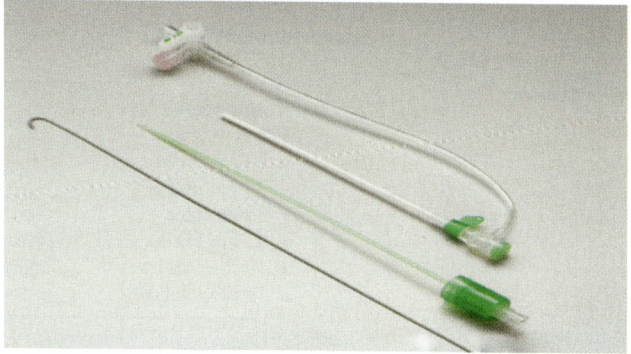

Fig. 6.1 Dilator, sheath conduit, three-way stop cock with a hemostatic valve

J. Kpodonu, *Manual of Thoracic Endoaortic Surgery*,
DOI 10.1007/978-1-84996-296-4_6, © Springer-Verlag London Limited 2010

the sheath kink resistant. This rather inflexible material has an extremely low coefficient of friction and is very torquable (turning the ex vivo portion results in rotation of the in vivo portion), making it ideal for establishing a conduit through which exchange of devices can occur. A radiopaque material is often incorporated into the distal end of the sheath, enabling clear visualization under fluoroscopy. Nearly all sheaths feature a hemostatic valve and side infusion port. The valve is of principal importance to the function of sheaths: it allows insertion of devices into the vessel while maintaining hemostasis. Hemostatic valves can be either the traditional slotted membrane or the rotating valve, which can be manually opened and closed. While both types are effective in preventing blood loss, the rotating hemostatic valve allows back-bleeding in the open position, which is thought to reduce the risk of air embolization. The sheath side port can be used for blood sampling, pressure monitoring, and contrast injection. Radiopaque tips allow operator ability to visualize the end of the sheath which is particularly important with stent placement. Differences in hemostatic valves account for difference in minimizing blood loss. Sheath lengths may vary from 5.5 to 90 cm.

Sheaths are measured by inner diameter and catheters measured by outer diameter. A general rule of thumb: generally there is a 2 Fr size difference between the inner diameter and the outer diameter of both sheaths and guiding catheters. Peripheral and coronary sheaths have a universal color code (Table 6.1).

Large diameter sheaths (20–24 Fr) (Fig. 6.2) are available for delivery of endografts in the treatment of aortic pathologies. Multiple valve construction configurations are available and generally have a braided shaft design offering strength and flexibility (kink resistant). A femoral cutdown is generally required for access although alternate sites may include axillary artery access or not uncommonly construction of a retroperitoneal conduit when the access femoral/iliac vessels are small, tortuous and or calcified. Occasionally serial dilatation of the iliac vessels can be performed using dilators (Fig. 6.3). These sheaths are often included in the endograft delivery systems. Sheath lengths range from 10 to 65 cm, but the 10–15 cm length is standard for most peripheral vascular interventions. Longer length sheaths are usually only needed for endograft placement or access to the contralateral side of the body. The majority of sheaths used in our endograft cases are 10 cm in length.

Table 6.1 Universal color coding sheaths measured in F sizes 0.1 Fr = 0.33 mm

- 4 Fr = red
- 5 Fr = gray
- 6 Fr = green
- 7 Fr = orange
- 8 Fr = blue
- 9 Fr = black
- 10 Fr = violet
- 11 Fr = yellow

Device	Dimensions	Company	Characteristics
Pinnacle Introducer	7–11 Fr × 10–25 (4 Fr with brachial access)	Terumo	Straight sheath with cross-cut hemostatic valve
Large (12–24 Fr) sheaths are incorporated in endograft delivery system			
Keller-Timmerman	18–24 Fr × 25–65 cm	Cook	Large, valved sheath
Large and Extra Large Check-Flo	10–24 Fr × 25–60 cm	Cook	Tapered sheath with hemostatic valve

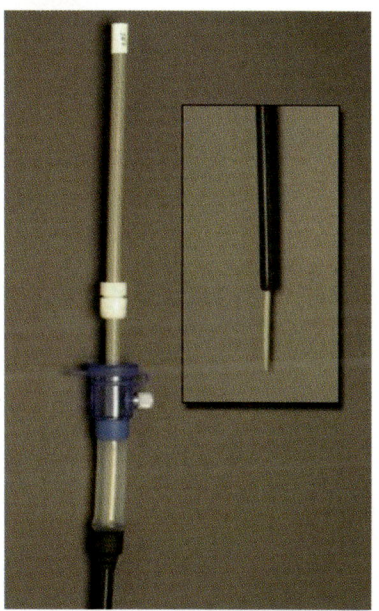

Fig. 6.2 Large sheath (20–24 Fr) used to deploy a Gore TAG thoracic endograft

Large sheaths range from 12 to 24 Fr in outer diameter, with lengths ranging from 10 to 85 cm. Multiple valve construction configurations are available and generally have a braided shaft design offering strength and flexibility (kink resistant). A femoral cutdown is generally required for device access although alternate sites including axillary artery access and construction of a retroperitoneal conduit are occasionally required for small, tortuous, and/or calcified femoral/iliac vessels. Occasionally serial dilatation of the iliac vessels can be performed using dilators when the iliac vessels are marginal (Fig. 6.3).

Fig. 6.3 Dilators for dilating iliac vessels

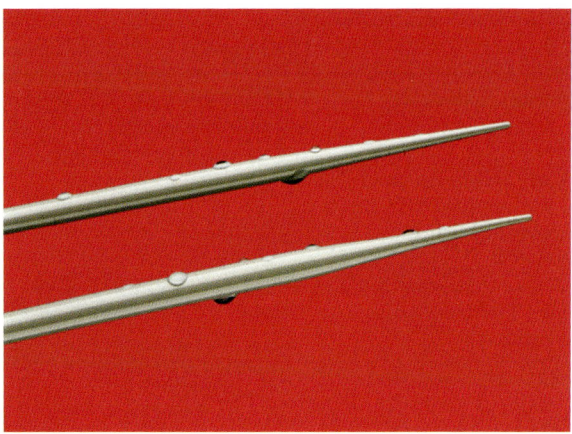

References

1. Rutherford RB. *Rutherford Vascular Surgery.* 6th ed. Philadelphia, PA: Elsevier Saunders; 2005.
2. Casserly IP, Sacher R, Yadav JS, eds. *Manual of Peripheral Vascular Intervention.* Philadelphia, PA: Lippincott Williams and Wilkins; 2005.
3. Moore WS. *Vascular and Endovascular Surgery: A Comprehensive Review.* 7th ed. Philadelphia, PA: Elsevier Saunders; 2006.

Chapter 7
Stents Used in Conjunction with Thoracic Aortic Endografting

7.1 Stents

Stents are metallic scaffolding used to permanently dilate a lesion to restore or preserve the patency of a vessel. Stents are primarily used to treat dissections after angioplasty, residual stenosis (>30%), pressure gradient (>10 mmHg systolic), target vessel occlusion, and recurrence of disease. Based on the method of deployment vascular stents are divided into two main categories: balloon-expanded or self-expanding.

Balloon-expandable stents (Fig. 7.1) are straight, rigid cylinders constructed of 316L stainless steel secured on an angioplasty balloon. Most balloon-expanded stents possess high radial force "hoop strength," but lack flexibility. With improvement in mesh design, smaller and thinner cell struts, flexibility of stents has improved with preservation of excellent radial strength. Guiding catheters and sheaths are necessary to advance the device through tortuosity of the vascular system in order to avoid dislodgement of the undeployed stent. The working qualities of the balloon-expanded stent make it a better choice for precise treatment of a focal lesion in an area with less tortuosity and without repetitive external trauma such as the inguinal ligament and across joints. The excellent hoop strength makes it the preferred device for ostial lesions. As a routine the device size is matched to the anticipated vessel diameter. Balloon-expanded stents can be dilated 2–3 mm beyond

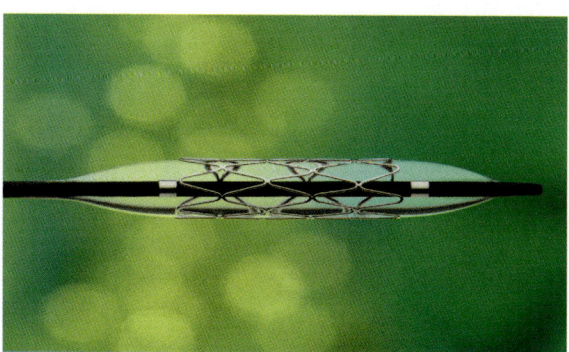

Fig. 7.1 Balloon-expandable stent

J. Kpodonu, *Manual of Thoracic Endoaortic Surgery*,
DOI 10.1007/978-1-84996-296-4_7, © Springer-Verlag London Limited 2010

Table 7.1 Commercially available balloon-expandable stents in the United States

Company name	Product name	Indicated use	Material used	Maximum guidewire size (in.)	Introducer French size (Fr)	Stent diameter (mm)	Stent length (mm)	Delivery system length (cm)
Atrium	iCAST stent	Tracheobronchial	316L stainless steel/PTFE	0.035	6 7 7	5–6 7 5, 7–9	16, 22 16, 22 38, 59	120 120 80, 120
Boston Scientific	Express Biliary LD	Biliary	316L stainless steel	0.035	6 7 7	5–8 8 9,10	17, 27, 37, 57 57 37	75, 135
Boston Scientific	Express Biliary SD (monorail)	Biliary	316L stainless steel	0.018	5	4–6	15, 19	90
Cook Medical Inc.	Formula 418	Biliary	316L stainless steel	0.018	5	5–7	16, 20, 24	80
Cordis Endovascular	Palmaz Genesis	Biliary (US) Peripheral (Europe)	316L stainless steel	N/A (unmounted)	7	5–9	59, 79	N/A (unmounted)
Cordis Endovascular	Palmaz	Biliary, iliac, renal	316L stainless steel	N/A (unmounted)	7 11, 12	4–9 10–28	20, 29, 39 31, 40	N/A (unmounted)
Cordis Endovascular	Palmaz Blue	Biliary (US) Peripheral (Europe)	Chromium cobalt	0.018	5	5–6	15, 18, 24	80
Cordis Endovascular	Palmaz Genesis	Biliary (US) Peripheral (Europe)	316L stainless steel	0.035	6 7	5–7 8	24, 29, 39 29, 39	80, 135
EV3	Intrastent LD	Biliary	316L stainless steel	0.035	10–16	12–18	58, 78	N/A (unmounted)
Medtronic Vascular	Bridge Assurant	Biliary	316L stainless steel	0.035	6 7	6–8 8	30, 40, 60 60	80
Medtronic Vascular	Racer	Biliary	Chromium cobalt	0.018	5	4–6	12, 18	80, 130

their nominal size with appropriate balloon oversize. Corresponding decrease in the length should be expected with balloon-expandable stents. The basic technique of stent deployment requires that the balloon catheter with the stent secured into place be advanced using fluoroscopy to the desired location. Once in good position across the lesion, the stent is expanded by inflating the balloon. The balloon first inflates at both ends of the stent followed by expansion in the center, allowing for precise positioning. Before deployment, it is critical to make sure that the stent is still correctly mounted on the balloon to avoid forward or backward misplacement.

Table 7.1 is a list of commercially available balloon-expandable stents in the United States

7.1.1 Self-Expanding Stents

Self-expanding stents are constructed of stainless steel or the nickel–titanium alloy called nitinol. The former is not MRI compatible (only up to 1.5 T), while the latter may be evaluated using MRI. Radiopacity is another feature of contemporary stents. Stainless steel devices are usually easy to identify. Nitinol stents on the other hand require radiopaque markers to facilitate accurate position and subsequent radiographic evaluation.

When the nitinol is chilled the metal can be compressed so the stent can be loaded into a delivery catheter system. This is done by the stent manufacturing company. When the stent is placed in the human body and the delivery system is deployed, the stent expands due to the body temperature. The interesting property of nitinol is that it has memory, so it can be crushed and it will recover its manufactured specifications. Self-expanding stents (Fig. 7.2) are placed in lesions where the vessels are more mobile, e.g., near joints or in limbs. Most self-expanding stents have radiopaque markers that increase their visibility. Device deployment is carried out by retracting the outer sheath while holding the stent in place with the inner tube. Due to its better flexibility self-expanding stents are preferred devices for tortuous

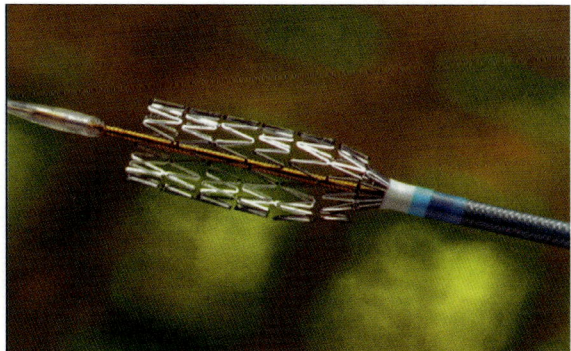

Fig. 7.2 Self-expandable stent

Table 7.2 Table of commonly used self-expandable stents on the market

Company name	Product name	Indicated use	Material used	Maximum guidewire size (in.)	Introducer French size (Fr)	Stent diameter (mm)	Stent length (mm)	Delivery system length (cm)
Abbott Vascular	Xceed	Biliary	Nitinol	0.035	6	5 6, 8	60, 80 80, 100, 120	120
Abbott Vascular	Xact	Carotid	Nitinol	0.014	8	7, 8, 9, 10 8/6, 9/7, 10/8	30 30, 40	136
Abbott Vascular/Guidant	Absolute	Biliary	Nitinol	0.035	6	6, 8	40, 60, 80, 100	80
Abbott Vascular/Guidant	Acculink	Carotid	Nitinol	0.014	6	5, 6, 7, 8 6/8, 7/10	30, 40	132
Bard	Luminexx	Transhepatic biliary	Nitinol	0.035	6	10, 12, 14	40, 60	80
Bard	Conformexx	Transhepatic biliary	Nitinol	0.035	6	6, 8	60, 80, 100, 120	135
Boston Scientific	Sentinol	Biliary	Nitinol	0.035	6	5 6, 8	60, 80 40, 60, 80	135
Boston Scientific	Monorail Wallstent	Biliary (Wallstent)	Elgiloy	0.014	5 5 6	6 8 10	22 21, 29, 36 24, 31, 37	135
Boston Scientific	Wallstent	Tracheobronchial, Transhepatic biliary, iliac	Elgiloy	0.035	8 9	12 14, 16	40, 60	100
Boston Scientific	Wallgraft	Tracheobronchial	Elgiloy Dacron	0.035	10 11 12	10 12 14	30, 50, 70 30, 50, 70 50, 70	75

Table 7.2 (continued)

Company name	Product name	Indicated use	Material used	Maximum guidewire size (in.)	Introducer French size (Fr)	Stent diameter (mm)	Stent length (mm)	Delivery system length (cm)
Cook Medical Inc.	Z-Stent	Tracheobronchial Gianturco	Stainless steel	0.035	16	25, 35	5 cm	Unmounted
Cook Medical Inc.	Zilver 635	Biliary	Nitinol	0.035	6	5, 6, 8	40, 60, 80	125
Cordis Endovascular	Precise	Carotid	Nitinol	0.014	6 7	7, 8 9	30, 40 30, 40	135
Cordis Endovascular	Smart Control	Transhepatic biliary, iliac	Nitinol	0.035	6	6, 8	30, 40, 60, 80, 100	80,120
EV3	Protégé/Everflex	Biliary/SFA	Nitinol	0.035	6 6	6, 8 14	30, 40, 60, 80, 120, 150 60, 80	120 120
W.L. Gore	Viabahn 5–8 mm heparin coated	Tracheobronchial, SFA	Nitinol, PTFE	0.035 0.035 0.025 0.025	7 8 11 12	5, 6 7, 8 9 11, 13	5, 10, 15 5, 10, 15 10, 15 10	120 120 110 110

vessels. They can cover longer lesions but are not practical for treating focal disease. These stents guarantee very precise placement only at the end to be deployed first (Wallstents deploy from distal to proximal). Definite advantage of the Wallstent is the ability to recapture the device until up to 85% of the stent is deployed. This may facilitate adequate repositioning. As a rule the leading end of the device is always maneuvered just past the planned landing zone, allowing for fine adjustments during its deployment. Self-expanding stents are better choices for tortuous vessels especially in areas of permanent external forces, i.e., across the inguinal ligament or across joints, etc. Because of the inability for additional dilatation of the device, as opposed to balloon-expanded stents, better device/target vessel size match is required. Most peripheral vessels can be stented through sheaths ranging from 6 to 10 Fr. Table 7.2 shows a list of commercially available self-expanding stents.

7.1.2 Covered Stents

Fabric-covered stents are intended to replace the inner lining of a vessel by endovascular graft placement. There are several commercially available covered stent grafts used for peripheral interventions, with different approved indications. They usually require 8–12 Fr access sheaths (Fig 7.3).

Aortic endografts are larger covered stent grafts used to treat aortic pathologies[1–3] (Table 7.3). The advances in the development of intravascular stents made possible the construction and approval of the currently available endovascular grafts for the treatment of abdominal and thoracic aortic pathology. Thoracic endograft devices are applicable in treating thoracic aortic pathology including aneurysms, traumatic aortic transection, complicated type B aortic dissection and

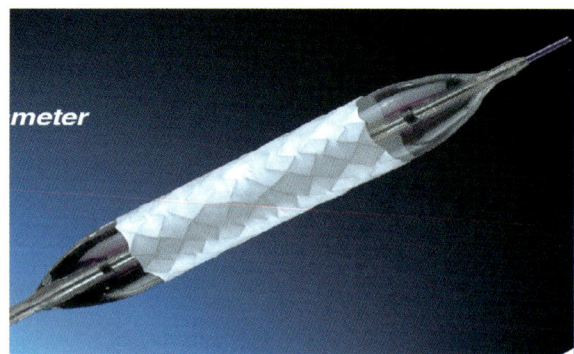

Fig. 7.3 Atrium iCAST balloon expandable covered stent

Table 7.3 Commercially available covered stents used for peripheral indications

Fluency Plus	(Bard)	Tracheobronchial	Self-expanding
Jostent	(Abbott)	Coronary perforation	Balloon-expanded
Viabahn	(Gore)	SFA	Self-expanding
iCAST	(Atrium)	Tracheobronchial	Balloon-expanded

also the different stages of the uncommon aortic wall abnormality of intramural hematoma, penetrating ulcer and pseudoaneurysm. In addition to the Gore TAG thoracic endoprosthesis The Talent Thoracic Device (Medtronic), The Valiant Thoracic Device (Medtronic), The Zenith TX2 TAA Endovascular Device, The Zenith TX2 Dissection Endovascular Device (Cook Medical), and The Relay Thoracic Stent Graft (Bolton Medical) are also available commercially in the United States and Europe and also as part of ongoing clinical trials.

References

1. Moore WS, Ahn SS. *Endovascular Surgery.* 3rd ed. Philadelphia, PA: W.B. Saunders; 2001.
2. Schneider PA. *Endovascular Skills.* St. Louis, MO: Quality Medical Publishing; 1998.
3. Endovascular Today 2007:6(12) GORE TAG IFU, Flagstaff, AZ: W.L. Gore & Associates, Inc.

Chapter 8
Vascular Closure Devices

Worldwide, between 7.5 and 8 million catheter-based vascular procedures are performed a year. Only around 20–25% of these procedures utilize a vascular closure device (VCD) for access site hemostasis. The use of larger sheaths and the widespread use of peri-procedural anticoagulation have increased the risk of bleeding complications, resulting in the need for better methods of hemostasis. Complication rates related to hemostasis for diagnostic angiograms range from 0 to 1.1%, and increase to 1.3–3.4% for therapeutic procedures. While the outcomes of VCD studies have shown increased patient satisfaction, early ambulation and decreased hospital resource utilization, compared with manual compression, there is limited evidence that hemorrhage and other puncture site complications are reduced by VCDs compared with manual compression. Indeed, the use of VCDs is associated with a new group of complications related to the devices themselves.

8.1 Manual Compression

The method considered the gold standard, described by Seldinger et al. in 1953, involves manual compression over the puncture site, for 10–30 min, followed by overnight bed rest. This method achieves hemostasis due to the formation of a fibrin and platelet plug following exposure of the blood to the collagen in the arterial wall at the puncture site. Traditional bed rest times after manual compression are set arbitrarily.

The evidence suggests that overnight bed rest is unnecessary. For example, in a study of early mobilization following manual compression of 6 Fr arterial punctures post-angioplasty, 90% of 128 patients were ambulant at 4 h following gradual mobilization after 2 h of supine bed rest. This was achieved with no major puncture site complications and no delayed complications.

8.2 Types of Vascular Closure Device

Vascular closure devices fall into two main categories.

J. Kpodonu, *Manual of Thoracic Endoaortic Surgery*,
DOI 10.1007/978-1-84996-296-4_8, © Springer-Verlag London Limited 2010

8.2.1 Active Devices

These achieve hemostasis immediately and involve some kind of mechanical seal.

Suture alone – Perclose AT and Prostar XL10 (Abbott Vascular, Redwood City, CA).
Extravascular collagen alone.
Suture–collagen combinations – Angio-Seal (St. Jude Medical, St. Paul, MN):
Surgical staple or clip.
StarClose (Abbott Vascular, Redwood City, CA).
EVS-Angiolink (Medtronic Co., Minneapolis, MN).

8.2.2 Passive Devices

These do not achieve immediate hemostasis.

Augmented manual compression:
External patches with prothrombotic coatings – Syvek Patch (Marine Polymer Technologies, Danvers, MA).
Wire-stimulated track thrombosis-Boomerang Closure Wire (Cardiva Medical, Mountain View, CA).

Mechanically assisted manual compression:
Femstop – (RADI Medical Systems, Uppsala, Sweden).
Clamp-ease (Pressure Products, Rancho Palos Verdes, CA).
Sandbags and pressure dressings.

8.3 Active Vascular Closure Devices

8.3.1 Prostar XL10 and Perclose A-T

Both are suture-mediated devices and create a purely mechanical seal.

8.3.1.1 Prostar XL10

The device consists of a 10 Fr shaft holding two pairs of needles connected by two braided polyester suture loops and a rotating barrel that is used to facilitate the positioning of the device before needle deployment and to guide the needles during their travel through the subcutaneous tract.

Device Deployment

1. At the end of the procedure, the sheath is removed and the device is inserted over a standard guidewire.
2. Dilatation of the subcutaneous tract is needed to accept the oversize barrel.

3. Correct positioning of the device with the barrel against the arterial wall is confirmed when pulsatile blood exits the marker lumen (this occurs when the distal end of the marker lumen enters the artery).
4. The needles are deployed, passing from within the device in the arterial lumen through the arterial wall and back into the barrel.
5. They take the suture ends with them and exit from the top of the device.
6. The needles are cut from the sutures that are then freed from the device.
7. The surgical knots are tied using a slipknot. The knots are slipped (pushed) down onto the arterial wall while the device is removed.
8. The knots are tightened with a knot pusher, achieving hemostasis, and the suture ends are cut short.

This device can be used to close very large arteriotomies and has been used to perform endovascular aneurysm repair using a totally percutaneous technique without the need for a surgical femoral arteriotomy.

The availability of the Prostar device varies widely worldwide. At the present time, it is very difficult to acquire the device in the United Kingdom.

8.3.1.2 Perclose A-T

This is a smaller device and is designed to be used to close puncture sites 6–8 Fr in diameter. With the Perclose A-T (auto-tie) a slipknot is already created within the device, which enables a more rapid, easier, and single-handed operation.

The device is inserted over a guidewire, which can be reintroduced during the procedure if a problem is encountered.

The device can also be used to close larger arteriotomies using the technique known as *pre-deployment.*

Pre-deployment involves inserting the suture into the arterial wall *at the start of the procedure.*

Provided the stitch is not "tied and locked," the puncture site can be dilated to a larger French size.

Once the procedure is completed, hemostasis is achieved by tightening the pre-deployed suture.

Thus the 6 Fr device can be pre-deployed prior to dilation of an arteriotomy up to 12 Fr. It is also possible to use more than one device at a time in order to close even larger arteriotomies. Similar to the Prostar XL10, the Perclose A-T can be used to perform endovascular aneurysm repair using a combination of the pre-deployment technique and more than one device. Perclose devices have been used successfully to close puncture sites in other locations such as the brachial and popliteal arteries.

The devices have also been used to close inadvertent subclavian artery punctures created during central venous catheter insertion.

8.3.2 Angioseal Closure Device

This device creates a mechanical seal by sandwiching the arteriotomy between a biodegradable polymer anchor, which remains inside the vessel, and an

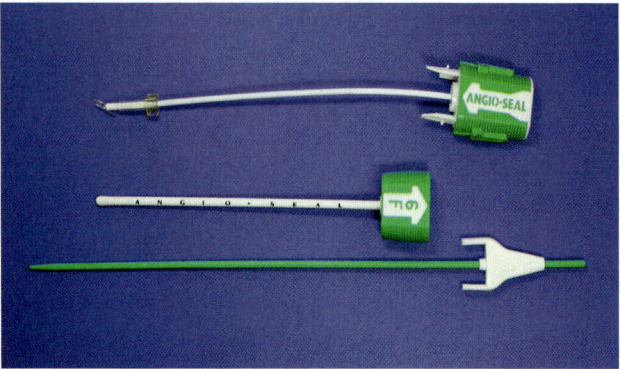

Fig. 8.1 Angioseal St. Jude Minnetonka MN vascular closure device used to achieve hemostasis

extravascular collagen sponge (Fig. 8.1). The collagen augments the mechanical seal by inducing platelet adhesiveness and is held in place by a self-tightening suture.

The device is available in 6 and 8 Fr versions. It consists of a delivery system and three bioabsorbable components. The delivery system consists of a 0.035 in. guidewire, an insertion sheath, and a dilator with a marker lumen (which locates the arteriotomy). The bioabsorbable components consist of a flat 10 mm × 2 mm × 1 mm anchor (footplate), a collagen plug, and a suture that maintains tension between these two components.

8.3.2.1 Device Deployment

1. At the end of the procedure the insertion sheath/dilator combination is inserted over a guidewire.
2. The sheath is inserted until blood exits from the marker hole at the proximal end of the dilator.
3. The entire system should be gently withdrawn over the guidewire until the passage of blood from the marker hole stops.
4. After this point has been reached, the device should be reinserted 1.5 cm into the artery.
5. The guidewire and dilator are removed.
6. While holding the sheath fixed in position, the carrier tube containing the anchor, plug, and suture is inserted into the sheath.
7. The anchor is deployed into the arterial lumen and is pulled back to abut against the wall of the artery over the arteriotomy site.
8. The carrier tube and the sheath are withdrawn to reveal a tamper tube that is used to tamp the collagen plug against the outer arterial wall and locks into place.
9. The suture is cut below the skin.

The anchor is reabsorbed in a process that is physically complete at approximately 30 days and chemically complete at approximately 90 days post-procedure. Arterial re-puncture within 90 days is not recommended because of the risk of displacement of the anchor. It may be possible to identify and avoid the anchor using ultrasound, if arterial puncture at the same site is required urgently before this interval. The current device is the Angioseal STS PLUS platform. A more recent development is the Angioseal VIP (V-twist Integrated Platform). This version features a larger collagen plug that conforms to the vessel by twisting down onto the arterial wall. Apart from this design change the deployment is the same as the STS device.

8.3.3 StarClose System

The StarClose system Fig. 8.2 (Abbott Vascular, Redwood City, CA) is designed to deliver a 4 mm diameter nitinol staple onto the outside of the vessel. The device can close a 6 Fr puncture site. The system is designed for single-operator use and closure time should be less than 60 s.

Fig. 8.2 The StarClose system (Abbott Vascular, Redwood City, CA)

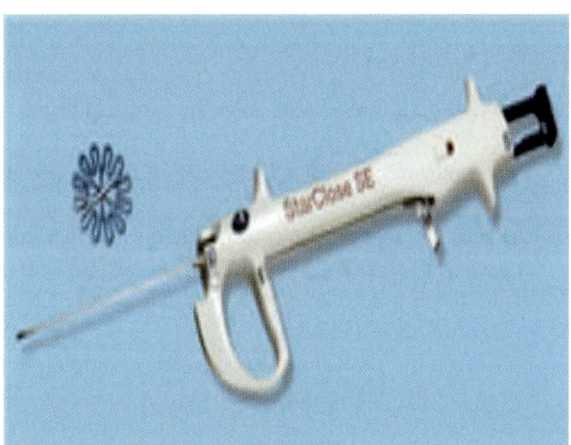

8.3.4 Passive Vascular Closure Devices (VCD)

8.3.4.1 Boomerang Closure Wire

This is a relatively new device. The Boomerang Closure Wire consists of a collapsed nitinol disc on an introducer/deployment wire (Fig. 8.3).

Fig. 8.3 Boomerang closure
device (Cardiva Medical Inc.,
Sunnyvale, CA)

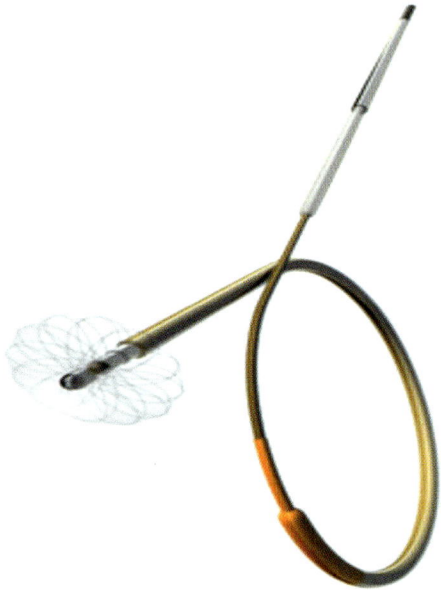

Device Deployment

1. The device is introduced into the artery through the sheath at the end of the
   procedure.
2. Once the wire is in place, the nitinol disc is opened to form a flat, low-profile
   disc within the vessel.
3. Upon removal of the arterial sheath, the Boomerang disc is positioned against the
   arterial wall forming a temporary hemostatic seal until the natural elastic recoil
   of the arteriotomy, known as the Boomerang Effect, returns the arteriotomy to
   the size of an 18 G needle.
4. Following the procedure, the device is completely removed leaving no residual
   foreign body and minimal scarring.
5. Final hemostasis is achieved by a few minutes of occlusive finger pressure.

A recent modification of the device, *the Boomerang Catalyst wire*, incorporates an active agent that can initiate hemostasis in the track. The surface of the
Boomerang Catalyst wire adjacent to the arteriotomy site has a negatively charged
proprietary compound which activates factor XII thereby promoting hemostasis.
The device has been used to close arteriotomies up to 10 Fr with only a few minutes
of manual compression required following removal of the device. The main draw-
back of the device is that elastic recoil at the arteriotomy site may take 20–30 min
and therefore hemostasis may be time consuming, arguably with no tangible benefit
versus conventional manual compression.

8.3.4.2 Patch Technology

In the past there has been some interest in the so-called patch technologies which encompass a group of products that augment manual compression. They consist of celluloid polymer patches coated with agents that are applied externally and accelerate the coagulation process when blood comes into contact with the patch, along the puncture tract. Manual compression is still required. However, they have a number of advantages: ease of use. They can be used in anticoagulated patients. They can be used in patients on anti-platelet therapy. No foreign body is left in situ. There are no stipulations regarding repeat arterial puncture at the same site of Antisocial. One size fits all. At present, there is no clinical evidence that the time to ambulation is reduced with these devices.

8.3.4.3 Syvec Patch

The Syvec Patch consists of a celluloid polymer patch coated with poly-N-acetyl glucosamine (pGlcNAc). Where it comes into contact with blood, it invokes both clot formation and local vasoconstriction as part of its overall hemostatic effect. Following the procedure the sheath is removed and the saline-moistened Syvec Patch is applied and held in place with manual compression for 4 min. Manual compression is maintained if blood continues to ooze. Once hemostasis is achieved, the patch is left in place with a non-occlusive dressing for 24 h.

8.3.4.4 D-Stat

D-Stat uses an adhesive dressing containing thrombin and is available for use in the United Kingdom. However, clinical information is limited. Application is the same as with the Syvek patch, although the company recommends an initial check after 5 min. Once hemostasis is achieved, the patch is left in place with a non-occlusive dressing for 12–24 h. The patch can be used for puncture sites up to 8 Fr, and in patients on anticoagulation and/or anti-platelet therapy.

8.3.4.5 ChitoSeal

As with the other devices, the ChitoSeal is a topical hemostasis pad. In this case, the active ingredient is chitosan gel. Application is the same as with the other two devices, although the company recommends an initial check after 2–3 min. Once hemostasis is established, a dressing is applied and removed within 24 h.

8.4 Benefits of VCDs

Patients are at an increased risk of hemorrhage when large sheath size, long complex procedures and the need for continued anticoagulation immediately post-procedure, e.g., post-carotid stenting. With the current closure devices (Perclose, Angioseal, and Starclose), hemostasis is usually achieved in minutes when the indication for use is adhered to.

Use of VCDs enables more procedures to be performed on a day-case basis. Patient comfort: these devices allow early mobilization and discharge.

8.5 Drawbacks of VCDs

Potentially long learning curve and device/deployment failure. Deployment success rates vary from 86 to 100%, with evidence of increased failure early in the learning curve. Perclose Prostar deployment failure rates vary from 3.6 to 12% of procedures. Small vessels (5 mm or less) are unsuitable for active VCDs. Non-common femoral artery (CFA) punctures or antegrade CFA punctures may not be suitable for a VCD. Peripheral vascular disease (PVD) is a frequent contraindication to use endoluminal components (e.g., Angioseal), as they may promote vessel thrombosis if the native vessel lumen is narrow. Device costs. Patients may still require bed rest post-closure. Impaired or delayed CFA re-puncture with some VCDs. Catastrophic complications (1–2%, but may be underreported). Detachment and distal embolization of the footplate of the Angioseal device. The retrograde movement of the needles of the Prostar Perclose devices can result in device entrapment in the heavily scarred groins of patients with prosthetic grafts, requiring surgical removal. As all of the collagen plug and suture-mediated closure devices involve leaving a foreign body at the puncture site, there is an increased risk of local infection, especially in the presence of a hematoma.

8.6 Outcomes

Published outcome data of closure devices in patients with peripheral vascular disease are relatively limited. Published outcomes for passive VCDs are negligible and the limited evidence involves active VCDs. Unfortunately, the use of arterial vascular closure devices has not eliminated the occurrence of puncture-site complications. In a review of the world literature of VCDs, the minor complication rates are 5.3 and 5.9%, and major complication rates are 1.3 and 4% for Angio-Seal and Perclose, respectively. In a prospective study of 1605 cardiology patients, the major complication rates were 3.2, 2.3, and 1% for Angio-Seal, Perclose, and manual compression, respectively. One of the main problems of such studies is the lack of consistency in the definition of complications, particularly hematoma formation. Most of the published data on closure devices relate to cardiology patients. However, complication rates are broadly similar in the few published series of patients with peripheral vascular disease. VCDs are used in only 20–25% of all catheter-based procedures and the decision to use them is generally based on the potential advantages and disadvantages in each case.

8.7 Conclusions

As with any situation where there are a number of solutions to a problem, no single method of achieving hemostasis is perfect. Without doubt, the most important step in reducing puncture site complications is good technique and operator experience, both with respect to the initial puncture and the use of the favored closure device. The available data make it difficult to recommend the use of closure devices for all patients, but there are certain circumstances and patient types for which their use may be particularly advantageous, such as day-case procedures, patients who are unable to lie flat post-procedure, patients who require immediate post-procedural anticoagulation, and patients who are unable to stop their anticoagulant medication before a procedure (e.g., patients with prosthetic heart valves). Interventional radiologists should become familiar with a few of the available devices and select each device on the basis of each individual patient.

Suggested Readings

1. Dauerman HL, Applegate RJ, Cohen DJ. Vascular closure devices: the second decade. *J Am Coll Cardiol*. 2007;50:1617–1626.
2. Doyle BJ, Konz BA, Lennon RJ, et al. Ambulation 1 hour after diagnostic cardiac catheterization: a prospective study of 1009 procedures. *Mayo Clin Proc*. 2006;81:1537–1540.
3. O'Sullivan GJ, Buckenham TM, Belli AM. The use of the Angio-Seal hemostatic puncture closure device in high-risk patients. *Clin Radiol*. 1999;54:51–55.
4. Duda SH, Wiskirchen J, Erb M, et al. Suture-mediated percutaneous closure of antegrade femoral arterial access sites in patients who have received full anticoagulation therapy. *Radiology*. 1999;210:47–52.
5. Shrake KL. Comparison of major complication rates associated with four methods of arterial closure. *Am J Cardiol*. 2000;85:1024–1025.
6. Warren BS, Warren SG, Miller SD. Predictors of complications and learning curve using the Angio-Seal closure device following interventional and diagnostic catheterization. *Catheter Cardiovasc Interv*. 1999;48:162–166.
7. Baim DS, Knopf WD, Hinohara T, et al. Suture-mediated closure of the femoral access site after cardiac catheterization: results of the suture to ambulate and discharge (STAND I and STAND II) trials. *Am J Cardiol*. 2000;85:864–869.
8. Eidt JF, Habibipour S, Saucedo JF, et al. Surgical complications from hemostatic puncture closure devices. *Am J Surg*. 1999;178:511–516.
9. Cooper CL, Miller A. Infectious complications related to the use of the Angio-Seal hemostatic puncture closure device. *Catheter Cardiovasc Interv*. 1999;48:301–303.
10. Rickli H, Unterweger M, Sutsch G, et al. Comparison of costs and safety of a suture-mediated closure device with conventional manual compression after coronary artery interventions. *Catheter Cardiovasc Interv*. 2002;57:297–302.

Part II
Imaging Required for Thoracic Endografting

Chapter 9
Fluoroscopy and Angiographic Imaging in Thoracic Aortic Endografting

Fluoroscopy provides real-time imaging during catheter and guidewire manipulation/continuous fluoroscopy is used "to shoot" an arteriogram at a higher frame rate and resolution and is used when optimal image quality is required. Fluoroscopy is the backbone for the workup, evaluation, and successful deployment of thoracic aortic stent grafts. Pulsed fluoroscopy is used when less detail is required like the passage of guidewires, catheters, and sheaths. A digital subtraction arteriography "DSA" is created by image software which first shoots a mask of the background objects, and subtracts the background and allows the column of contrast in the angiogram to be displayed without interference of the background. "Road mapping" permits real-time catheter guidance with a contrast background. Road mapping is established by digitally subtracting the initial non-contrast background; then contrast is injected into the vessel of interest and a new combined image of the contrast injection is superimposed on the real-time fluoroscopic image. All of these techniques are available with the most basic vascular package software on a portable C-arm unit. When using fluoroscopy for measurements, a marker catheter, with 1 cm radiopaque markers, is useful to avoid parallax error. Parallax error is the difference in length measurements that occur when the C-arm is moved toward or away from the patient and the relative relationships of landmarks and lesions are altered.

9.1 Contrast Power Injection Versus Hand Injection

Contrast can be injected using an automated power injector or hand injector. Most cases use a combination of the two methods to complement one another. Hand injection is fast and can be used to guide the advancement of catheters in the iliacs and aorta. However, power injection is needed to opacify large volume arteries such as the aorta. Common injection settings for contrast injection of the aorta are "20 for 40" which correlates to 20 ml/s for a total of 40 ml. Standard contrast solutions contain iodine and are offered in a variety of osmolarities and in both ionic and non-ionic forms. The lower the osmolarity, the less physiological damage to the patient but the more expensive. Non-ionic contrast is associated with fewer complications because of its associated lower osmolarity. Both Omnipaque and Visapaque are non-ionic contrast agents at different osmolarities.

J. Kpodonu, *Manual of Thoracic Endoaortic Surgery*,
DOI 10.1007/978-1-84996-296-4_9, © Springer-Verlag London Limited 2010

9.2 Basic Fluoroscopic Projections

Angulation of the C-arm is essential for fluoroscopic evaluation of the arterial tree. The basic projections are listed in Table 9.1. These suggested projections optimize full visualization of the artery and are necessary for correct assessment of angulation, tortuosity, and length measurements.

Table 9.1 Common C-arm fluoroscopic angulations

Artery of interest	C-arm angulation suggestion
Aortic arch	45–60° left anterior oblique (LAO)
Innominate artery	Right anterior oblique (RAO)
Left subclavian artery	LAO
Aortic valve	20–30° cranial angulation
Left renal artery	LAO with cranial angulation 10–20°
Right renal artery	RAO with cranial angulation 10–20°
Left Iliac bifurcation	RAO
Right Iliac bifurcation	LAO
Right SFA/profunda	RAO
Left SFA/profunda	LAO
Celiac artery	RAO steep angulation

9.2.1 Angiography for Evaluation of Access Vessels

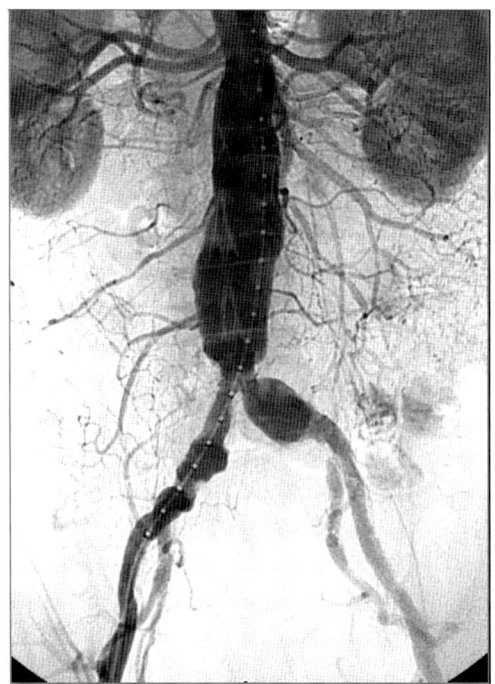

Angiography of the common iliac, external, femoral is useful to evaluate the access sites to determine if devices which are fairly large, 20–25 Fr, are deliverable to the target site. About 15–25% of patients require an iliac or aortic conduit due to small, calcified, or tortuous iliac vessels.[1–3]

9.2.2 Fluoroscopy as Applied to the Thoracic and Arch Aorta

The normal arch aorta consists of the innominate artery which divides into the right subclavian artery and the right carotid artery (RCA), the left carotid artery (LCA), and the left subclavian artery.

9.2.3 Normal Arch Aorta

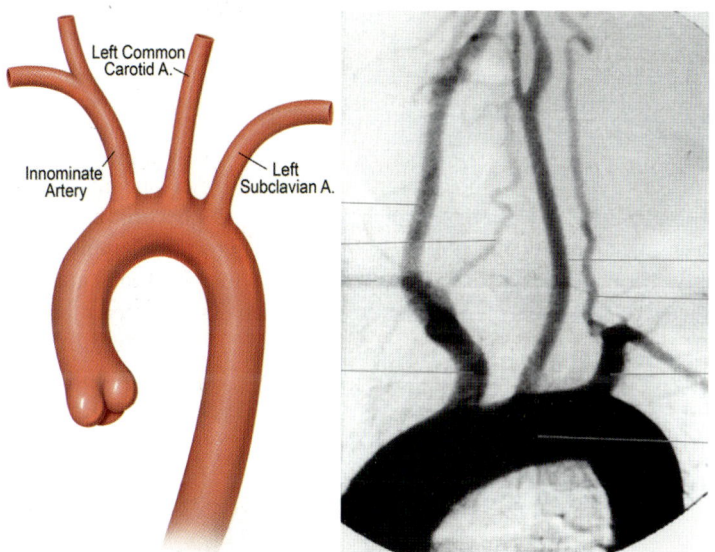

9.2.4 Variations of Aortic Arch

Sixty-five percent of individuals have a normal arch aorta with three separate origins of the arch vessels. Twenty-five percent have a "bovine" arch; left common carotid artery arises from the innominate artery (Fig. 9.1). Other important anomalies include separate origin of left vertebral and aberrant origin of right subclavian (distal to left subclavian artery) (Fig. 9.2). It is important to image the intracerebral circulation (Fig. 9.3) when anomalies of the aortic arch are suspected.

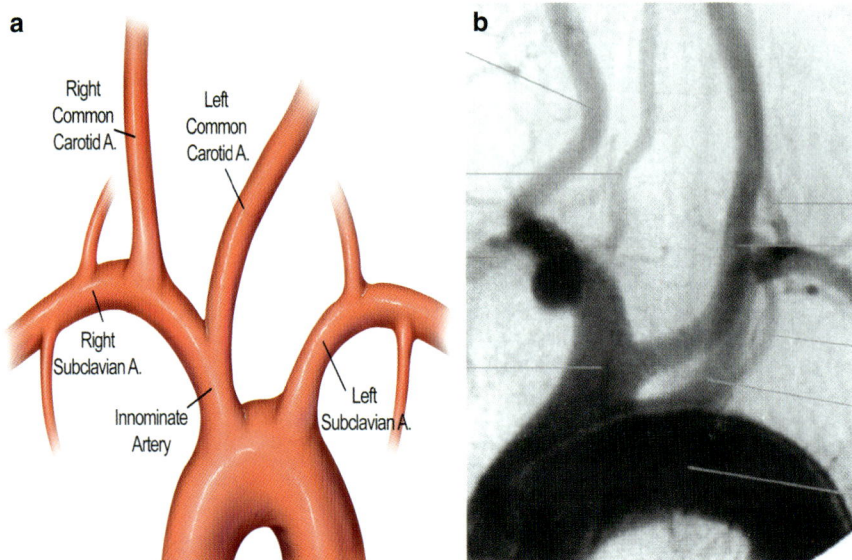

Fig. 9.1 (**a**, **b**) Illustration with an intra-operative angiogram demonstrating a bovine aortic arch with the innominate and left common carotid artery originating from a common ostium

Optimal imaging of the thoracic aorta is obtained by advancing a 90 cm pigtail catheter to the level of interest, which is usually in the proximal aortic arch. The power injector is connected using sterile tubing and all tubing in de-aired thoroughly. Thoracic aortic contrast is set to 20 ml/s for 40 ml total and the patients are instructed to hold their breaths and the aortogram is performed.

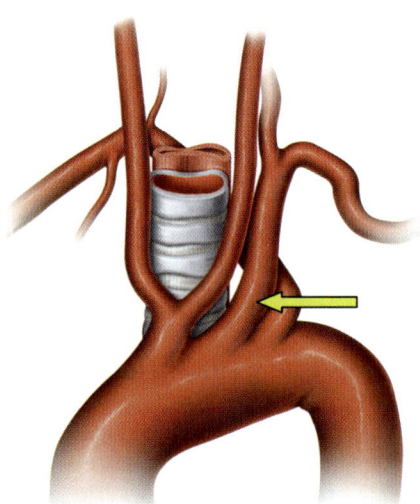

Fig. 9.2 Illustration with arrow demonstrating an aberrant right subclavian artery

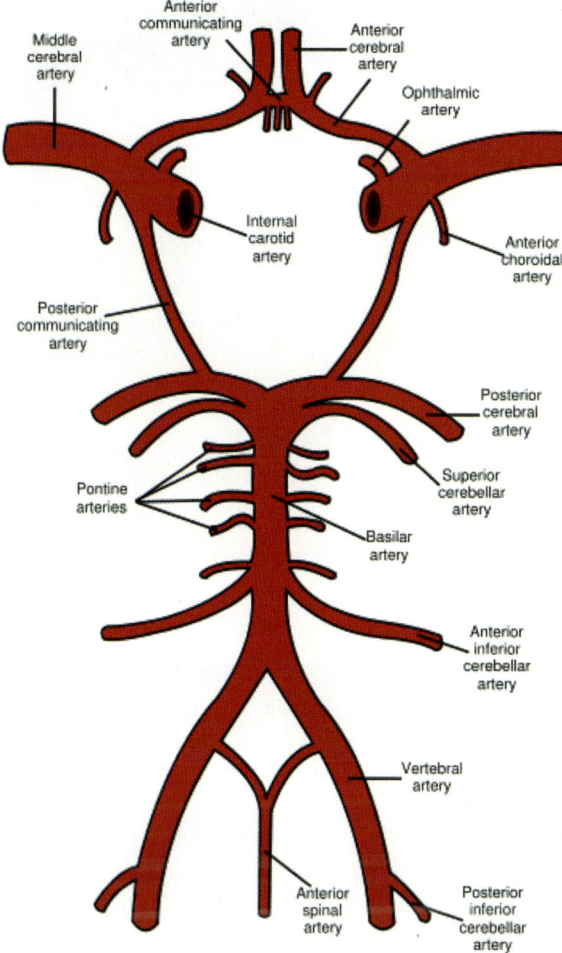

Fig. 9.3   Illustration demonstrating intracerebral circulation

9.3 Thoracic Aneurysms

Thoracic aneurysms are defined as a localized or diffuse dilation of an artery with a diameter at least 50% greater than an adjacent normal size artery. Appropriate angiographic images are necessary to confirm size (Figs. 9.4 and 9.5), extent of aneurysm as well as angulation of arch (Fig. 9.6), proximal and distal neck length and diameter. The consensus size for intervention is generally 5.5 cm in the ascending aorta and somewhere in the range of 6.0–7.0 cm in the descending aorta.

Fig. 9.4 Thoracic aortogram performed with a pigtail catheter demonstrating a large thoracic aortic aneurysm with diameter >6.0 cm

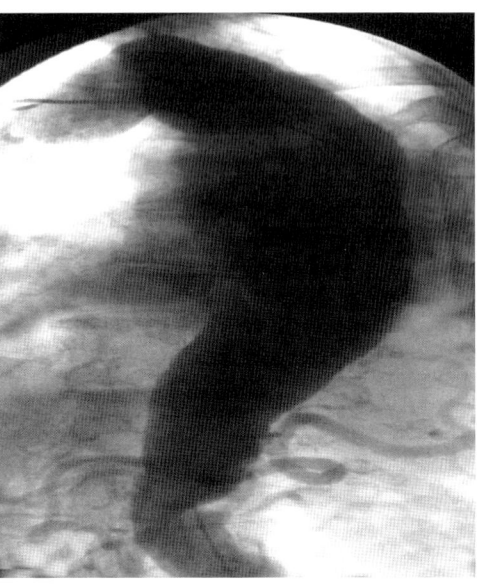

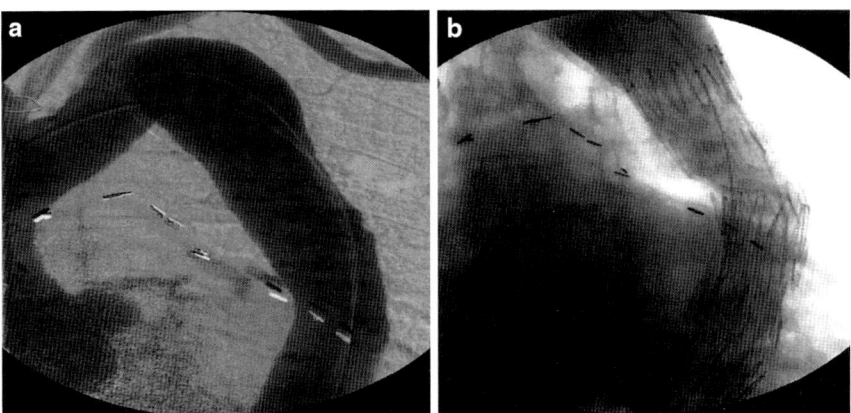

Fig. 9.5 Angiogram images demonstrate a thoracic aortic aneurysm (**a**) treated with a thoracic aortic stent graft to exclude the aneurysm (**b**)

9.4 Thoracic Arch Aneurysms

Thoracic arch aneurysms (Fig. 9.7a, b) are more complex to treat with a thoracic aortic stent graft as proximal landing zones are usually short, arch is usually angulated, and occasionally coverage of the left subclavian artery is warranted with or without revascularization.

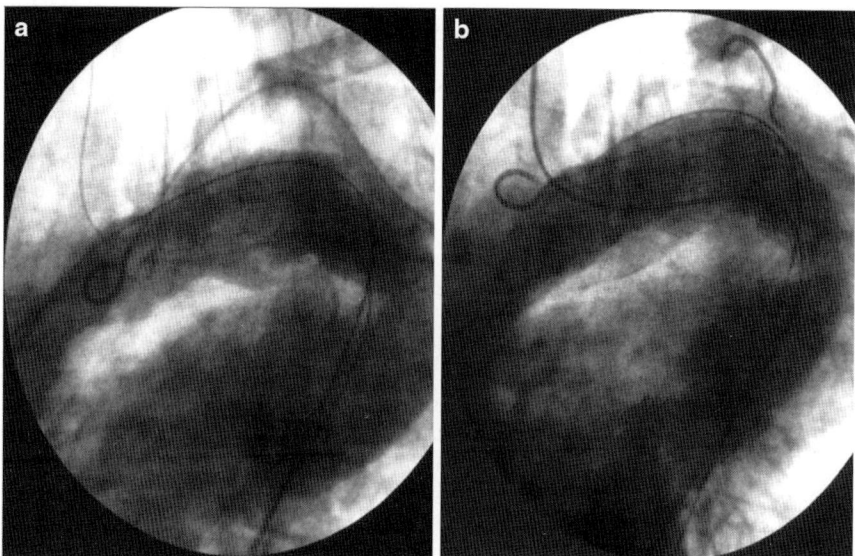

Fig. 9.6 Angiogram of a patient with a much angulated arch (**a**) and a thoracic aortic aneurysm successfully managed with an endoluminal graft with no endoleak (**b**)

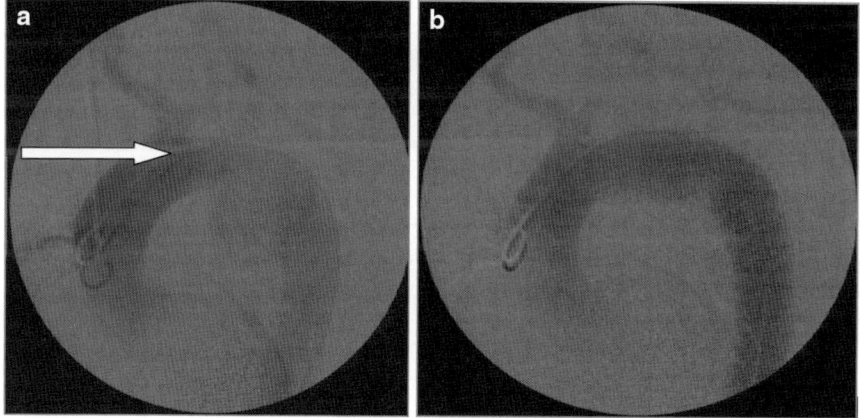

Fig. 9.7 (**a**) Angiogram performed demonstrates an angulated bovine arch with a saccular aneurysm of the arch aorta. (**b**) Angiogram post-stent deployment with satisfactory exclusion of aneurysm and no identifiable endoleak and patent bovine arch vessels. Subclavian artery is purposely covered by the endoluminal graft to achieve a satisfactory landing zone for deployment of endoluminal graft

9.5 Aortobronchial Fistula

Aortobronchial fistula is a communication between the airway and the aorta. It is commonly seen in patients with previous aortic repair and presents with hemoptysis. Confirmation of diagnosis is commonly made with an angiogram or occasionally bronchoscopy or transesophageal echocardiography (Fig. 9.8).

Fig. 9.8 Angiogram in a patient presenting with hemoptysis which demonstrates (*white arrow*) a communication between the aorta and the airway

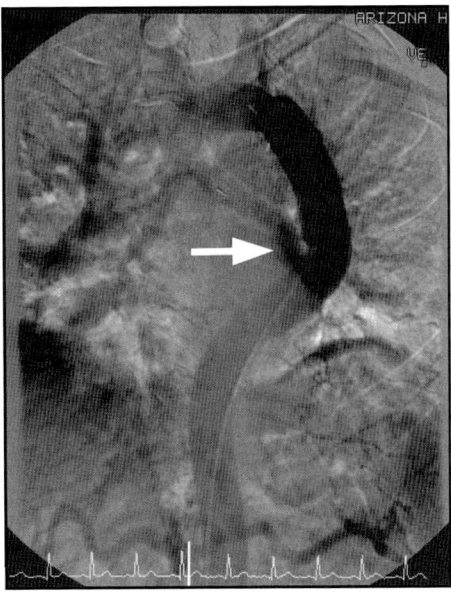

9.6 Coarctation of the Aorta

Adult coarctation is characterized by a shelf-like narrowing within the lumen of the aorta with closed ducts forming the ligament arteries. Presentation may vary from chest pain to hypertension (Figs. 9.9 and 9.10).

9.7 Type B Dissections

Acute Type B dissection results from a tear in the intima with resulting true and false lumen flow. Clinical symptoms depend on the extent of dissection as well as on the characteristics of the true lumen and false lumen flow. Diagnosis is well established with an angiogram and stent graft can effectively be used to treat symptomatic patients with improvement in clinical condition (Figs. 9.11a, b and 9.12a, b).

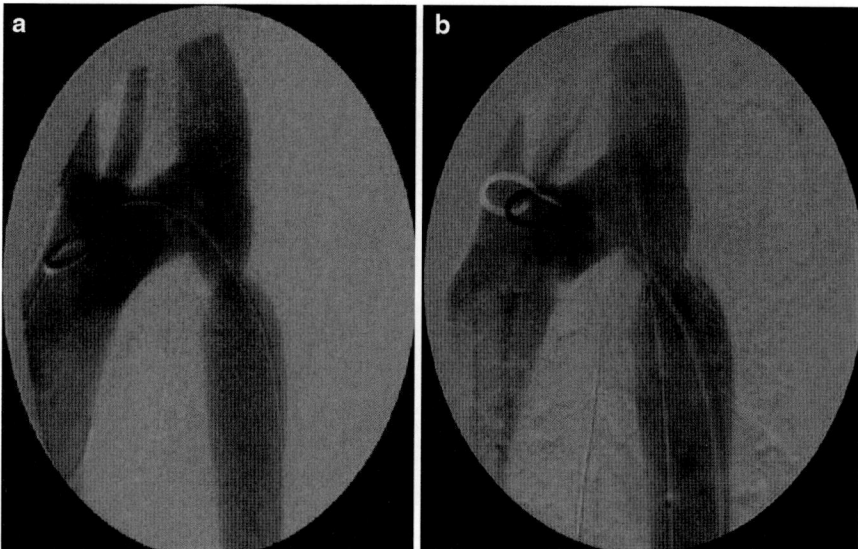

Fig. 9.9 Angiogram in a patient who presented with uncontrolled hypertension (**a**) demonstrates a coarctation of the aorta treated with a Palmaz1040 XL stent with a resulting increase in the luminal diameter (**b**)

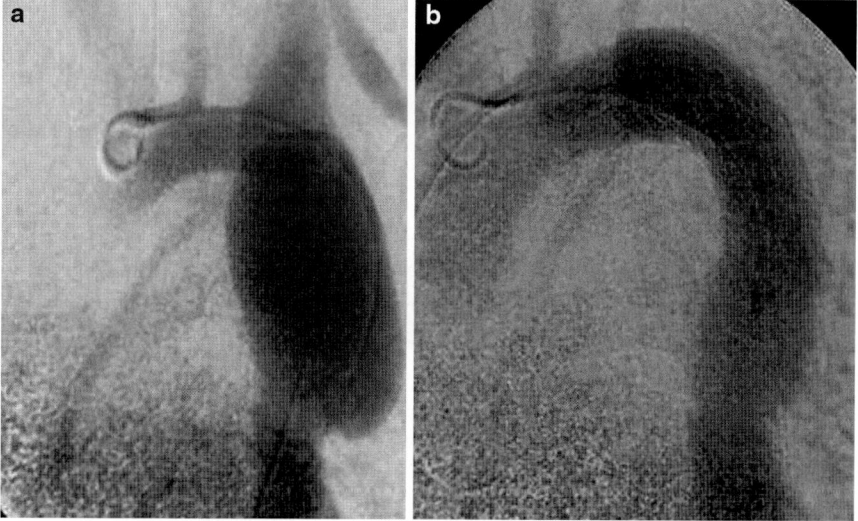

Fig. 9.10 (**a**) Angiogram of a patient with a post-coarctation repair pseudoaneurysm. Patient underwent a left carotid to left subclavian transposition with deployment of an endoluminal graft with complete exclusion of the post-coarctation pseudoaneurysm (**b**)

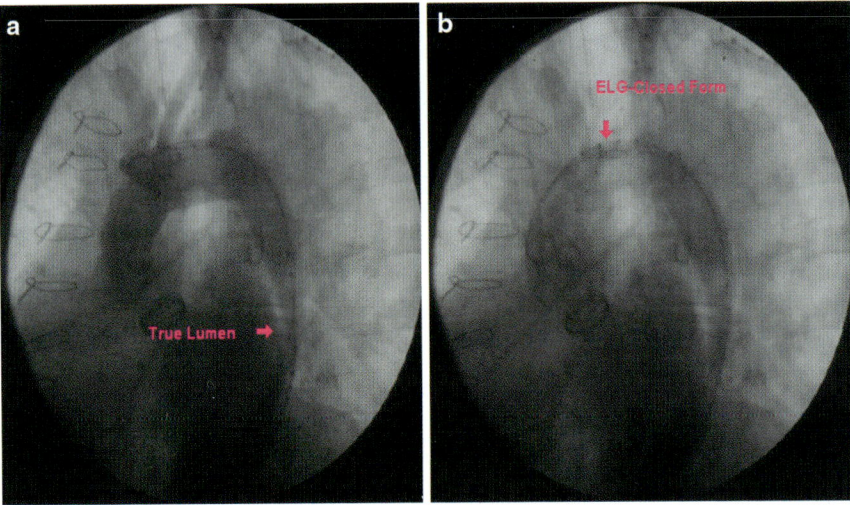

Fig. 9.11 (**a**, **b**) Angiogram of a patient with back pain which demonstrates a type B dissection with a compressed true lumen

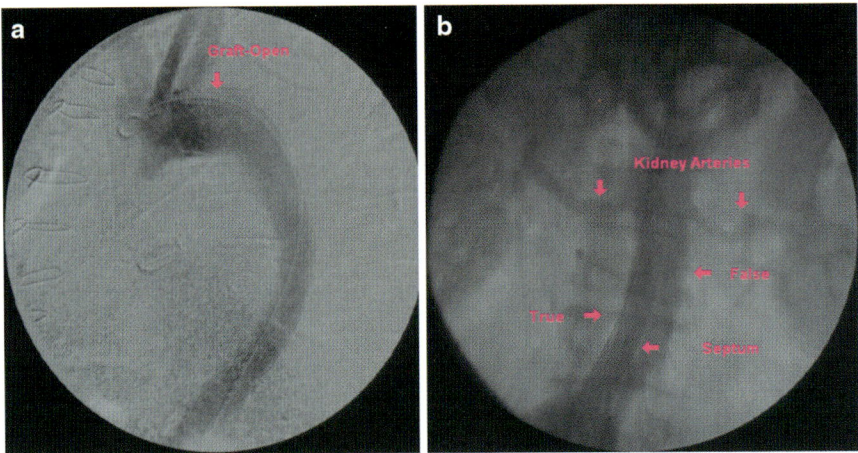

Fig. 9.12 (**a**) Angiogram post-deployment of stent with exclusion of entry point, re-expansion of true lumen. (**b**) Angiogram post-deployment of endoluminal graft with expansion of true lumen with visceral and renal perfusion maintained by both true and false lumen flow

9.8 Penetrating Aortic Ulcers

Patients with penetrating aortic ulcers often present with a sharp back pain characteristic of acute dissection (Fig. 9.13).

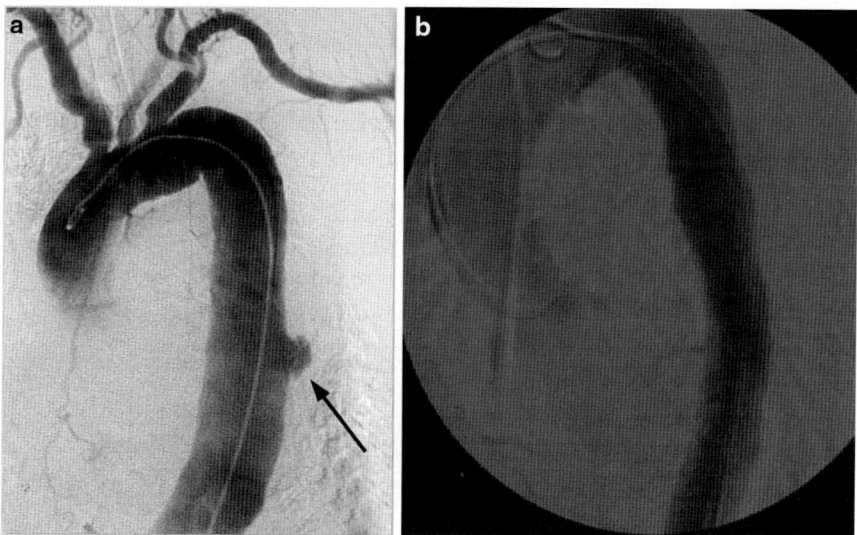

Fig. 9.13 (**a**) Angiogram often will demonstrate a penetrating aortic ulcer of the descending thoracic aorta. (**b**) An endoluminal graft can be effectively deployed to exclude the penetrating aortic ulcer with satisfactory results

9.9 Aortic Pseudoaneurysm

Pseudoaneurysms result from anastomotic dehiscense of a previous repair and may result from an infection, fistula, trauma, or poor surgical technique. Redo surgery is often risky as patients have extensive scar from previous repair. Angiogram

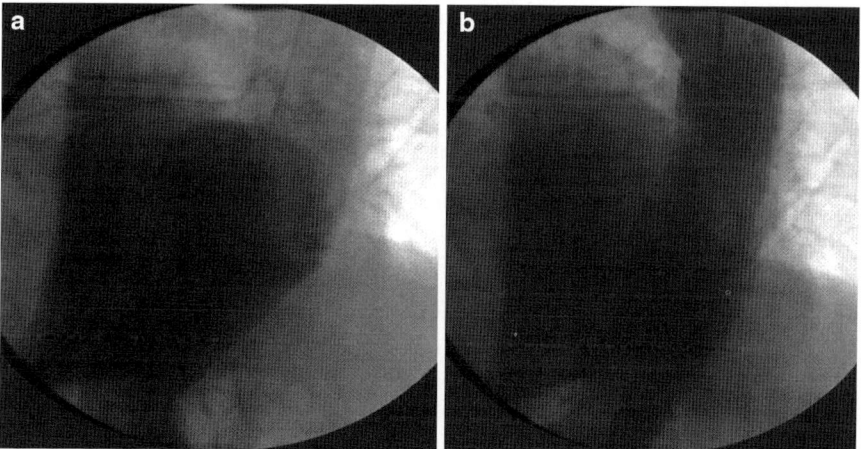

Fig. 9.14 Angiogram of patient (**a**) demonstrates a large pseudoaneurysm of the thoracic aorta which was successfully managed with an endoluminal graft (**b**)

can confirm the diagnosis (Fig. 9.14a) and oftentimes the pseudoaneurysm can be repaired with an endoluminal stent graft (Fig. 9.14b).

9.10 Mycotic Pseudoaneurysm

Mycotic pseudoaneurysms result from infection and may be native or result from infection of a previous repair. Surgery is often required to remove infected graft but occasionally the risk is so high that there may be a role for a stent graft (Fig. 9.15a–c).

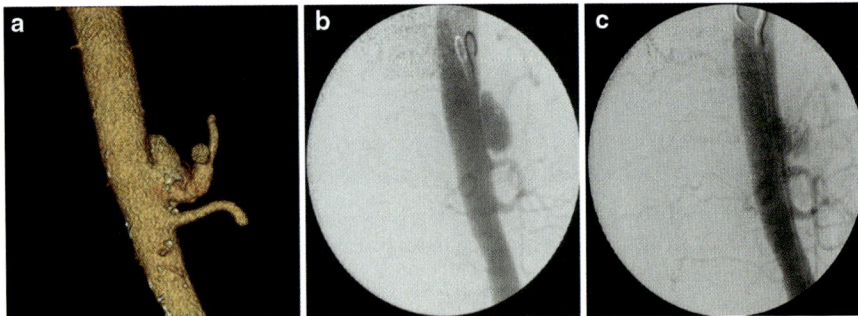

Fig. 9.15 A 71-year-old male with recent neurosurgical intervention on his disc for a paraspinal abscess who presented a couple of weeks later with fever, chills, and MRSA in blood. CT scan (**a**) demonstrated a saccular mycotic aneurysm of his thoracoabdominal aorta. An angiogram (**b**) demonstrates the saccular aneurysm originating close to the ostium of the celiac trunk which was successfully treated with coil embolization of the celiac trunk followed by deployment of an endoluminal graft (**c**)

References

1. Diethrich EB, Ramaiah VG, Kpodonu J, Rodriguez JA. *Angiographic Images and Illustrations Courtesy of Endovascular and Hybrid Management of the Thoracic Aorta. A Case Based Approach*. 1st ed. West Sussex: Wiley Blackwell; 2008.
2. Schneider PA. *Endovascular Skills: Guidewires and Catheter Skills for Endovascular Surgery*. 2nd ed. New York, NY: Marcel Dekker; 2003.
3. Moore WS. *Vascular and Endovascular Surgery: A Comprehensive Review*. 7th ed. Philadelphia, PA: Saunders; 2005.

Chapter 10
Case-Specific CT Imaging to Evaluate Thoracic Aortic Pathologies

CT angiography has become the main imaging method used for the assessment of the thoracic aorta (Fig. 10.1). It is preferable that any patient being evaluated for a thoracic aortic procedure have imaging of the entire aorta commencing above the aortic arch and extending inferiorly to include the abdominal aorta and the iliac arteries as far as the inguinal ligament. Use of multiplanar reconstructions (MPR) and maximum intensity projection (MIP) images on the CT workstation enables review of the location and extent of the aortic lesion, the presence of proximal and

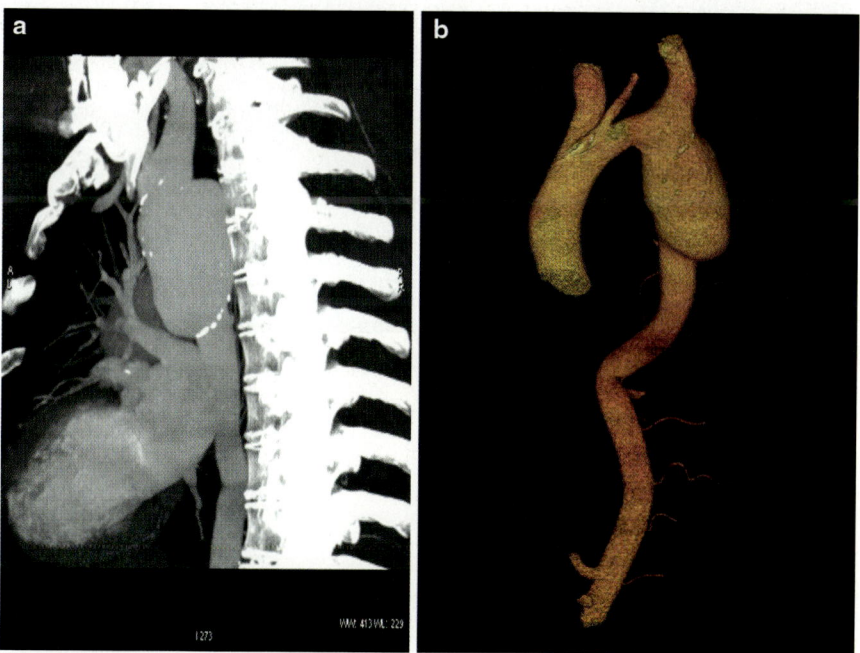

Fig. 10.1 (**a, b**) CT scan demonstrates a post-coarctation pseudoaneurysm with involvement of the left subclavian artery

J. Kpodonu, *Manual of Thoracic Endoaortic Surgery*,
DOI 10.1007/978-1-84996-296-4_10, © Springer-Verlag London Limited 2010

distal landing zones for an endograft(s), the configuration of the aorta and iliac vessels with regard to tortuosity and kinking which might cause problems in delivery of the endograft to the required site and review the access site and iliac arteries for their diameter and amount of calcification.

10.1 Coarctation of the Thoracic Aorta

A 49-year-old male with a history of hypertension, status post-coarctation repair 20 years ago, was noted to have a mediastinal mass upon routine workup prior to undergoing knee surgery. Past surgical history is notable for previous coarctation repair, cholecystectomy, and appendectomy. Sixty-four slice CT angiography demonstrates a post-coarctation pseudoaneurysm (Fig. 10.1a, b). Repair was achieved with an endoluminal graft (Figs. 10.2a, b, 10.3, 10.4, 10.5, and 10.6).

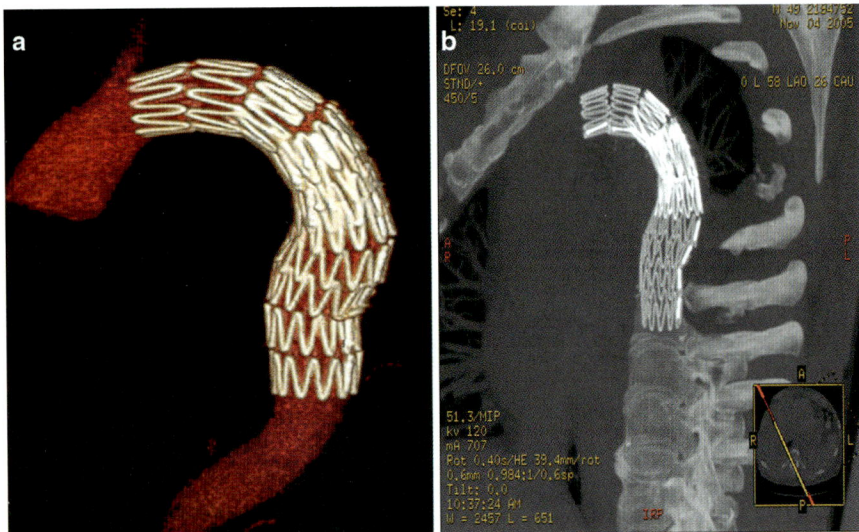

Fig. 10.2 (**a, b**) Sixty-four slice CT scan post-exclusion of pseudoaneurysm with a customized endoluminal graft with no identifiable endoleak

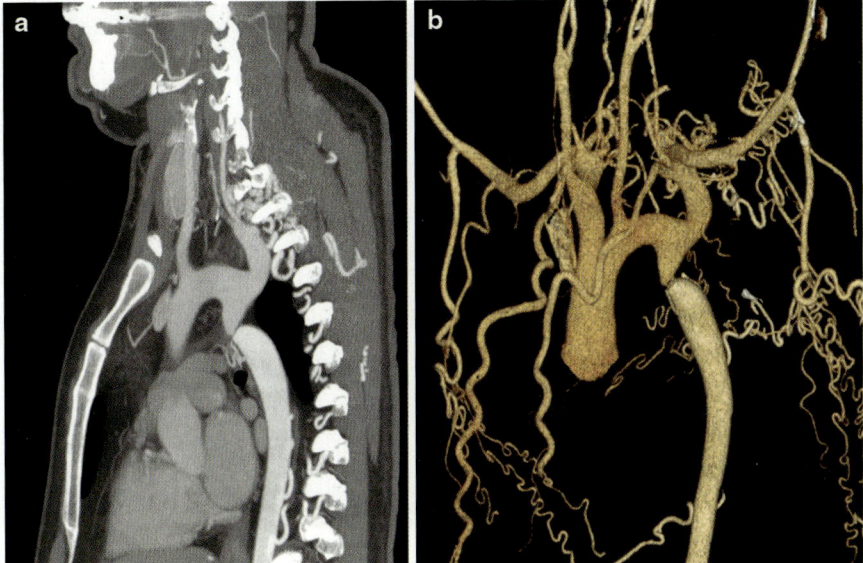

Fig. 10.3 (**a, b**) Sagittal CT scan images in a patient with a primary coarctation of the aorta. The area of carctation was measured at 4 mm on intravascular ultrasound. Note the abundant collateral circulation and large internal mammary arteries

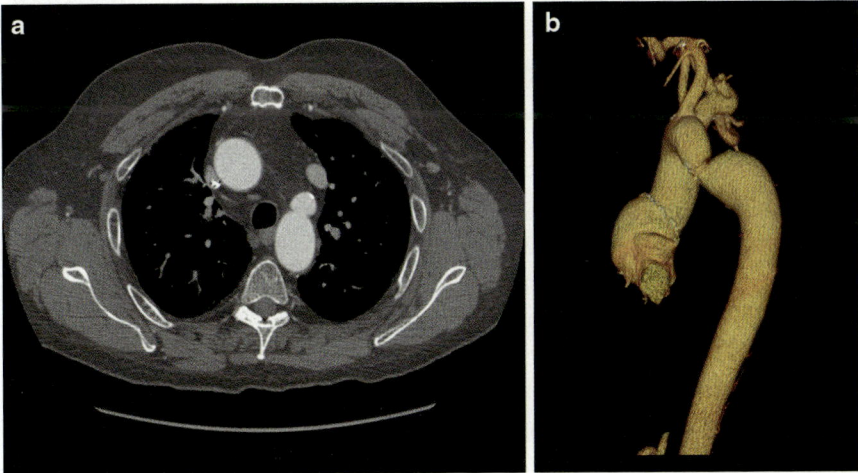

Fig. 10.4 (**a**) Axial and (**b**) reconstructed CT scan images in a patient with hypertension and chest pain demonstrating coarctation of the aorta with post-stenotic dilatation of the aorta

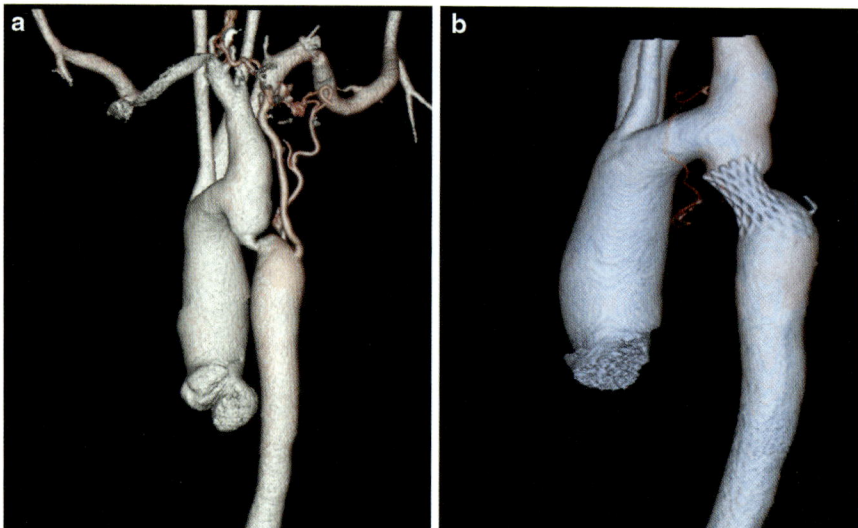

Fig. 10.5 (**a**) Sixty-four slice CT scan of a patient with primary coarctation pre- and (**b**) post-Palmaz stent deployment. There is an increase in luminal gain after stent deployment. The proximal and distal ends of the stent have been flared with balloon angioplasty to conform to the aorta

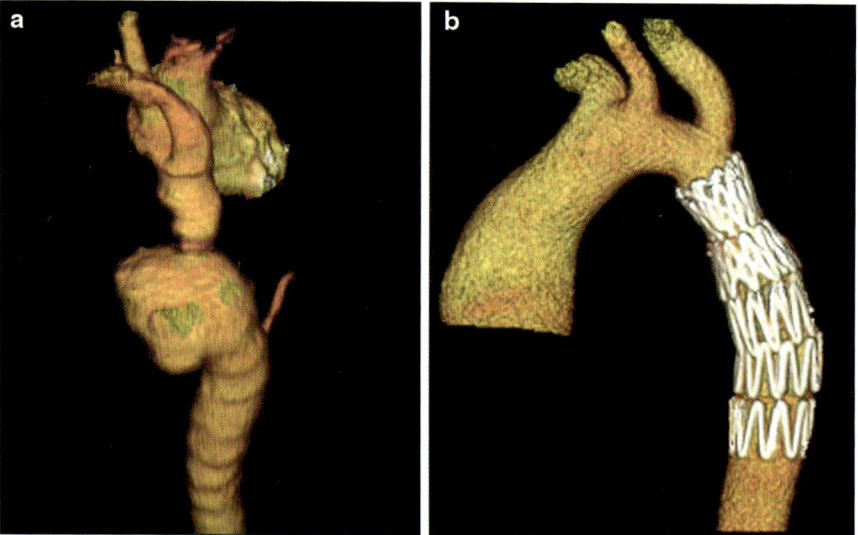

Fig. 10.6 (**a**) Sixty-four slice CT scan in a patient with a coarctation pseudoaneurysm after primary surgical repair managed with an endoluminal graft. (**b**) The is no identifiable endoleak with satisfactory exclusion of the coarctation pseudoaneurysm

10.2 Penetrating Aortic Ulcer

A 66-year-old male with a history of coronary artery disease, hypertension, Type II diabetes mellitus and morbid obesity had been experiencing back pain for a period of a month. CT imaging demonstrated a penetrating aortic ulcer (Figs. 10.8a, 10.9a) which was succesfully treated with an endoluminal graft (Figs. 10.8b, 10.9b).

Fig. 10.7 Sixty-four slice CT image in a patient with previous endoluminal graft with a symptomatic penetrating aortic ulcer (*arrow*)

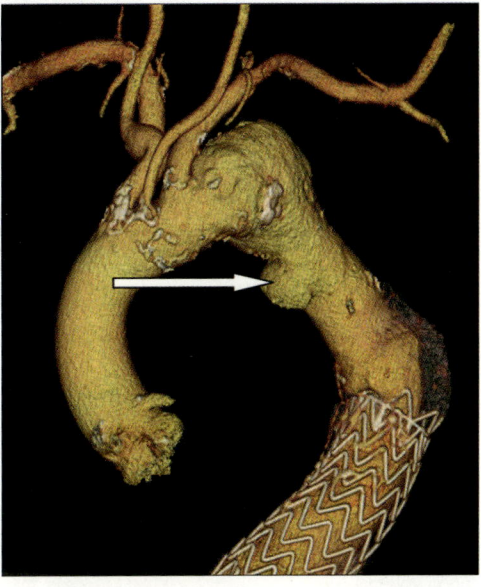

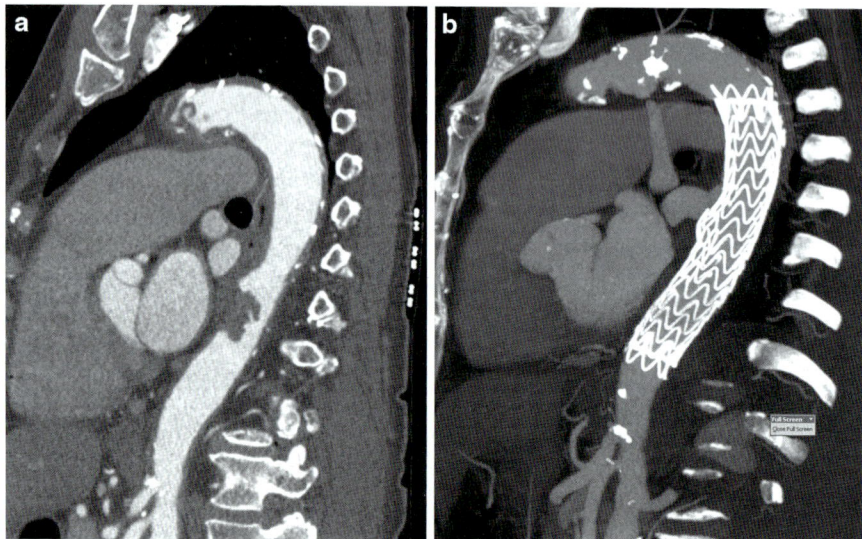

Fig. 10.8   A patient with severe back pain (**a**) CT scan of the aorta demonstrates a penetrating aortic ulcer treated with an (**b**) endoluminal graft

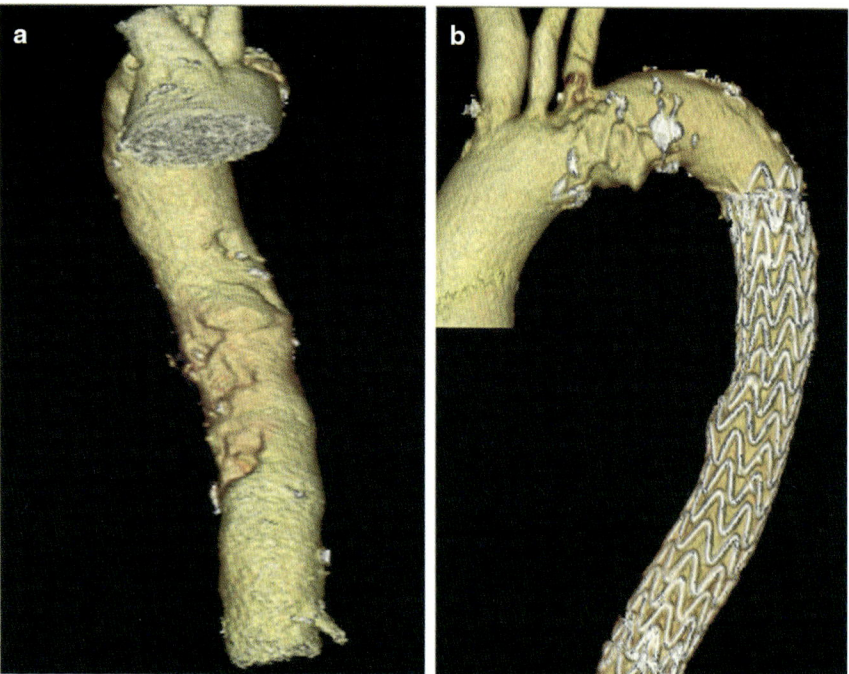

Fig. 10.9   (**a, b**) Sixty-four slice CT views demonstrate descending thoracic aortic penetrating aortic ulcers treated with an endoluminal graft

10.3 Thoracic Aortic Aneurysm

A 79-year-old male with a prior history of abdominal aortic aneurysm develops chest pain. CT scan of the chest reveals a large thoracic aortic aneurysm (Fig. 10.10a, b). Illiac vessels (Fig. 10.10c) are of adequate diameter for management with an endoluminal graft.

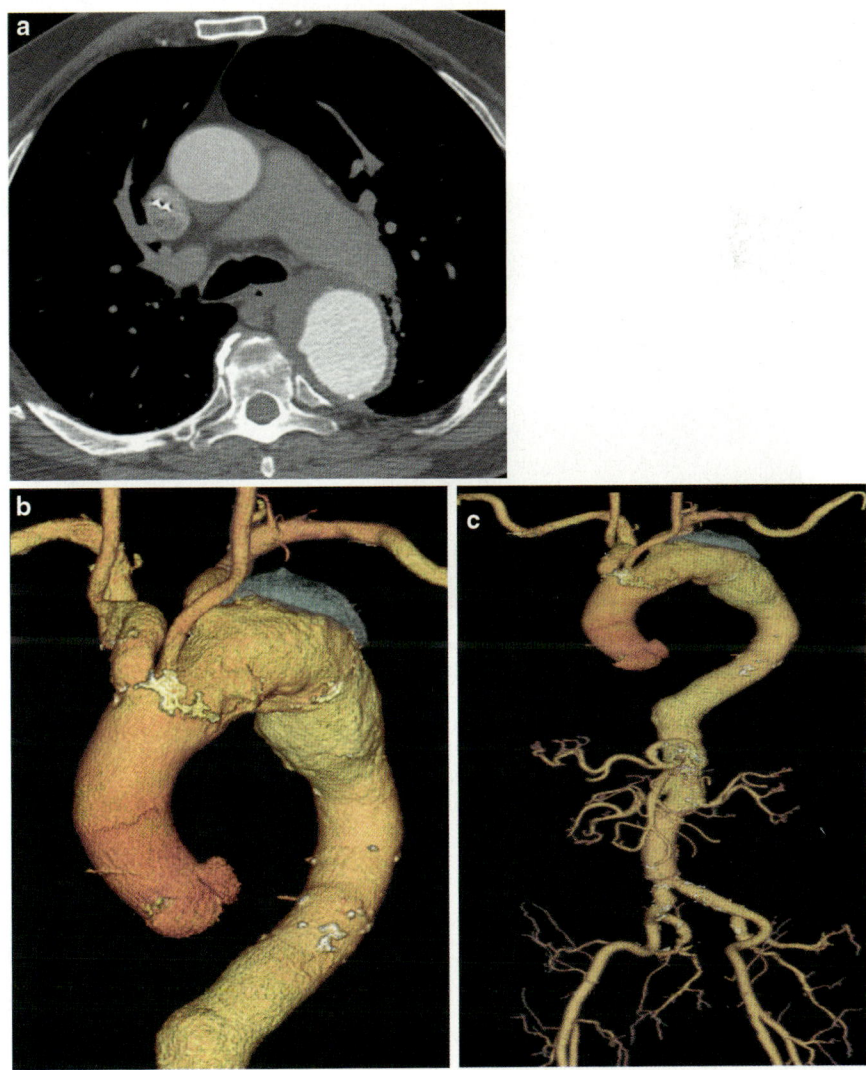

Fig. 10.10 (**a**) Axial CT image demonstrating a descending thoracic aneurysm with thrombus in the aneurysm sac. (**b**) Sixty-four slice CT image confirms the descending thoracic aneurysms. (**c**) Iliac vessels on CT scan are tortuous with mild calcification

10.4 Type B Aortic Dissection

10.4.1 Acute Type B Aortic Dissection

A 50-year-old man presenting with type B aortic dissection presenting with a painful, pulseless lower extremity. An open thrombectomy of the right common femoral artery was performed and a right axillary – to right femoral and a right to left femoral bypass to restore perfusion to the lower limbs who now presents with chest pain. Sixty-four slice CT image demonstrates a patent right axillary to right femoral bypass graft and a right to left femoral bypass graft used to provide perfusion to the lower extremities (Figs. 10.11a, b, 10.12a, b).

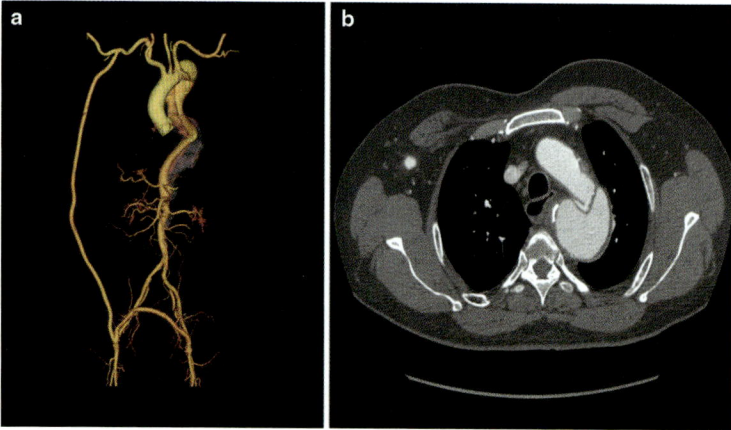

Fig. 10.11 (**a, b**) Sixty-four slice CT scan performed in a patient who developed acute type B dissection 5 years ago with malperfusion of bilateral lower extremities requiring a right axillary – to right femoral and a right to left femoral bypass to restore perfusion to the lower limbs who now presents with chest pain. Sixty-four slice CT image demonstrates a patent right axillary to right femoral bypass graft and a right to left femoral bypass graft used to provide perfusion to the lower extremities. Axial CT image demonstrates a dissecting aneurysm with true and false lumen flow

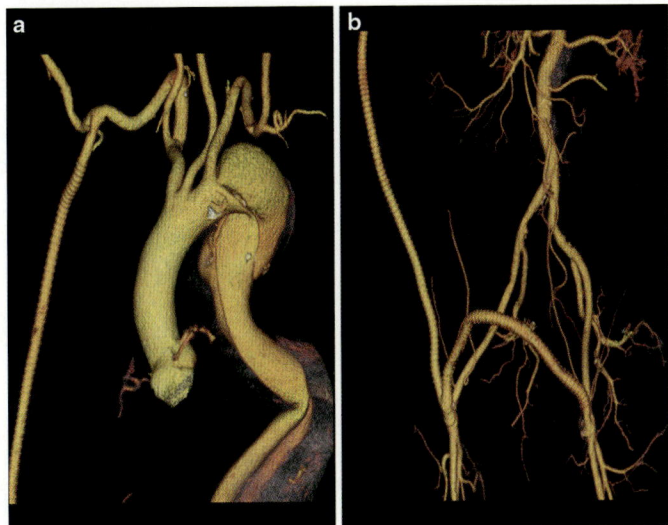

Fig. 10.12 (**a**, **b**) Sixty-four slice CT Image demonstrates a type B dissecting aneurysm with the entry point distal to the left subclavian artery. True lumen collapse with flow in the false lumen can be seen. There is aneurysmal expansion of the false lumen resulting in a false lumen diameter approaching 6.0 cm at the entry point of the dissection flap. Thrombus can be seen in the distal aorta false lumen

10.4.2 Chronic Type B Dissection

A 63-year-old male presents with a 5.7 cm aneurismal dilatation of a chronic descending thoracic dissection as demonstarted on 64 slice CT scans (Figs. 10.13, 10.14). He was subsequently managed with an endoluminal graft with successful repair as confirmed with CT scan (Fig. 10.15).

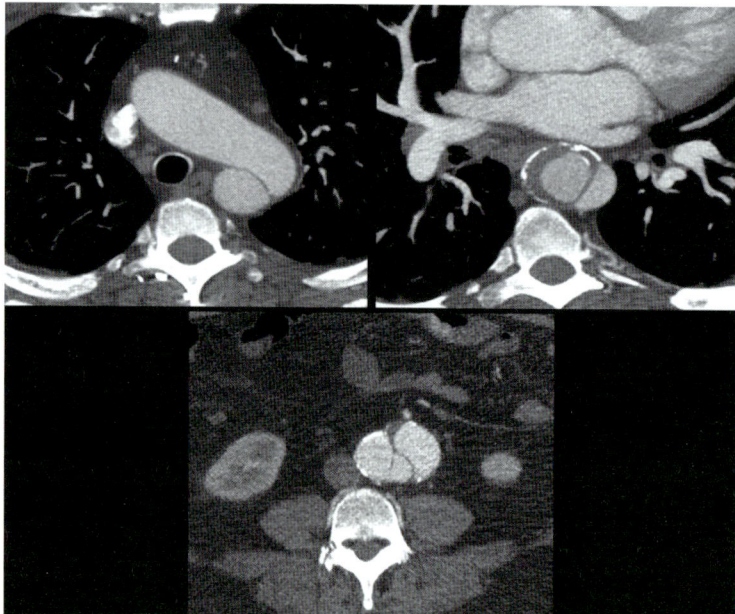

Fig. 10.13 Axial and sixty-four slice CT scan images of a patient with a chronic type B dissection. There is true and false lumen flow. Iliac vessels are of adequate caliber for deployment of endoluminal graft

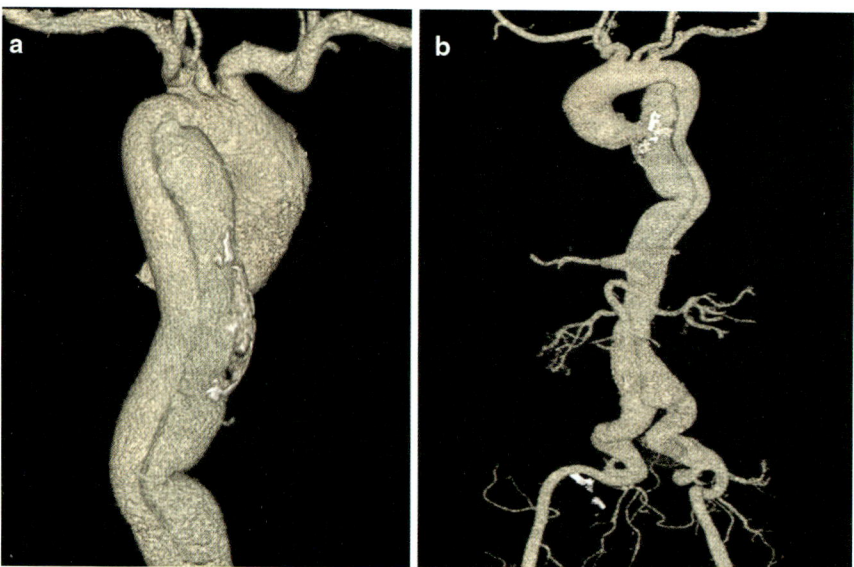

Fig. 10.14 (**a**, **b**) CT image demonstrates a type B dissection with dissection extending into the right iliac artery

Fig. 10.15 Management of type B dissection with an endoluminal graft with CT image demonstrating true lumen expansion

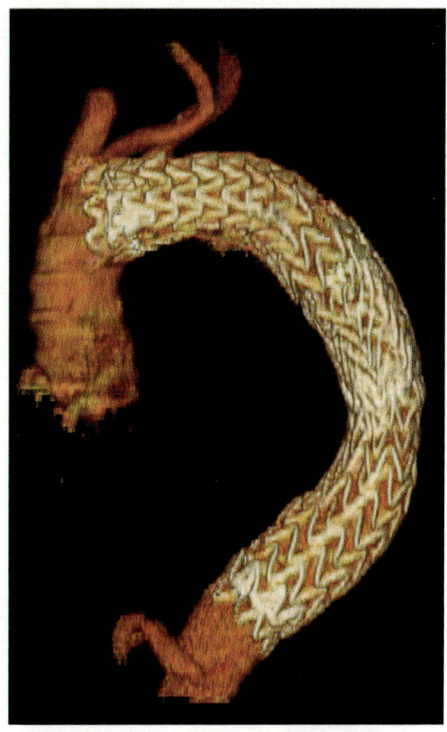

10.5 Saccular Arch Pseudoaneurysms

A 54-year-old male with a past history of CABG X3 and no notable history of trauma presents with vocal cord paralysis and shortness of breath. A saccular aneurysm of 4 cm was identified on his initial chest CT scan. Serial evaluations by CT scan reveal that the saccular aneurysm had enlarged and now measured 7.6 cm (Figs. 10.16, 10.17, and 10.18).

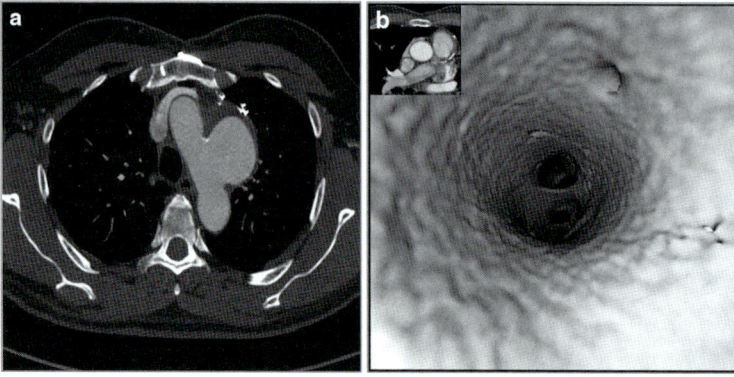

Fig. 10.16 (**a**) Axial CT scan of the chest demonstrates a saccular pseudoaneurysm of the arch aorta. (**b**) Virtual angioscopy demonstrates patent arch vessels

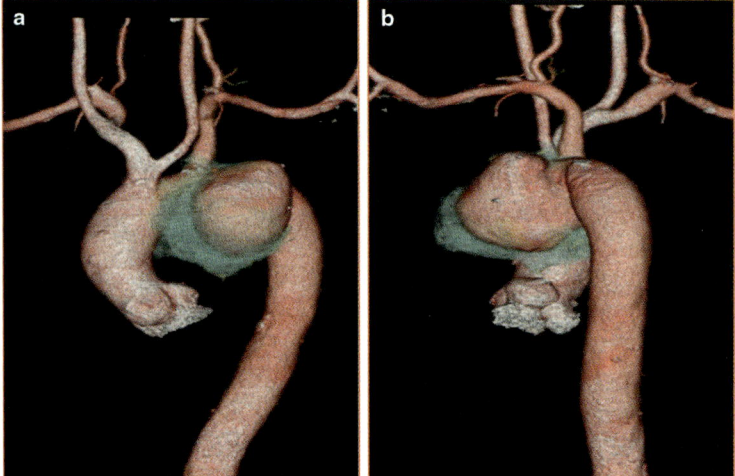

Fig. 10.17 (**a**, **b**) Sixty-four slice CT scan of the chest demonstrates a saccular pseudoaneurysm of the arch with thrombus. Note the severe angulations of the arch aorta. Virtual angioscopy demonstrates patent arch vessels

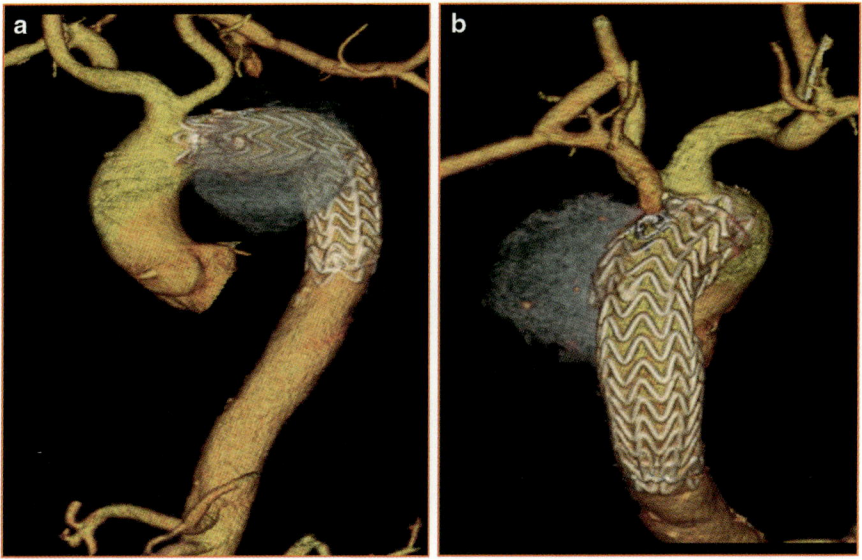

Fig. 10.18 (**a**, **b**) Sixty-four slice CT scan of the chest after stent deployment demonstrates satisfactory exclusion of arch aneurysm with no demonstrable endoleak. Patent bovine arch vessels with demonstrable thrombus in excluded pseudoaneurysm sac

10.6 Innominate Artery Pseudoaneurysm

A 54-year-old gentleman with chest pain and no recollection of trauma in the past presents with a CT scan finding of an innominate artery pseudoaneurysm (Figs. 10.19 and 10.20).

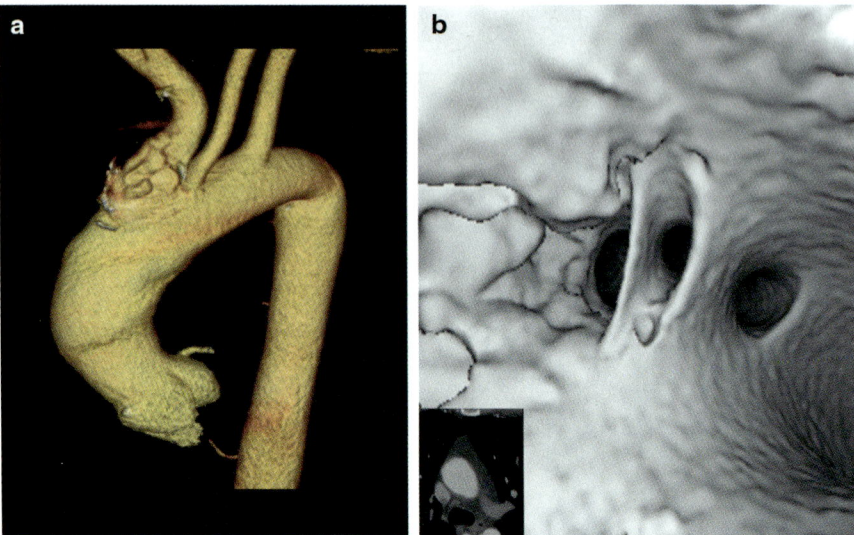

Fig. 10.19 (**a**) Sixty-four slice CT scan images demonstrate an innominate artery pseudoaneurysm. (**b**) Virtual angioscopic image demonstrating the arch vessels with areas of irregularity at the level of the innominate artery

Fig. 10.20 Sixty-four slice CT image demonstrates a thoracic debranching of the arch vessels with patent grafts and exclusion of the innominate artery aneurysm with an endoluminal graft

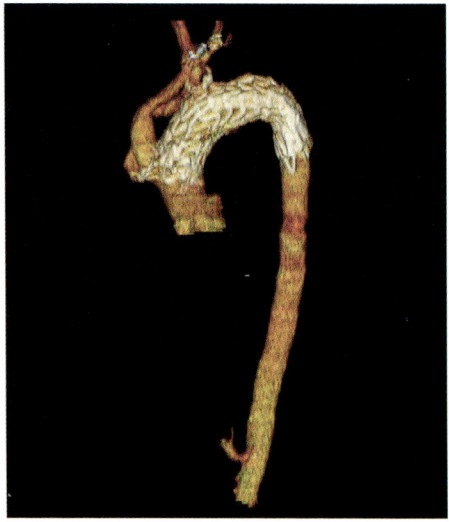

10.7 Thoracic Arch Aneurysm

A 68-year-old lady presents with chest discomfort A. CT scan of the chest demonstrates an arch aneurysm (Fig. 10.21a) which is managed with a thoracic arch debranching and an endoluminal graft deployment (Figs. 10.21b, 10.22a) with coiling of the left subclavian artery to treat a type II endoleak (Fig. 10.22b).

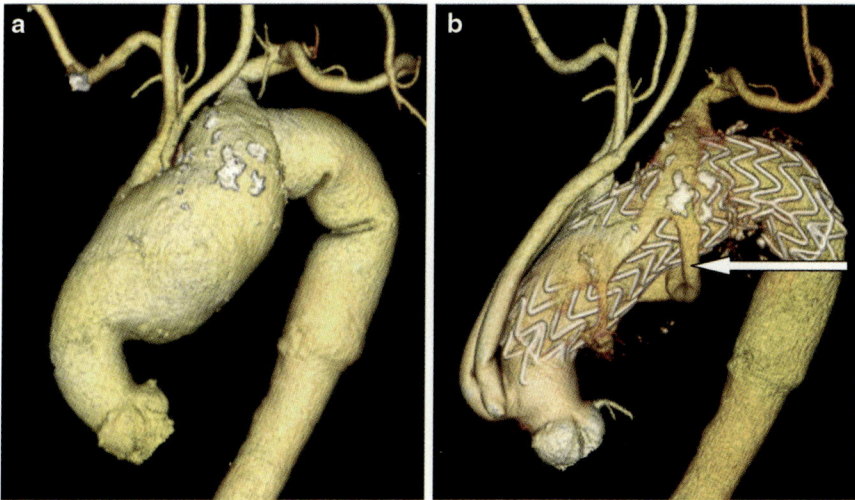

Fig. 10.21 (**a, b**) Sixty-four slice CT scan of a patient with an arch aneurysm managed with a thoracic debranching of the arch vessels. One can identify the patent debranched arch vessels with exclusion of the arch aneurysm with an endoluminal graft. There is an identifiable type II endoleak from the left subclavian artery post-procedure (*white arrow*)

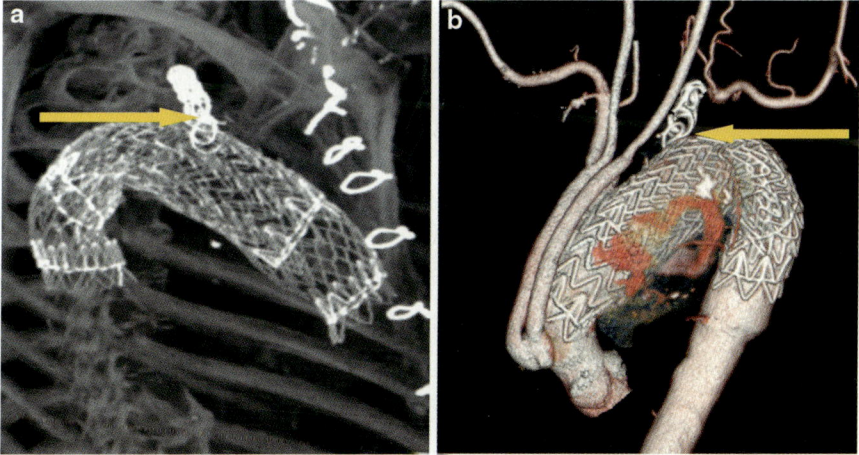

Fig. 10.22 (**a, b**) CT images post-coiling of the left subclavian artery to treat a type II endoleak of the same patient. Embolization coils in the left subclavian artery are seen on the CT images (*yellow arrow*)

10.8 Thoracoabdominal Aneurysms

A 71-year-old female presented with worsening back pain. Past medical history was significant for chronic obstructive lung disease and hypertension. She is an active smoker. Physical examination was non-contributory (Figs. 10.23 and 10.24).

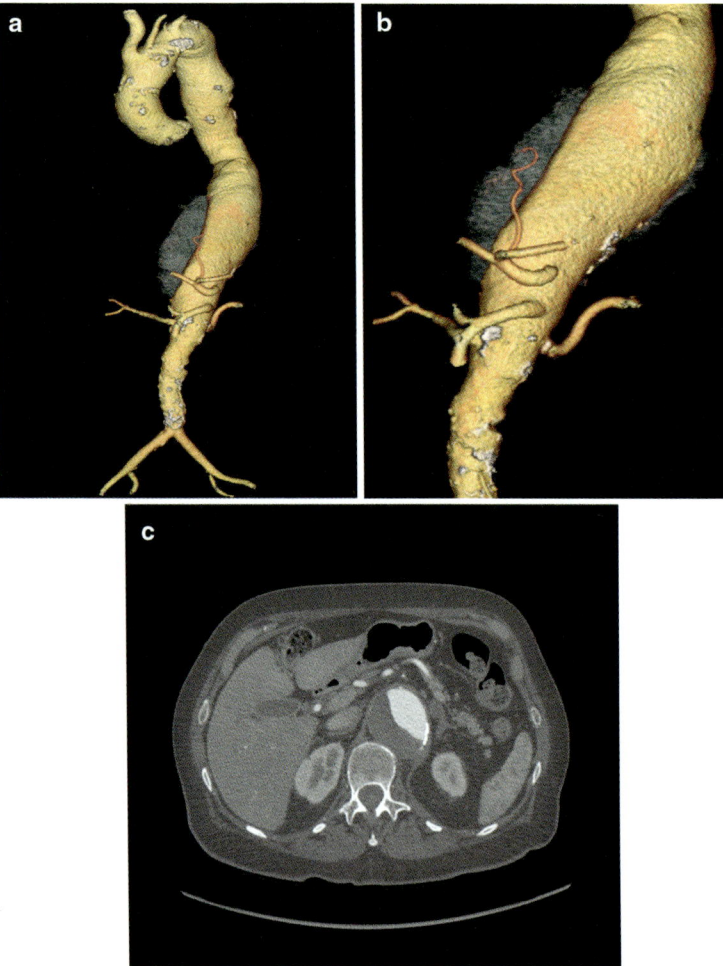

Fig. 10.23 (**a–c**) Sixty-four slice and axial CT scan demonstrates a type III thoracoabdominal aneurysm measuring 6.1 cm × 5.7 cm involving the celiac, superior mesenteric, and renal arteries; distal abdominal aorta measures 4.3 cm × 3.8 cm. Iliac vessels are very tortuous and small in caliber

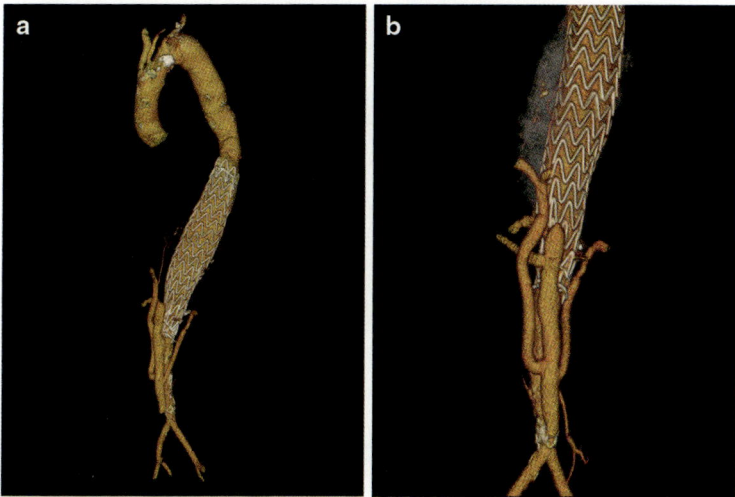

Fig. 10.24 (**a, b**) Post-operative CT scan demonstrates satisfactory exclusion of thoracoabdominal aneurysm with an endoluminal graft. There are patent debranched vessels with inflow graft coming off the distal abdomnal aorta. No endoleak is identified

10.9 CT Imaging of the Thoracic Aorta for Pre-operative Planning

CT angiography has become the main imaging method used for the assessment of the thoracic aorta. Use of multiplanar reconstructions (MPR) and maximum intensity projection (MIP) images on the CT workstation to assess the location and extent of the aortic lesion, the presence of proximal and distal landing zones for an endograft(s), the configuration of the aorta and iliac vessels with regard to tortuosity and kinking which might cause problems in delivery of the endograft to the required site, the access site and iliac arteries for their diameter, amount of calcification and the presence of aneurysms.

Diameter measurements of the aorta should always be made orthogonal to the vessel. This is most easily done using the reformatted images. If only axial images are available, the diameter of the short axis of the vessel should be measured. The following diameter measurements should be obtained: the maximum diameter of the aorta, the diameter of potential landing zones for an endograft proximal and distal to the aortic lesion, the diameter of the access vessels – i.e., the iliac and common femoral arteries. Length measurements are best made using oblique sagittal or curved reformatted images. CT imaging of the access vessels is important in preplanning to decide vessels' size, degree of tortuosity, and calcification (Fig. 10.25).

Based on a pre-operative worksheet (Fig. 10.26) various measurements can be obtained from the reformatted CT scan of the chest for deciding if patient is a candidate for an endovascular repair. The access vessels' sizes are determined by the CT

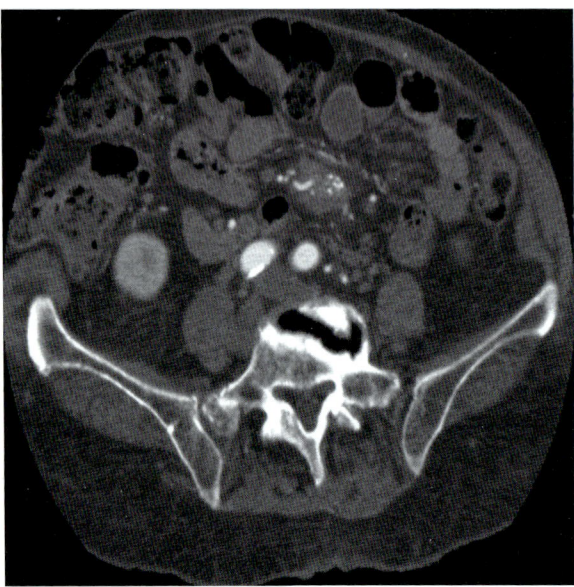

Fig. 10.25   An axial CT image demonstrating adequate-sized iliac arteries with mild calcification in the posterior wall of right iliac artery

Fig. 10.26   A pre-operative worksheet to evaluate the candidacy for stent graft placement: A, proximal implantation site; B, 1 cm proximal to implantation site; C, 2 cm from implantation site; D, aneurysm diameter; E, secondary aneurysm; F, 2 cm distal to implantation site; G, 1 cm from distal implantation site; H, distal implantation site; M, aneurysm length; N, distal neck, distance from aneurysm to celiac axis; O, total treatment length

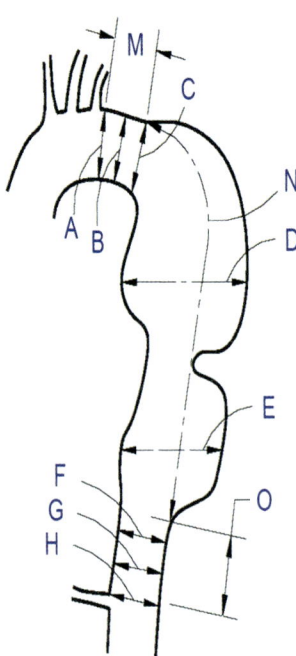

Fig. 10.27
Three-dimensional
reformatted scan to determine
iliac vessel size, tortuosity,
and degree of calcium

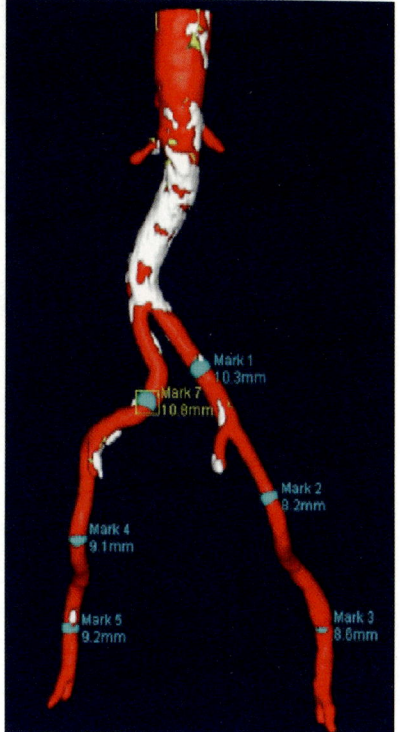

reformatted scan (Fig. 10.27) and the iliac diameters are matched to the appropriate sheath device. If the access vessels are smaller than the anticipated delivery sheath (Table 10.1), then a retroperitoneal conduit should be entertained (Table 10.2).

Descending thoracic aneurysms with a diameter ≥5 cm. Descending thoracic aneurysms with a history of growth ≥.5 cm per year. Descending thoracic aneurysms with degenerative or atherosclerotic ulcers ≥10 mm in depth and 20 mm in diameter.

Table 10.1   Gore TAG sizing chart

Device diameter (mm)	Vessel diameter (mm)	Oversizing (%)
26	23–24	8–14
28	24–26	8–17
31	26–29	7–19
34	29–32	9–16
37	32–34	9–16
40	34–37	9–18

Table 10.2 Recommended iliac diameter for the introduction of delivery sheaths

Size (Fr)	ID (mm)	OD (mm)
20	6.7	7.6
22	7.3	8.3
24	8.1	9.1

ID, inner diameter; OD, outer diameter

Reference

1. Diethrich EB, Ramaiah VG, Kpodonu J, Rodriguez JA. *Figures and Text Courtesy of Endovascular and Hybrid Management of the Thoracic Aorta. A Case Based Approach.* 1st ed. West Sussex: Wiley Blackwell; 2008.

Chapter 11
Intravascular Ultrasound Applications to the Thoracic Aorta

Unlike traditional cardiac ultrasound that uses an exterior probe and is limited to imaging between the patient's ribs or a transesophageal probe, intravascular ultrasound uses a miniature ultrasound transducer mounted on the tip of a catheter. Due to its intraluminal perspective, IVUS imaging provides information that supplements angiography. Standard IVUS catheters use a 9 Fr delivery sheath and a 0.035 in. guidewire, but smaller catheters do exist like the eagle-eyed gold catheter which uses a 0.014 in. guidewire. The ultrasound transducer emits and receives signals at 12.5, 20, or 30 MHz, producing an axial image (or frame) similar to the cuts from computed tomography and magnetic resonance imaging. Increase in MHz results in a more detailed image ("Near vision") with a decrease in MHz resulting in more penetration with larger field of view.

Two-dimensional IVUS images are obtained by passing an ultrasound catheter over a guidewire into the area of investigation. The axial view is a 360° real-time image obtained by rotating the ultrasound beam rapidly around the axis of the catheter. The radius of detection can be altered to suit the diameter of the vessel. In the normal artery, ultrasound waves are reflected differently by various vessel wall components. The reflections from collagen and elastin are stronger than smooth muscle cells, revealing the muscular media as a hypo-echoic circle, distinct from the reflective intima and adventitia. The use of 3D IVUS technology is of particular importance in preventing sub-optimal intraluminal device deployment that may not be appreciated on angiography as well as selecting the size of the endovascular device to use. IVUS 3D images are created by the computer using an edge tracking formula (algorithm). Consecutive axial 2D images are aligned and stacked longitudinally during a "pull-back" of the ultrasound catheter through the vessel. Each picture element (pixel) of the 2D image is assigned a digital position on an X and Y axis. By adding a Z axis, or a third dimension, each square pixel becomes a cubic picture element (voxel). When all the stacked frames are put together, the 3D reconstruction is complete and can then be examined by the computer software to view the vessel from any angle, slice, or rotation. Three-dimensional reconstruction can assemble the stack of serial 2D axial frames into both a "longitudinal" image and a "volume" image. For acquisition of high-quality longitudinal and volume views, a smooth pull-back of the catheter at a steady rate is required. This may be done

J. Kpodonu, *Manual of Thoracic Endoaortic Surgery*,
DOI 10.1007/978-1-84996-296-4_11, © Springer-Verlag London Limited 2010

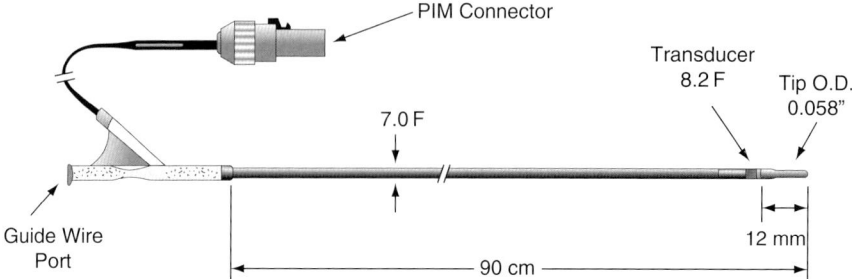

Fig. 11.1 0.035 Visions PV IVUS catheter system

manually or using a motorized device. In general, 1 mm/s with a 30 frames/s rate is recommended for shorter lesions. For longer areas of interrogation (>7 cm), the frame rate needs to be lowered to 10 frames/s because the computer can handle only 2048 frames in one pull-back. Currently in clinical practice there are three types of IVUS catheters which are currently in use for coronary/aortic interventions, the 0.035 Visions PV catheter systems (Fig. 11.1), the 0.014 eagle-eyed gold catheter system, and the 0.018 Visions PV catheter systems.

The 0.035 visions PV IVUS catheter is an over-the-wire catheter-based ultrasound with an 8.2 Fr crossing profile at the level of the transducer and a 7.0 Fr shaft diameter. The minimum sheath internal diameter is 9 Fr. The working catheter length is 90 cm and the imaging diameter is 60 mm and it is an over-the-wire catheter. The 0.014 Eagle Eye Gold IVUS catheter is a monorail based system with a 2.9 Fr crossing profile at transducer and a 2.7 Fr shaft diameter. The minimum guide catheter internal diameter is 5 Fr. The working length is 150 cm and the imaging diameter is 16 mm. The transducer however cannot be flushed and is compatible VOLCANO Trak Back II and R-100 Pullback devices. The 0.018 Visions PV IVUS catheter system is also a monorail-based system with a 3.5 Fr crossing profile at transducer, an imaging diameter up to 24 mm, and a working length of 135 cm. The minimum guiding catheter inner diameter is 6 Fr and the transducer cannot be flushed. IVUS provides precise anatomical information on the relationship between the aortic side branches and the aneurysm, as well as the dimensions of the proximal and distal fixation sites. A strong correlation has been identified between arterial lumen diameter measurements performed on histological specimens and IVUS. In addition to providing precise measurements, IVUS also provides important qualitative information on luminal morphology, including the presence of atherosclerotic plaque, calcification, fibrous lesions, and intraluminal thrombus.

11.1 Universal IVUS Applications

IVUS permits imaging of the vessel wall with identification of branch vessel landmarks. Using the pull-back techniques, luminal diameters, cross-sectional area

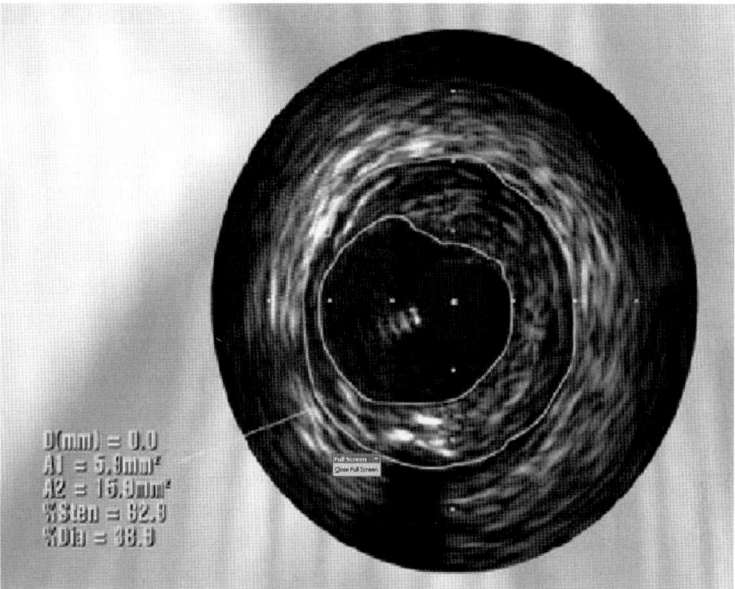

Fig. 11.2 Calculating area and percentage stenosis flow lumen diameter divided by vessel diameter

(Fig. 11.2), wall thickness, lesion length, shape and volume, lesion position within the lumen – concentric versus eccentric, lesion type – fibrous (soft) versus calcific (hard), presence and extent of flap, dissection, or ulceration, presence and volume of thrombus and vessel pathology can be determined. Tracing of the circumference of a vessel can also be performed to calculate vessel area, size, flow lumen area and size, as well as percentage stenosis. Settings on IVUS include Grayscale which determines level of blackness and whiteness (contrast). The gain enhances the details of the mage and the pixel determines increase/decrease matrix. IVUS has multiple advantages, such as imaging of calcification or stenosis, which may affect stent graft placement. IVUS is critical during the treatment of aortic dissections to confirm guidewire location in the true or false lumens. IVUS catheters also have the advantage of measuring lengths, which are often underestimated by CT scans. IVUS is also helpful in the identification of the exact location of an aneurysm when intraluminal thrombus may create a normal angiographic arterial lumen at either landing zone. IVUS may be critical in the identification of saccular aneurysm or arterial ulcerations filled by thrombus, and atheromatous sources of arterial emboli may at times be identified only by IVUS. Despite the numerous advantages of IVUS, there are two distinct concerns with the use of IVUS measurements. The first is off-center measurements that distort the image and may mislead the observer. The second is tangential measurements on a curve, which would not reflect a true centerline diameter. Instead, the 2D representation may be an oblique slice through the aorta.

11.2 Selective Applications of IVUS to the Abdominal Aorta

IVUS is an important tool that can be applied for endovascular management of infra-renal abdominal aneurysms. IVUS can be used to confirm measurements of the aneurysm size as measured on a routine CT scan of the abdomen. Using IVUS technology allows one to identify the renal vein as our landmark (figure) and subsequently identification of the diameter and length of the neck to determine suitability for endovascular technology as well as choice of graft. Presence of thrombus at the neck may be a relative contraindication for deployment of an endograft and this can easily be detected with the help of IVUS. The renal vessels can be identified and flow assessed (Fig. 11.3). The diameter of the aneurysm is also confirmed (Fig. 11.4) and sizes of the iliac vessels (Fig. 11.5) are determined to determine suitability for femoral deployment of an endoluminal graft. The IVUS catheter is useful for measurement of length from distal main body to internal iliac artery to confirm limb selection and also to visualize the guidewire in "the gate" after the main body is deployed and before iliac extension limbs are deployed. Confirmation of the true diameter of proximal neck and common iliac arteries is determined with the help of IVUS in choosing the appropriate-sized balloon(s) for percutaneous balloon angioplasty. IVUS is also helpful for determination of apposition of the stent graft to the aortic wall. A significant advantage of IVUS over angiogram is that it may be used instead of angiograms to save contrast on a patient that has renal insufficiency. The endoluminal graft diameter and length can be determined and deployed using only IVUS technology.

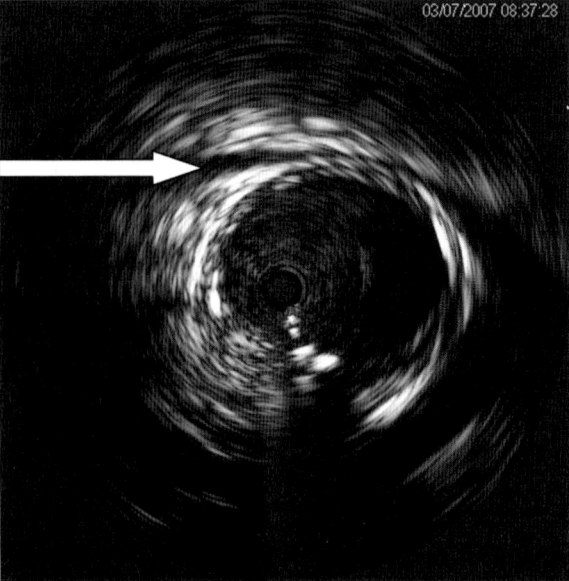

Fig. 11.3 Renal vein crossing the aorta (*arrow*)

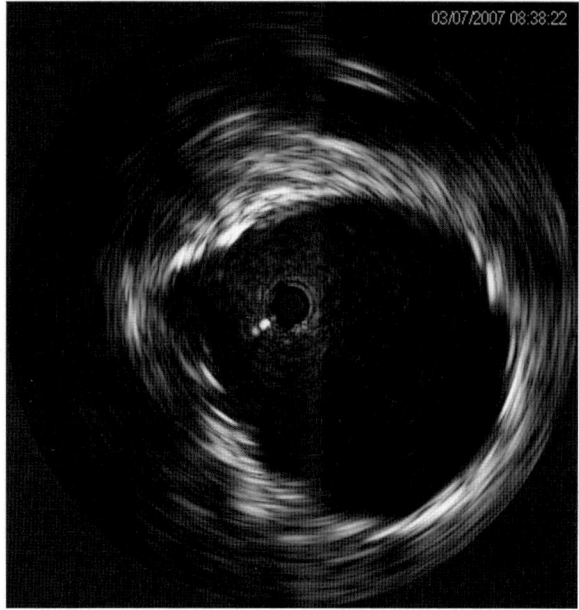

Fig. 11.4 IVUS demonstrates abdominal aortic aneurysm with thrombus in wall

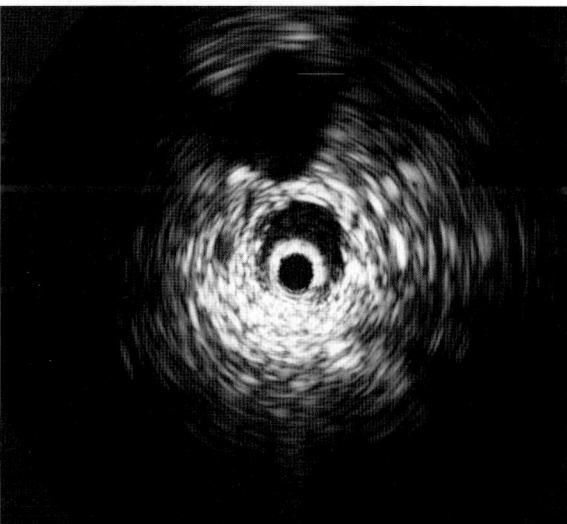

Fig. 11.5 Intravascular ultrasound (IVUS) demonstrating a common iliac artery measuring 8.5 mm with no thrombus and mild calcification amenable to deployment of a stent graft

11.3 Selective Application of IVUS in the Management of Thoracic Aortic Aneurysms

IVUS is useful for the treatment and evaluation of thoracic aortic aneurysms[1]. IVUS confirms measurements from CT scan and maps different diameters in the proximal aortic and distal aortic neck (Fig. 11.6a, b) as well as determines actual neck length. Pull-back measurements with IVUS enables accurate measurement of length and size of aneurysm, proximal and distal neck diameter and lengths. The anatomy can be well demarcated with demonstration of the branched arch vessels without the need for an angiogram. Thrombus can be detected in the aneurysm sac and the proximal and distal landing zones well characterized. Prior to deployment of an endograft the following information which includes luminal area and length of proximal and distal necks, length of aneurysm or arteriovenous fistula, and wall morphology, i.e., calcifications, thrombus, etc., at site chosen for endoluminal graft fixation are determined to help select the appropriate size and length of endoluminal graft. Position of collateral vessels that could produce distal ischemia if they were excluded from the

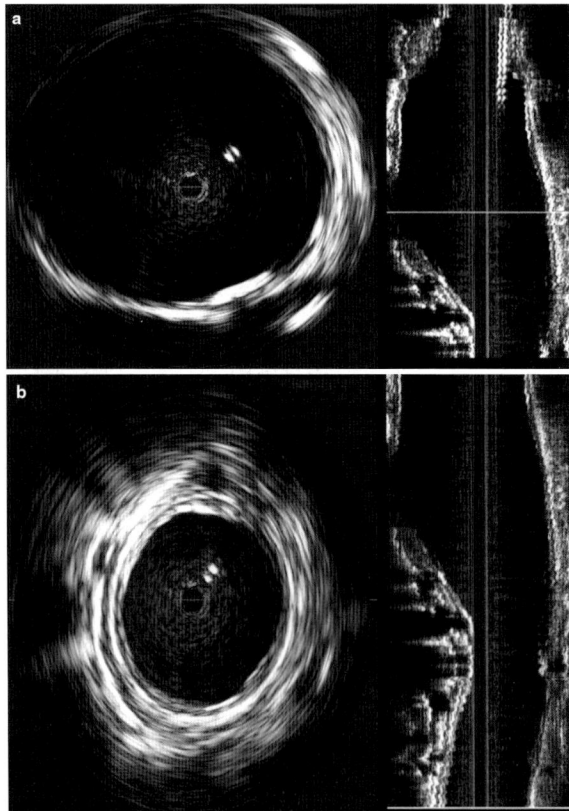

Fig. 11.6 (a) IVUS images in an axial and longitudinal view demonstrates a thoracic aortic aneurysm with a conical proximal neck, aneurysm, and a distal aortic neck with minimal thrombus. (b) IVUS demonstrating distal neck of thoracic aortic aneurysm with no demonstrable thrombus

lumen by the endograft can be accurately determined at deployment. Appropriate endoluminal graft position, appropriate expansion of fixation devices, and proper alignment of graft can be determined. After deployment device fixation is determined to prevent migration as well as confirmation of exclusion of the aneurysm from blood flow as well as identify the presence or absence of graft kinking, folding, or abnormal motion that might predispose to luminal narrowing, embolization, or graft thrombosis.

11.4   IVUS Application to Thoracic Aortic Dissections

IVUS is an important tool in identifying and confirming the presence of a type A or B dissection. The applicability of managing type B dissections with an endovascular graft depends on the location of the intimal tear, which determines whether one needs to cover the left subclavian artery or not, the dynamics of true lumen flow with respect to the false lumen as a result of the dissecting flap, and the state of visceral and renal vessels whether they are involved in the dissection or not (Fig. 11.7). IVUS is able to give us all this information as well as confirm the true lumen index flow, diameter of the thoracic aorta for device selection. IVUS can be used to confirm branch vessel dissection (Fig. 11.8) and also to treat branch vessel dissection with a stent to increase true lumen flow and restore perfusion to the branch vessel organ (Fig. 11.9).

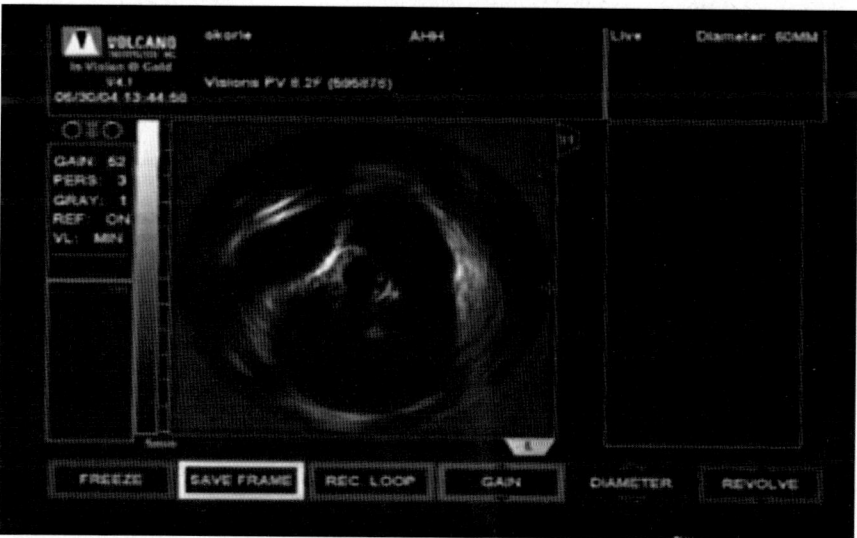

Fig. 11.7 IVUS demonstrates a type B dissection with a dissecting flap separating a compressed true lumen

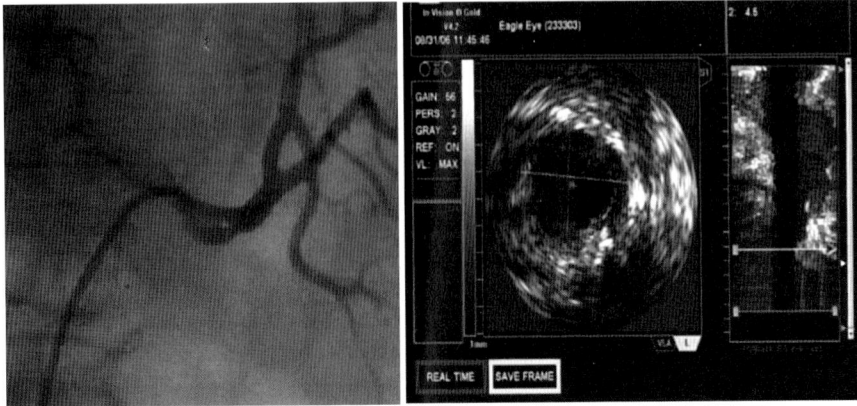

Fig. 11.8 Angiogram in a patient with a type B dissection with renal malperfusion confirmed with IVUS

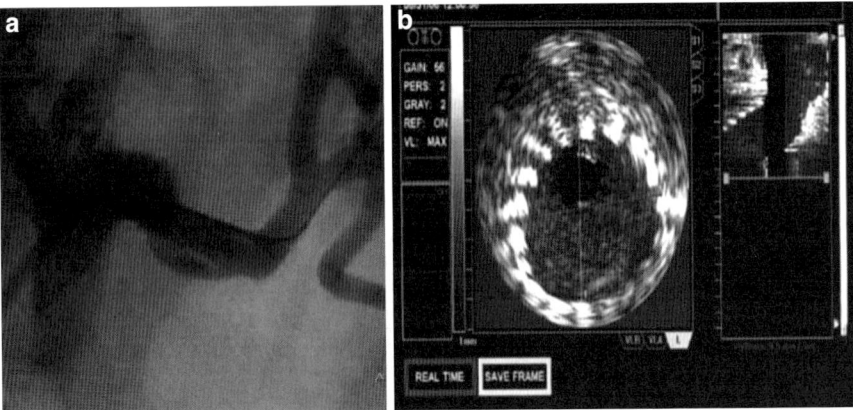

Fig. 11.9 (**a**) Angiogram post-stent deployment in the true lumen to re-expand the true lumen with improvement in renal flow. (**b**) IVUS demonstrates increased renal lumen diameter with demonstration of a well-apposed renal stent

11.5 IVUS Application for the Management of Coarctation of the Aorta

IVUS technology can also be applied to diagnose and treat endovascularly primary coarctation, recurrent coarctation, and post-coarctation pseudoaneurysms (Fig. 11.10). IVUS can be used to measure the diameter of the area of coarctation, the proximal aorta diameter and the post-stenotic aorta diameter, as well as the length of the area of coarctation. The choice of stent or stent graft can then be chosen and deployed accurately based on the IVUS measurements. IVUS also can determine proper stent apposition to the aortic wall after balloon angioplasty and provide post-stent measurements to determine success of the procedure (Fig. 11.11).

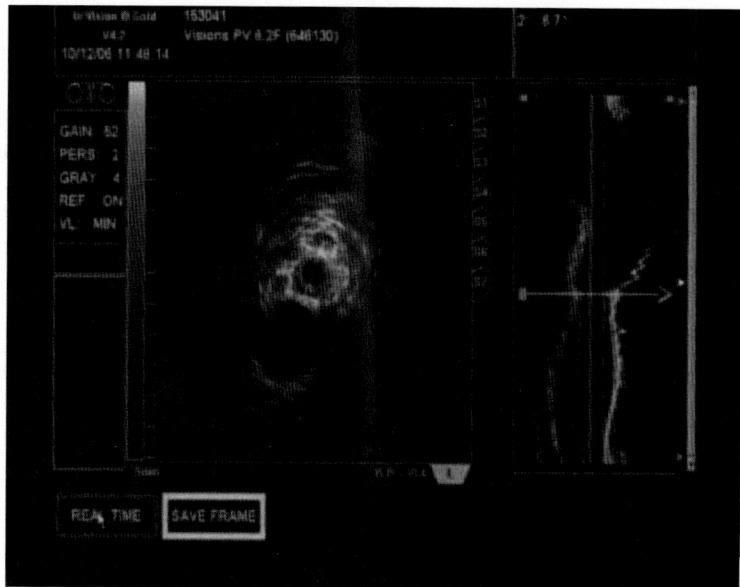

Fig. 11.10 Intravascular ultrasound demonstrating coarctation with a post-stenotic dilatation

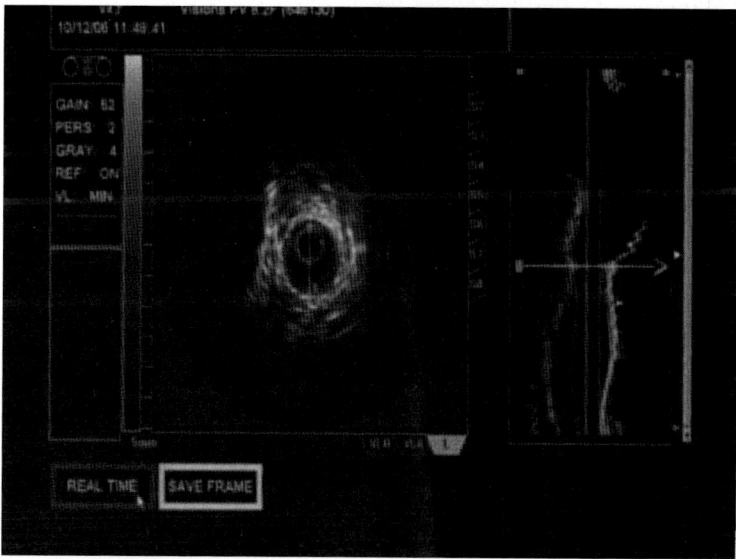

Fig. 11.11 Intravascular ultrasound post-stent deployment demonstrating an increase in luminal gain

11.6 IVUS Management for the Management of Penetrating Aortic Ulcers

Penetrating ulcers (PAU) of the thoracic aorta arise when atherosclerotic lesions rupture through the internal elastic lamina of the aortic wall with subsequent hematoma formation between the media and the adventitia. The ulcers are most often found in the distal descending thoracic aorta but can occur throughout the thoracic and abdominal aorta and have a characteristic appearance on computed tomography (CT) (Fig. 11.12) and magnetic resonance imaging. PAU may represent one pathology in the spectrum of acute aortic diseases but it may be associated with aortic dissection and aneurysm formation, although it is distinct from those conditions. I VUS is accurately able to diagnose aortic penetrating ulcers by demonstrating the break in the internal elastic lamina (Fig. 11.13). IVUS can further demonstrate the extent of ulcers and presence of any hematoma or dissection and is also important in the selection of device size and length needed to treat PAU. Once the endoluminal graft is deployed, accurate deployment and good apposition of the stent graft to the aortic wall can be determined.

Other applications of IVUS to aortic pathologies include diagnosis and therapeutic interventions for pseudoaneurysms, aortic transections, shaggy aorta, aorto-bronchial fistulas, and aorto-esophageal fistulas.

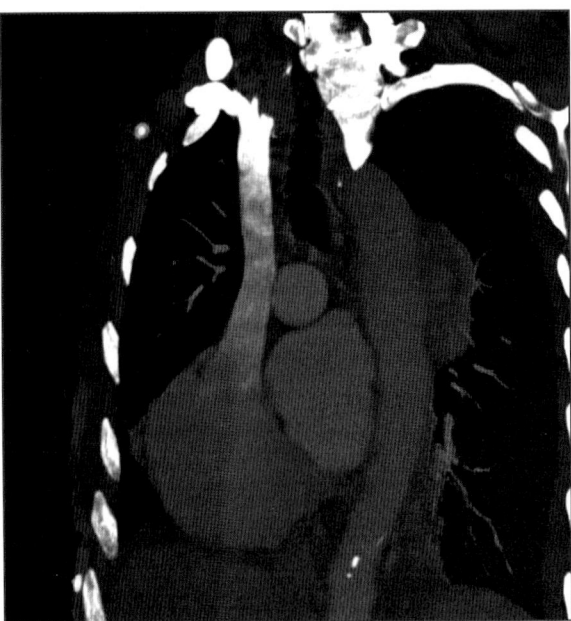

Fig. 11.12 CT scan demonstrates a penetrating aortic ulcer of the descending thoracic aorta with contained rupture

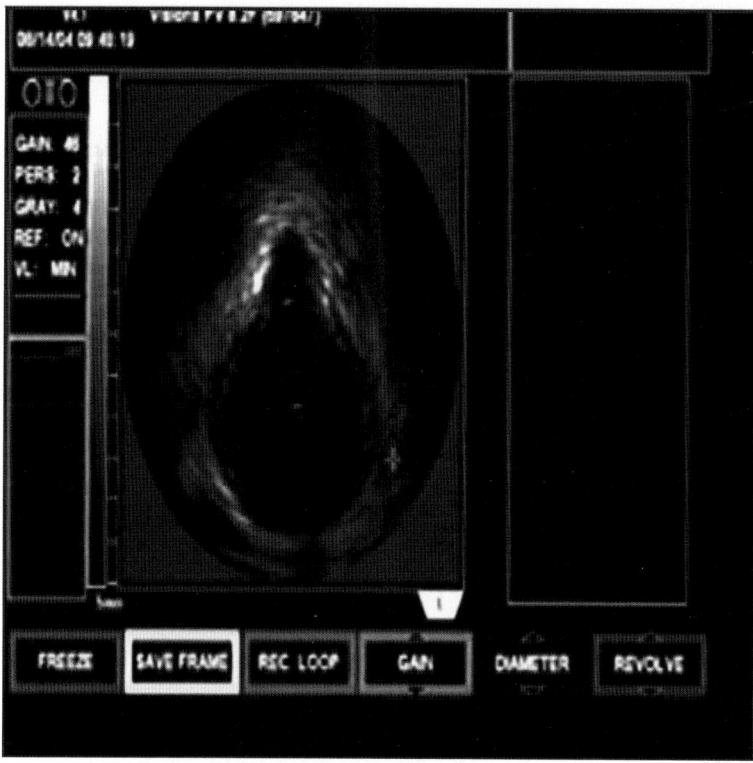

Fig. 11.13 IVUS image demonstrates a break in the intima of the descending thoracic aorta compatible with a penetrating aortic ulcer

Reference

1. Kpodonu J, Ramaiah VG, Diethrich EB. Intravascular ultrasound imaging as applied to the aorta: a new tool for the cardiovascular surgeon. *Ann Thorac Surg*. 2008;86(4):1391–1398.

Chapter 12
Endovascular Imaging, Planning, and Sizing for Treatment of Thoracoabdominal Aortic Aneurysms

12.1 Introduction

Endovascular aortic aneurysm repair is now the preferred treatment modality for patients with anatomy suitable to commercially available devices.[1,2] Aneurysms involving visceral and/or arch vessels not amendable to these devices are increasingly treated with investigational fenestrated and branched devices within all segments of the aorta. Once a patient is identified as a candidate for non-traditional endovascular aortic repair, a detailed pre-operative assessment directed at patient anatomic and physiologic variables is initiated to fabricate a customized device. Unlike traditional open aortic surgery where anatomic variances can be assessed and dealt with intra-operatively, the success of endovascular aortic repair is greatly contingent on careful pre-operatively planning. Careful consideration is given to patient anatomy and device design as well as the complex interaction between these two. Success is dependent on the ability of imaging modalities to accurately and reliably obtain this critical information. Once the raw image data is obtained, pre-operative planning is further enhanced by post-acquisition processing techniques. Necessary dimensions quantifying the aneurysm anatomy are determined from the compiled images. Once the patient data is gathered, the process of device design begins to generate a blueprint that will serve as the framework for the anticipated repair. Ideally and perhaps in the near future, the link between data acquisition and device design will be automated and the role of clinicians will be to oversee the process.

12.2 Patient Selection

Since this technology is still early in its development and the durability data are being accrued, it should be relegated to those patients considered high risk for conventional repair. Patients whose co-morbidities predict a life expectancy less than a year or two probably do not warrant aneurysm repair.

Eric Roselli is the editor of this chapter.

For endovascular therapy of these patients, several anatomic criteria must be met.

1. Presence of an aortic aneurysm at higher risk for rupture than the risk of repairing it using a fenestrated or branched graft. This is usually 6 cm or greater and a more detailed discussion of this determination is not appropriate in this chapter. However, it is important that the maximum aneurysm size is determined accurately with the use of 3D reconstructions to assure a measurement that is orthogonal to the course of the aorta.
2. Anatomy deemed unfavorable to endovascular repair with commercially available stent grafts because of one of the following:

   a. Proximal aortic neck length less than 15 mm
   b. Conical-shaped aortic neck
   c. Extensive thrombus-lined aortic neck
   d. Severe angulation
   e. Thoracoabdominal aortic aneurysm

3. Anatomy conducive to fenestrated or branched stent grafting including all of the following:

   a. Normal caliber visceral aortic segment (juxtarenal aneurysms) or other thoracic aortic segment relatively free of thrombus for proximal device landing zone
   b. Parallel landing zone segment

4. Iliac anatomy:

   a. Adequate luminal diameter to allow for device delivery (typically >7–8 mm)
   b. Lack of severe tortuousity or severe circumferential calcification precluding device passage

Furthermore, there are certain patient variables that may be contraindications for endovascular therapy.

1. Allergies to device materials.
2. Severe dye allergy or renal dysfunction inhibiting proper imaging.

12.3 Pre-operative Data Acquisition and Reconstructions

The development of multi-slice, helical computed tomography (CT) has markedly improved the ability to image the aorta [3,4] without the need for invasive angiography. However, accurate sizing is dependent on the quality of the images obtained. Surgeon familiarity with image acquisition can facilitate the development of the proper protocols in conjunction with radiologists and technicians. Typically, high-resolution helical CT of the chest, abdomen, and pelvis is performed utilizing a narrow collimation set between 0.5 and 1 mm intervals, with gantry rotation of

0.5 s, and table feed of 12 mm to allow for the acquisition of the appropriate data. Specific detail regarding acquisition protocols can be found in Table 12.1. The CT scan should be performed *without* oral contrast and with an intravenous contrast (low osmolar, non-ionic) bolus timed for the arterial phase. Non-contrast and venous phase (5 min delay) images are also obtained when performing post-operative studies directed at assessing endoleaks and device integrity. ECG gating is another important tool used to eliminate cardiac pulsation artifact when visualization of the ascending aorta and aortic root is necessary.[5] Reconstructions with 1–1.5 mm slices are helpful to accurately select patients, design the device, and plan the operation.

Table 12.1

Routine Gated Thoracoabdominal Aorta

CONTRAST

Intravenous:
130 ml contrast – 3.0 ml/s flow rate
                            Bolus tracking, trigger descending aorta
                            125HU Sensation 64/Definition
                            150HU Phillips 64

PATIENT DOSE

FOR CHEST
Sensation 16, Sensation 64/ Definition and Phillips 64
        120 kVp
        350 mAs **Increase mAs for larger patients**

RANGE

Chest: Scan from apices through the bottom of the heart.
Abdomen: Start with small overlap from the chest scan through the pelvis

CT SCANNER

Sensation 64/16 or Definition
Spiral – 1.2 mm collimation, 3 mm × 3 mm
        Kernel   B26
        Window   Cardiac
Phillips 64
Spiral – 0.625 collimation, 3 mm × 3 mm
        Filter (Kernel) Cardiac Standard (CB)
        Window   C: 90   W: 500

ECG Gating – 3–4 lead configuration ∗always use dose modulation

Table 12.1 (Continued)

CAP STENT (Chest/Abdomen/Pelvis)

CONTRAST

IV Contrast:
120 ml Ultravist 370 Sensation 64, Definition or Philips Brillance 64

Timing: 1st: Unenhanced scan of the chest, abdomen and pelvis **only if the patient has an endovascular stent**

2nd: Timing determined by Bolus Tracking at carina

150HU on Siemens Sensation 64 or Definition

150HU on Phillips Brillance

3rd: If the patient has a stent graft, scan delay

at **5 min** from the start of injection

CT SCANNER

Sensation 64 and Definition
0.6 mm collimation

Diagnostic images: 3 mm slice thickness, 3 mm interval (Send: MV1000)

Kernel: B31 Medium/Smooth   Window: Abdomen

Reconstruction: 0.75 mm slice thickness, 0.7 mm interval (Send: CT4_MS)

Through the stent only on the non contrast if scanned.

Kernel: B60 Sharp   Window: Abdomen

Thin slices through entire arterial scan.

Kernel: B31 Medium/Smooth   Window: Abdomen

Philips Brillance 64
64 × 0.625 mm collimation

Diagnostic images: 3 mm slice thickness, 3 mm interval

Window C: 90   W: 500

Filter   Standard B (B)

Reconstruction: 0.75 mm slice thickness, 0.7 mm interval (Send: CT4_MS)

Through the stent only on the non-contrast if scanned

Window C: 90   W: 500

Filter   Y-Detail (YB)

Enhancement – 0.5

Thin slices through entire arterial scan

Window C: 90   W: 500

Filter   Standard B (B)

To take full advantage of the large datasets acquired by multi-slice CT, and optimize accuracy in planning, use of a powerful post-processing software system such as Aquarius Workstation (TeraRecon, Inc, San Mateo, CA), M2S (M2S, Inc, West Lebanon, NH), or one of the other manufacturers is paramount. Traditional axial

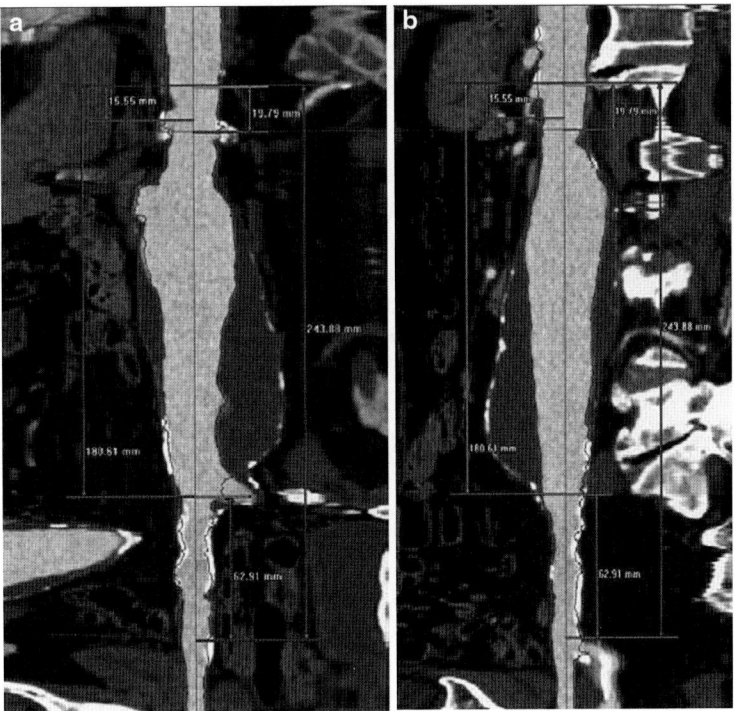

Fig. 12.1 Stretched views of a center line of flow reconstruction with longitudinal measurements in both (**a**) anterior view and (**b**) laterally rotated view

reconstructions cannot provide the details and accuracy needed to properly plan a complex endovascular procedure. Multiplanar reformations (MPR) in sagittal, coronal, and oblique cross-sections plus 3D volume rendered and maximum intensity projections (MIP) augment the surgeon's/interventionalist understanding of the anatomy. One of the most important visualization tools is the curved planar reformatting (CPR) algorithm which allows for the use of center line of flow analysis. This technique provides a straightened view of the vessels along the center line to facilitate accurate measurements of length along the vessel (Fig. 12.1a, b).

12.4 Planning

A clear understanding of the aortic, branch vessel, iliac, and femoral artery anatomy based on pre-operative imaging is critical to proper patient selection, device design, and accurate delivery. Employing a step-wise approach serves to simplify and build efficiency into the planning process.

12.4.1 Plan the Seal Zone

You should choose a seal zone at least ≥15 mm proximal to the aneurysm. The seal zone should be within a relatively normal and parallel segment of aorta which is an important factor for durability. This is especially important when the proximal seal is in the aortic arch or in an otherwise angulated neck where complete aortic apposition may be compromised by the tortuosity of the vessel. Also choose the lowest segment of aorta that will provide an adequate seal. The proximal diameter for the graft body is determined by diameter of the aorta within the seal zone. The graft is usually oversized by 15%, and the sizing forms provided by each of the device manufacturers offer guidance with sizing charts in this regard.

12.4.2 Select Side for Graft Body Introduction

Access vessels are assessed for size, stenosis, tortuosity, and calcification. The side that will allow for easiest passage of the device is usually selected. Keep in mind that calcification and stenosis can limit rotational ability which is especially critical to accurate delivery with fenestrated or branched devices which need to be aligned in the axial plane with the target vessels.

12.4.3 Choose Fenestration and Branch Configuration

First, there are several design guidelines pertaining to fenestrations that must be considered when planning a graft:

- Grafts may include no more than two of any one type fenestration (small, large, or scallop) within a single sealing stent (Fig. 12.2).
- The distance between fenestrations must be more than 5 mm in a longitudinal axis (generally approximately 2 h of clock position, depending on graft diameter).

Fenestration planning begins with generating a stretch vessel view via CPR. The reference point for measurement then becomes the proximal edge of the device within the seal zone. From this point, the following applicable measurements are taken in the stretch vessel view:

- Middle of celiac to reference point
- Middle of SMA to reference point
- Middle of highest renal to reference point
- Middle of lowest renal to reference point
- Middle of any accessory renal to reference point

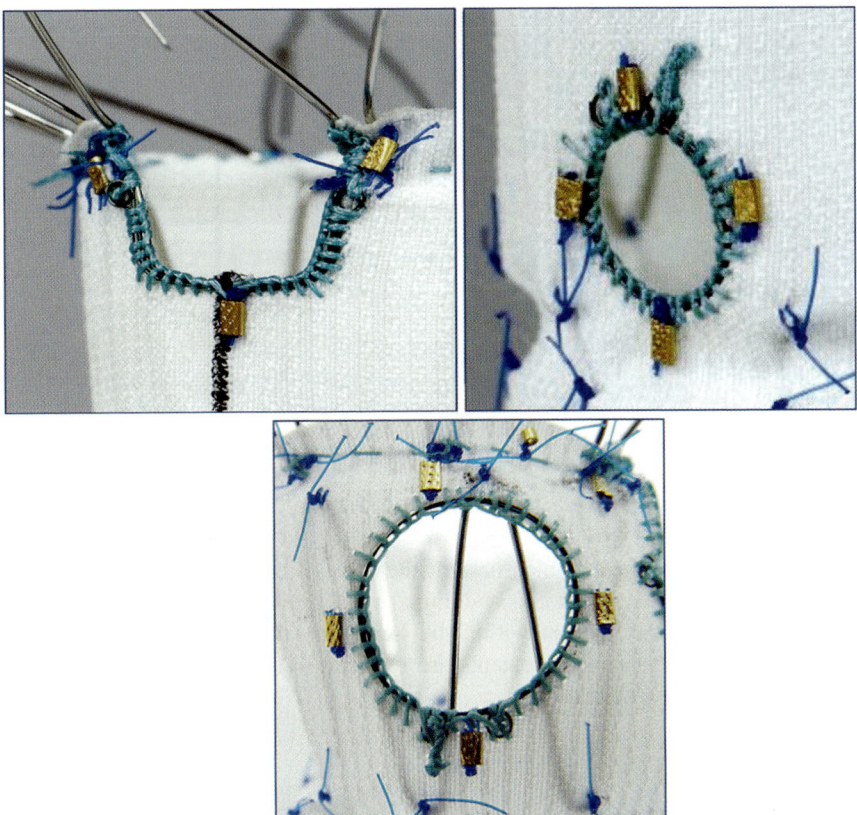

Fig. 12.2 Customizable target vessel access options: (1) scallop, (2) small reinforced fenestration, (3) large reinforced fenestration (notice stent limb across orifice), and (4) helical branch

After the applicable length measurements are taken, fenestration position upon the circumference of the graft, which is depicted as a clock face, must be determined from the axial MPR images (Fig. 12.3). Two measurements, longitudinal distance from the proximal point of reference and the clock position, are determined for each vessel of interest.

When designing a device with directional branches, similar descriptions of the location for each are provided and the devices are constructed accordingly. When feasible, directional branches are preferred over fenestrations for the celiac and superior mesenteric arteries since they provide the theoretic advantage of longer durability because of the longer sealing zones between the mated devices and the distribution of stress across a greater area. However, the use of directional branches is limited by the minimum caliber of aortic lumen required for their manipulation and expansion.

Fig. 12.3 Description of
target branch vessel
orientation in the axial plane

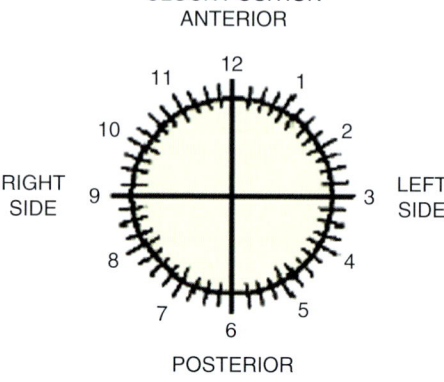

CLOCK POSITION
ANTERIOR

RIGHT
SIDE

LEFT
SIDE

POSTERIOR

Clock positions are in 15 min increments.

12.4.4 Determine Inner Aortic Vessel Diameter

The inner aortic diameter is measured at the level of each of the planned fenestrations or branches of the thoracoabdominal aorta (renals, celiac and mesenteric) (Fig. 12.4). Thrombus present within the lumen should not be included in this measurement. Accurate measurements are required to avoid posterior or anterior displacement of the fenestrations.

12.4.5 Choose Proximal Graft Length

In patients where the distal landing zone extends into the iliac arteries, the length of the graft will be determined by the distance from the proximal edge to a point 20–35 mm above the aortic bifurcation. This will serve to maximize the amount

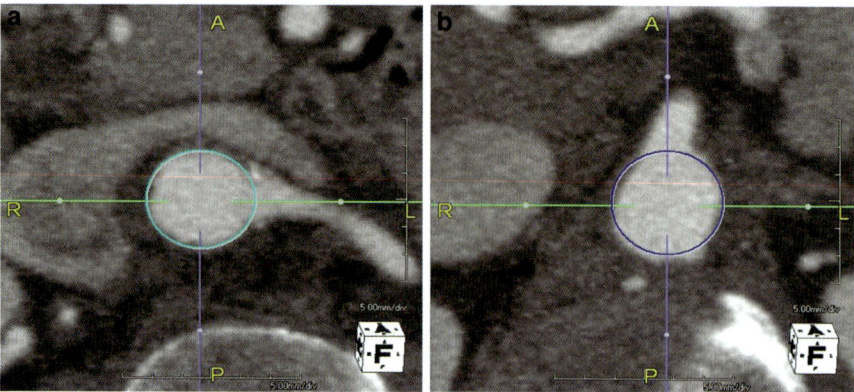

Fig. 12.4 Axial views of the (**a**) left renal artery at 3 o'clock position and (**b**) superior mesenteric artery at 12 o'clock position

of overlap between the proximal graft and distal body. In patients where the distal landing zone lies within the infra-renal aorta patency and location of the inferior mesenteric artery play an important role in determining length of the device.

The following rules applied to patients in the distal landing zone extend to the level of the iliac arteries.

12.4.6 Choose Distal Body Length

Distal body length should be determined observing the following principles:

– A minimum of two stent overlap is required while 3–4 stent overlap is preferred.
– The chosen length should keep the contralateral limb 5–10 mm above the aortic bifurcation.
– The proximal edge of the distal body should be below the lowest fenestration.

12.4.7 Choose Ipsilateral Leg Length

Ideally the ipsilateral leg will be designed to land just above the iliac bifurcation or other planned seal distal zone while maintaining the contralateral limb 5–10 mm above the aortic bifurcation.

12.4.8 Choose Ipsilateral Leg Diameter

Iliac vessel outer diameter is measured on axial CT images within the planned distal seal zone. Graft diameter is then oversized by 15–25%.

12.4.9 Choose Contralateral Leg Length

Ideally the contralateral leg will be designed to land just above the iliac bifurcation or other planned seal distal zone and allow for a minimum of one stent overlap with the distal body contralateral limb.

12.4.10 Choose Ipsilateral Leg Diameter

Iliac vessel outer diameter is measured on axial CT images within the planned distal seal zone. Graft diameter is then oversized by 15–25%.

12.5 Limitations of Branched Grafts

At this point in time, the need for customization of branched and fenestrated devices does not allow for their use in urgent or emergent indications. Although these devices have been used in patients with aortic dissections, particular details of the anatomy must be met to allow for successful deployment and use of this approach to repair. First of all, the target vessels must originate or communicate with the true lumen. The true lumen must be equal to or greater than 15 mm in diameter to allow for axial rotation and manipulation of these devices. Finally, in patients with aortic dissections it is especially important to have a secure proximal landing zone for fixation to optimize the durability of these devices.

12.6 Summary

Endovascular therapies are increasingly being used to treat more complex anatomy and pathology including extensive aneurysmal disease and complex dissections. The development and refinement of fenestrated and branched devices and techniques are further expanding the application of endovascular surgery to patients who previously were not candidates for repair with proven their safety and efficacy.[6] Procedural success for complex disease is entirely dependent on proper step-wise pre-operative planning. The process begins with high-resolution CT imaging with post-acquisition image processing. Accurate data gathering is then coupled with a sound understanding of device technology and the nuances of the procedure. This careful pre-operative planning approach can minimize unexpected events during deployment and allows for the preemptive preparation of rescue strategies to deal with intra-procedural problems when they do occur.

References

1. Greenhalgh RM, Brown LC, Kwong GP, et al. Comparison of endovascular aneurysm repair with open repair in patients with abdominal aortic aneurysm (EVAR trial 1), 30-day operative mortality results: randomized controlled trial. *Lancet*. 2004;364:843–848.
2. Prinssen M, Verhoeven EL, Buth J, et al. A randomized trial comparing conventional and endovascular repair of abdominal aortic aneurysms. *N Engl J Med*. 2004;351:1607–1618.
3. Flohr T, Schaller S, Stierstorfer K, Bruder H, Ohnesorge B, Schoepf J. Multi-detector row CT systems and image-reconstruction techniques. *Radiology*. 2005;235:756–773.
4. Ohnesorge B, Hofmann L, Flohr T, Schoepf J. CT for imaging coronary artery disease: defining the paradigm for its application. *Int J Cardiovasc Imaging*. 2005;21:85–104.
5. Fleischmann D, Mitchell RS, Miller DC. Acute aortic syndromes: new insights from electro-cardiographically gated computed tomography. *Semin Thorac Cardiovasc Surg*. 2008;20(4): 340–347.
6. Roselli EE, Greenberg RK, Pfaff K, Francis C, Svensson LG, Lytle BW. Endovascular treatment of thoracoabdominal aortic aneurysms. *J Thorac Cardiovasc Surg*. 2007;133(6):1474–1482. Epub 2007 May 2.

Part III
Access Techniques Required for Thoracic Endografting

Chapter 13
Brachial Access Techniques Used in Thoracic Aortic Endografting

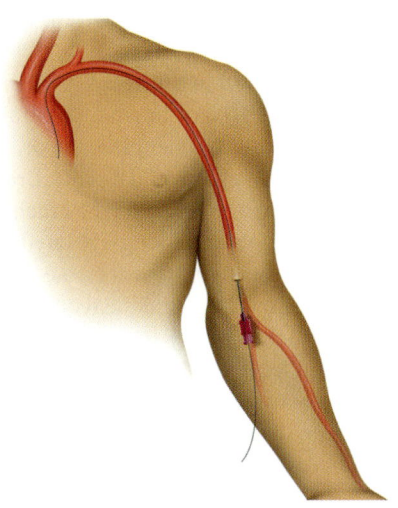

Percutaneous access techniques of the proximal vessels are occasionally performed to aid in proximal deployment of thoracic stent grafts, allow for easy identification of the left subclavian artery, coil embolization of the left subclavian artery for repair of type II endoleaks, as well as performance of an arch angiogram in severely tortuous thoracic aorta.

The arteries of the upper extremity have an enveloping fascial sheath. Therefore when a hematoma does occur, brachial plexopathies are more common. In addition, upper extremity vessels tend to spasm more frequently during manipulation, making access more challenging. Brachial access does carry the added risk of distal ischemia and embolization over radial access. Although sheaths up to 6 or 7 Fr may be percutaneously placed in either vessel, radial access should be preferred over brachial because of a lower complication profile and open access used for larger sheaths or on smaller patients.

Brachial and radial access techniques allow the utilization of angiographic catheters to assist with proximal deployment of thoracic stent grafts.[1] They allow for easy identification of the left subclavian artery, and angiography can be performed

J. Kpodonu, *Manual of Thoracic Endoaortic Surgery*,
DOI 10.1007/978-1-84996-296-4_13, © Springer-Verlag London Limited 2010

to avoid coverage with the proximal end of a thoracic stent. When coverage of the left subclavian artery is required for an adequate proximal landing zone, subclavian to carotid bypassing may be required. The radial or brachial access can therefore accommodate subclavian artery coil embolization to minimize the risk of type II endoleaks.

The left brachial artery is preferred over the right so as to avoid the origin of the right common carotid artery. The technique requires that the arm be abducted on an arm board with the arm circumferentially prepped. The artery is palpated just proximal to the antecubital fossa where the biceps muscle thins out to its tendinous insertion. Percutaneous retrograde puncture of the brachial artery with a 21 G micro-puncture kit is preferred to the 18 G due to the smaller size of the vessel (Fig. 13.1a). Catheter-over-wire exchange can then be performed to the desired sheath. Sheaths up to 6 Fr can be placed with relative safety (Fig. 13.1b). Long sheaths can help deal with the inherent vasospasm.

Deployment of an endoluminal graft in a tortuous aorta may be difficult requiring the use of a brachio-femoral wire. Use of brachio-femoral access wires can help straighten the most angulated of vessels. The presence of a tortuous aorta requires brachio-femoral access to deploy an endoluminal graft. Brachial access is obtained by a percutaneous retrograde puncture of the right brachial artery with an 18 G needle or a micro-puncture needle. An extra-long 450 cm 0.035 in. angled glide wire is advanced through the brachial sheath into the tortuous thoracic aorta, snared, and pulled out through the groin sheath. The technique requires that a protective guiding catheter be placed over the brachial artery to protect the subclavian artery from injury. It is important to have at least a 260 cm long wire and constant tension must be placed on both ends of the wire as the delivery sheath is passed into the aorta.[2,3] By pulling on both ends of the wire an endoluminal graft can be advanced up into the tortuous arch aorta with precise deployment of the endoluminal graft.

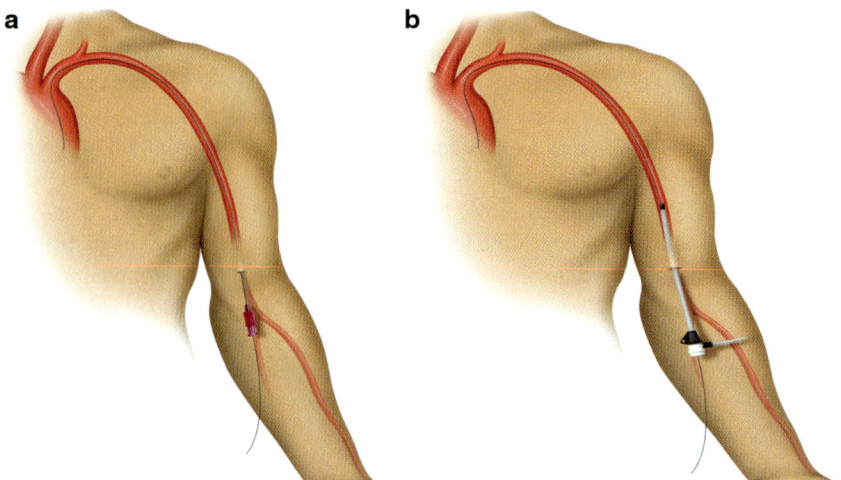

Fig. 13.1 (**a**, **b**) Retrograde percutaneous puncture of the brachial artery with placement of an introducer sheath

13.1 Case Scenario

A 75-year-old man with a past medical history significant for hypertension, hyperlipidemia, coronary artery disease, chronic obstructive lung disease, and prostate cancer post-radiation therapy was found to have a 7.0 cm thoracic aortic aneurysm for symptoms of back pain[3] (Fig. 13.2). He was considered high risk for open surgical repair and offered an endovascular approach to manage the aneurysm.

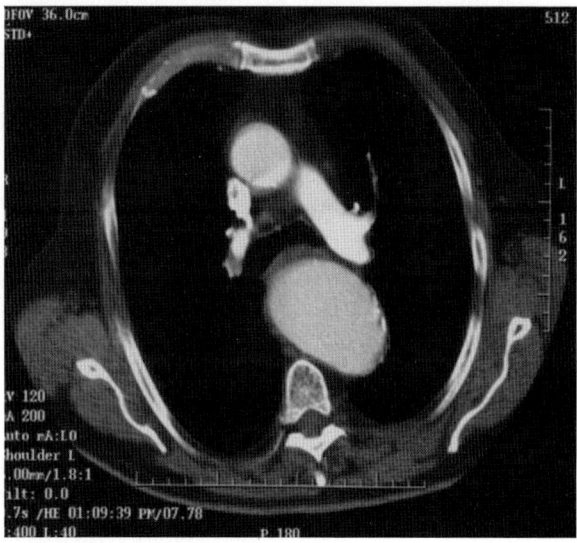

Fig. 13.2 CT scan of the chest demonstrating a thoracic aortic aneurysm with a diameter of 7.0 cm

13.2 Endovascular Technique

Placement of bilateral arterial radial arterial lines, open retrograde of the right common femoral artery with placement of a 9 Fr sheath, and percutaneous retrograde access of the left common femoral artery with a 5 Fr sheath were performed. 5000 units of heparin was given and ian liac angiogram was performed, which demonstrated diffuse stenosis and calcification of both common and external iliac arteries which was successfully managed with balloon angioplasty. An oblique thoracic aortogram performed through a 5 Fr angiographic pigtail catheter demonstrated a thoracic aortic aneurysm juxta distal to the left subclavian artery with a very tortuous angled arch (Fig. 13.3a). Using intravascular ultrasound the proximal neck diameter at the level of the left carotid artery measured 31 mm × 24 mm and a distal neck diameter at the level of the celiac trunk measured 27 mm × 24 mm. Due to the extreme tortuosity of the thoracic arch aorta, it was evident that a thoracic endograft would not be able to negotiate the aortic arch curve and a brachiofemoral wire conduit technique would be required to help navigate the tortous aortic arch. A retrograde percutaneous right brachial approach was therefore performed

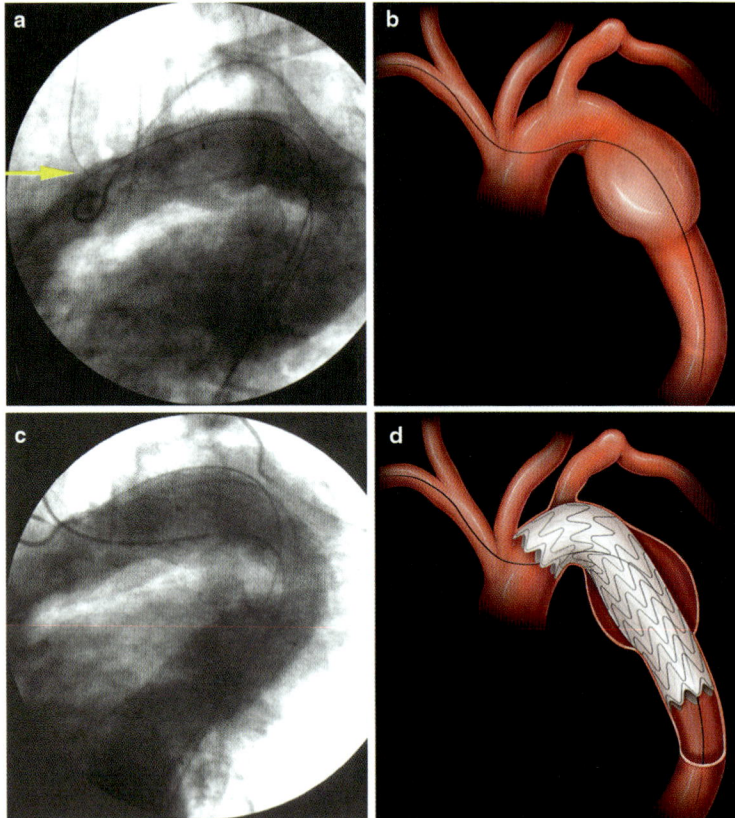

Fig. 13.3 (**a**, **b**) Advancement of a right brachio-femoral wire in a tortuous thoracic aorta. (**c**, **d**) Deployment of an endoluminal graft to exclude a thoracic aortic aneurysm by pulling on both ends of the brachio-femoral wire

with a 6 Fr 35 cm sheath and a 5 Fr Bernstein catheter was used as a guiding catheter to navigate a 260 cm length 0.035 in. angled glide wire into the tortuous descending thoracic aorta under fluoroscopic guidance (Fig. 13.3b). The wire was subsequently secured through the right groin sheath with the help of a snare. A glide catheter was used as an exchange catheter and the 260 cm length 0.035 in. glide wire was exchanged to a stiff 260 cm length 0.035 in. Lunderquist wire (Cook Bloomington, IN, USA). The 9 Fr sheath in the right groin was exchanged for a 22 F Gore sheath, which was advanced into the distal abdominal aorta. A road map angiogram was obtained through the left groin sheath pigtail catheter. By keeping a constant tension on the brachio-femoral wire conduit from the right brachial end and the right common femoral end, a 34 mm × 20 cm Gore TAG (W.L. Gore & Associates, Flagstaff, AZ, USA) device was advanced through the tortuous descending aorta into the arch and deployed distal to the left carotid artery partially covering the left subclavian artery (Fig. 13.3c). A 31 mm × 15 cm Gore TAG

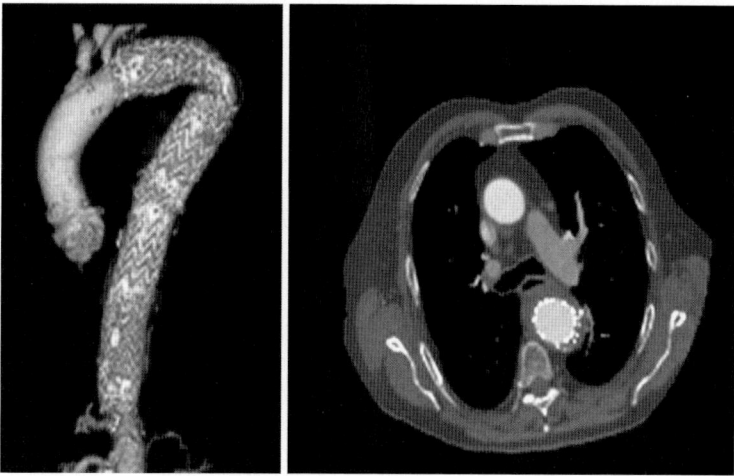

Fig. 13.4 Post-operative CT scan demonstrating exclusion of thoracic aortic aneurysm with no visualized endoleak

device was subsequently deployed distally just above the celiac trunk after an aortogram had been performed to demarcate the distal landing zone on the road map. A third device, 34 mm × 15 cm Gore TAG device, was necessary to cover the area of overlap between the proximal and distal endografts. A completion angiogram demonstrated successful exclusion of the thoracic aortic aneurysm with no endoleak (Fig. 13.3d). The 22 Fr sheath was then exchanged for a 9 Fr sheath and bilateral iliac angiograms demonstrated no extravasation of contrast. Bilateral 10 mm × 37 mm self-expandable stents were subsequently deployed at the area of previous iliac artery balloon angioplasty. Completion angiogram demonstrated satisfactory angiographic pictures with brisk flow through the iliac vessels and no pressure gradient. Sheaths and wires were removed and the right common femoral artery repaired and a closure device deployed to the left common femoral artery. The patient was extubated and transferred to the recovery room. A post-operative CT scan (Fig. 13.4) demonstrated no endoleak with exclusion of thoracic aortic aneurysm.

References

1. Schneider PA. *Endovascular Skills: Guidewire and Catheter Skills for Endovascular Surgery.* 2nd ed. New York, NY: Marcel Dekker Inc.; 2003.
2. Diethrich EB, Ramaiah VG, Kpodonu J, Rodriguez JA. *Images and Figures Courtesy of Endovascular and Hybrid Management of the Thoracic Aorta. A Case Based Approach.* 1st ed. West Sussex: Wiley Blackwell; 2008.
3. Kpodonu J, Rodriguez JA, Ramaiah VG, Diethrich EB. Use of the right brachio-femoral wire approach to manage a thoracic aortic aneurysm in an extremely angulated and tortuous aorta with an endoluminal stent graft. *Interact Cardiovasc Thorac Surg.* 2008;7:269–271.

Chapter 14
Transfemoral Access Techniques in Thoracic Aortic Endografting

14.1 Retrograde Percutaneous Access

The most common percutaneous access sites for thoracic endografting are the femoral and brachial arteries. When choosing which site to access the vascular tree, one must consider not only the intended procedure but also the size of the sheath and distance to the pathology. The goal for percutaneous access is to create the smallest incision, which provides safe and effective entry, without creating vascular trauma. Sheaths up to 12 Fr (4.0 mm) can be safely placed percutaneously. Larger sheaths require a cut down to ensure vascular hemostasis and minimize traumatic injury. If the physician is not adaptive to utilizing alternative access sites, then the procedure will be compromised.

14.2 Percutaneous Retrograde Femoral Artery Access

Most right-handed physicians will prefer the patient's right groin for femoral access, although both groins should be prepped in case of inaccessibility. After the pulse is identified, the inguinal ligament is found by tracing a line between the anterior iliac spine and the pubic tubercle. Often, especially in obese individuals, the inguinal crease is inferior to this landmark. Access should be made below the inguinal ligament corresponding to the common femoral artery. One will find that if access is made too high, corresponding with the external iliac artery, hemostasis is difficult to achieve with manual pressure. In this case hemorrhage can occur after removal of devices and a retroperitoneal hematoma can develop. This is often insidious in onset. In addition, the risk of pseudoaneurysm formation is higher in an external iliac stick, again because direct manual pressure cannot be applied this superiorly.

A properly equipped endovascular suite will allow fluoroscopic imaging of the groin to identify all anatomic landmarks. In addition to surface landmarks, most physicians use the medial half of the femoral head to guide femoral artery access; this ensures common femoral artery entry and avoids the complications of a higher stick. It is also useful in the pulseless femoral artery. Most vascular access kits

J. Kpodonu, *Manual of Thoracic Endoaortic Surgery*,
DOI 10.1007/978-1-84996-296-4_14, © Springer-Verlag London Limited 2010

Fig. 14.1 18 G 7 cm Cook
percutaneous needle

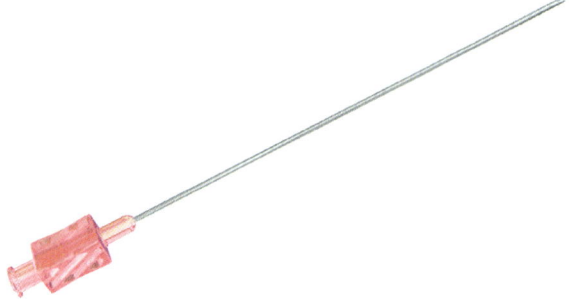

include an 18 G straight angiographic entry needle (Fig. 14.1). This is inserted
using the dominant hand at a 45° angle while using the non-dominant hand for
guidance using a Seldinger technique. Percutaneous arterial femoral access is usually obtained by the Seldinger technique. A careful palpation of the femoral pulse
is performed and a beveled needle (usually 18 G) is introduced through the arterial
wall. The needle is slowly withdrawn until the return of arterial blood is achieved
signifying the intraluminal position of the needle. The presence of poor blood flow

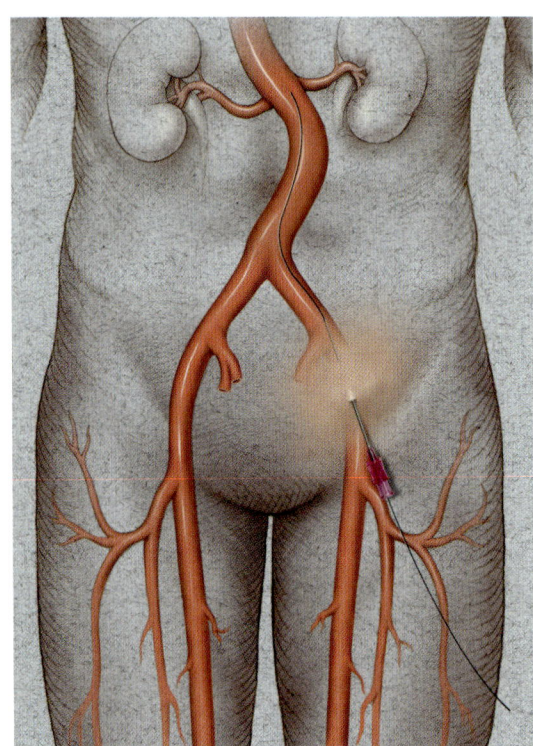

Fig. 14.2 Introduction of an
angled glide wire through the
18 G needle

signifies that the tip is misplaced or the needle is to close to the arterial wall. A soft tip angled 0.035 in. guidewire is then introduced through the central lumen of the needle under fluoroscopic guidance (Fig. 14.2). Progress of the guidewire intraluminally should be monitored with fluoroscopy to avoid diversion into branched vessels and dissection of the vessel. The presence of resistance in passing a guidewire signifies possible misdirection or dissection of the vessel wall. In instances where the vessel may be small, calcified, or tortuous, a smaller access needle may be desirable. A micro-puncture kit (Cook, Inc., Bloomington, IN) exists which includes a 21 G needle for initial access. Once access is achieved a small nick is made in the skin with a #11 blade and a dilator and an introducer sheath is then advanced over the glide wire with the dilator preceding the introducer sheath by a few inches again under fluoroscopic visualization (Fig. 14.3). Once the introducer sheath is positioned the dilator is removed. A hemostatic valve at the end of the introducer sheath prevents leakage of blood. The introducer sheath permits various guidewires, balloons, and stents to be introduced safely within the arterial lumen. The introducer sheath can subsequently be upgraded to a larger delivery sheath for the deployment of an endograft. In patients with a femoral to femoral graft, percutaneous access can be performed either through the inflow limb of the femoral–femoral graft or above the inflow limb.

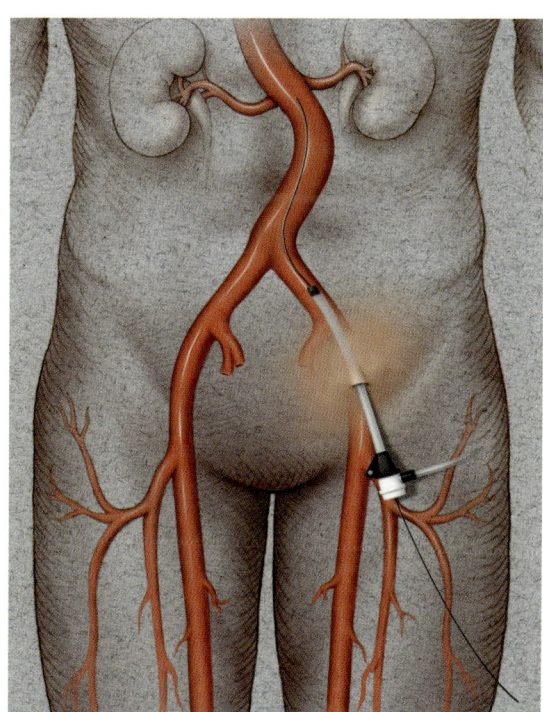

Fig. 14.3 Introduction of a 9 Fr 11 cm sheath in a retrograde percutaneous fashion through the common femoral artery

14.3 Contraindication to Percutaneous Femoral Access

In patients with significant peripheral vascular disease, imaging studies using an angiogram or a CT scan are necessary for sizing, determination of calcification, as well as tortuosity of vessels which would make the femoral delivery of an endograft hazardous. Large sheaths introduced in femoral vessels that are calcified, tortuous, small caliber, or a combination are predisposed to rupture.

14.4 Open Retrograde Access

The common femoral artery is usually exposed and accessed for retrograde cannulation with introduction of various large-sized introducer sheaths, balloons, self-expandable, balloon-expandable stents, and endoluminal grafts.

A curvilinear incision is made 2 finger breaths above the groin crease and over the palpable femoral pulse. The incision is carried down to the femoral sheath. Retraction is performed with a Gelpe retractor or a Wietlander retractor. The femoral sheath is incised to expose the common femoral artery. Heavy silk sutures are passed circumferentially round the various side branches. Adequate mobilization of the common femoral artery is achieved to be able to achieve adequate proximal and

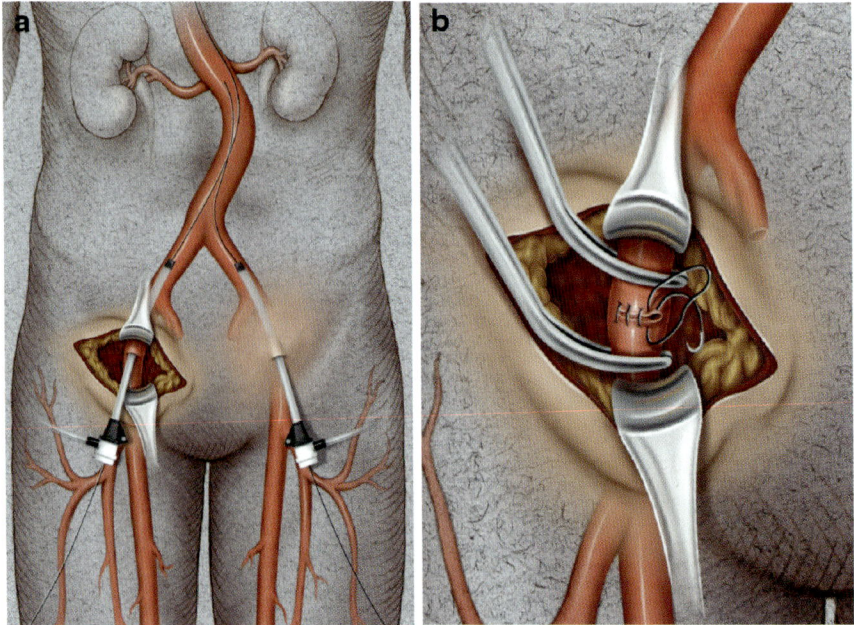

Fig. 14.4 (**a**) Open retrograde cannulation of the right common femoral artery and percutaneous retrograde cannulation of the left common femoral artery. (**b**) Closure of the arteriotomy after removal of guidewire and introduction sheath

distal control of the vessel. A Rummel tourniquet is applied to the common femoral artery to serve as a proximal control.

The fluoroscopic C-arm is then positioned over the exposed femoral artery. Retrograde cannulation of the common femoral artery is then performed with a beveled needle (18 G) until pulsatile blood flow is visualized. A soft angled tip guidewire is then advanced in the vessels under fluoroscopy. The needle is then exchanged for a selected sized dilator and introducer sheath. The dilator is the removed and the sheath flashed with heperanized saline. Open cannulation or retrograde percutaneous access can be similarly performed in the contralateral common femoral artery (Fig. 14.4a).

Once the procedure is completed, all wires and sheaths are removed under fluoroscopic guidance to ensure no injury is caused to the vessel wall. The arteriotomy is then closed with a 5-0 prolene suture after proximal and distal control is achieved (Fig. 14.4b).

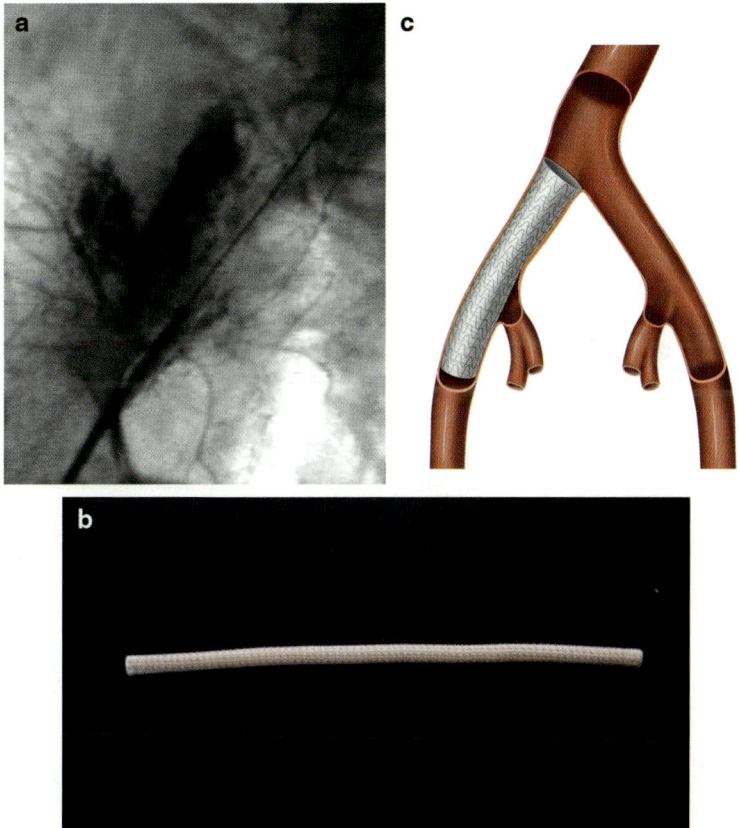

Fig. 14.5 (**a**) Angiogram demonstrates rupture of the right external iliac artery. (**b**) An illustration of a covered stent graft (Viahbahn, Gore & Associates) used to exclude site of rupture. (**c**) Illustration of a covered stent graft deployed across a ruptured iliac artery

14.5 Complications of Femoral Access

Rupture: Attempts to introduce a delivery sheath in a small, tortuous, calcified artery, or a combination will lead to rupture of the access vessel typically at the junction of the external and internal iliac artery or at the aorto-iliac bifurcation. Rupture of an access vessel should be suspected if there is a drop in the blood pressure during advancement of the delivery sheath or during removal of the delivery sheath. The guidewire should be maintained at all times prior to removal of a delivery sheath and an iliac angiogram performed prior to removal of introducer sheaths to confirm extravasation of contrast (Fig. 14.5a). Once rupture is confirmed an appropriate covered stent graft length and diameter should be chosen (Fig. 14.5b) and deployed across the area of rupture (Fig. 14.5c). In most instances coverage of the hypogastric artery is required.

Dissections: Introduction of guidewires and delivery sheaths may result in dissection of the access vessels. Similarly balloon angioplasty of calcified access vessels may also result in a dissection flap of the resulting access vessels. Once a dissection is identified on angiogram, gentle balloon angioplasty may be performed to seal off the dissecting septum or a covered r uncovered balloon deployable stent may be deployed to seal off the dissection. Failure to recognize a dissection may result in thrombosis of the access vessels with resulting ischemia of the involved lower extremity.

Reference

1. Diethrich EB, Ramaiah VG, Kpodonu J, Rodriguez JA. *Figures Courtesy of Endovascular and Hybrid Management of the Thoracic Aorta. A Case Based Approach*. 1st ed. West Sussex: Wiley Blackwell; 2008.

Chapter 15
Retroperitoneal Access for Thoracic Aortic Endografting

15.1 Introduction

Safe performance of thoracic endovascular procedures including thoracic stent grafting of aneurysms, dissections, retrograde delivery of transcatheter aortic valves, and other complex endovascular procedures for structural heart disease requires zero tolerance for major access-related complications. Thorough pre-operative planning, understanding the pathology of aorto-iliac occlusive disease, advanced endovascular skills, and ability to perform an iliac conduit via a retroperitoneal approach are necessary to achieve excellent results. Furthermore, deliverability of complex thoracic endovascular devices through tortuous anatomy or old graft material may be improved by the more proximal access provided by an iliac conduit.[1]

15.2 Indications and Pre-operative Planning

15.2.1 Patient Selection

Patients undergoing thoracic aortic endografting require access with devices ranging between 18 and 25 Fr in caliber. The external iliac artery is the size limiting segment and depending on the size of sheath required, a minimum diameter of 9 mm (3 Fr ~ 1 mm) may be necessary for safe access via the common femoral arteries. Patients with calcified, tortuous, small vessel size, or a combination (Fig. 15.1a–d) may not be candidates for delivery of these large sheaths through femoral arterial access and any attempts to deliver an introducer sheath or an endoluminal graft may result in an increased risk of iliac artery rupture or the "artery on a stick" phenomenon. Iliac artery diameters of 7.6–9.2 mm are required to deliver most devices through the femoral approach safely without the requirement of a conduit (Tables 15.1 and 15.2). Retroperitoneal exposure with construction of a 10 mm ilio-femoral conduit permits delivery of large sheaths in patients with tortuous, calcified, and small iliac vessels or vessels with severe ilio-femoral vascular occlusive disease.

J. Kpodonu, *Manual of Thoracic Endoaortic Surgery*,
DOI 10.1007/978-1-84996-296-4_15, © Springer-Verlag London Limited 2010

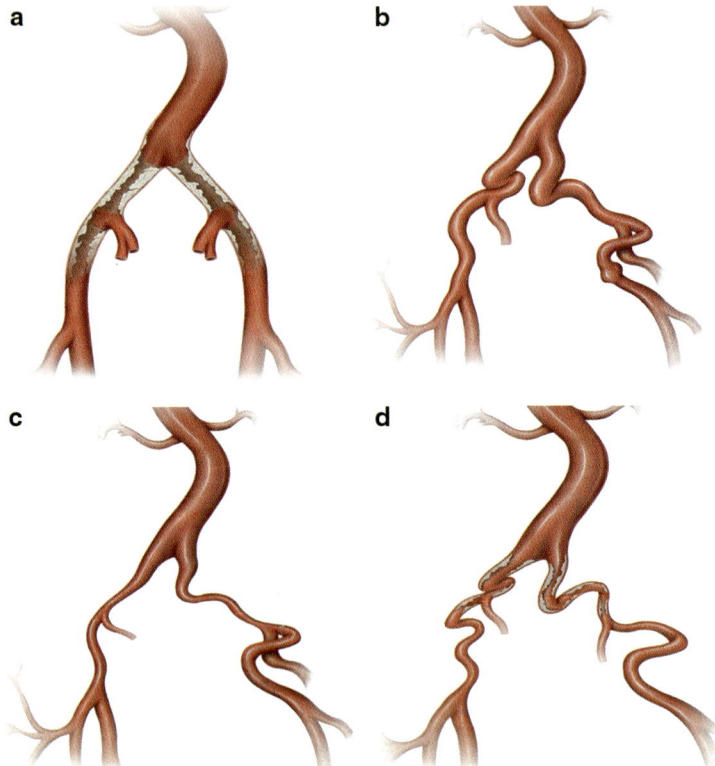

Fig. 15.1 Illustrations demonstrating (**a**) calcified, (**b**) tortuous, (**c**) small tortuous, and (**d**) small calcified tortuous iliac arteries which are contraindication for femoral access requiring a retroperitoneal exposure with sewing of an iliac conduit for delivery of endograft

Table 15.1 Graft and delivery sheath sizes for descending thoracic aortic stent grafts currently available in the United States

Endograft	Graft size available (diameter) (mm)	Sheath size required (diameter)
Gore TAG	26–40	20–24 Fr (7.6–9.2 mm)
Zenith TX1/TX2	28–42	20–22 Fr (7.6–8.3 mm)
Talent	22–46	22–25 Fr

Table 15.2 Recommended iliac diameters ID (inner) and OD (outer) for the introduction of Gore sheaths

Size (Fr)	ID (mm)	OD (mm)
20	6.7	7.6
22	7.3	8.3
24	8.1	9.1

15.2.2 *Construction of a 10 mm Retroperitoneal Conduit*

A 15 cm semi-lunar right flank incision is made 4 finger breaths above the groin crease. Division of the external oblique, internal oblique, and transversus abdominus muscle is performed in the direction of their fibers. Extra-peritoneal fascia and peritoneum are then retracted medially and dissection is carried out in the avascular plane of the retroperitoneum down to the level of the psoas muscle. All of the abdominal contents are then retracted medially with the help of a handheld retractor or an omni retractor. providing excellent exposure of the lower infra-renal aorta, common iliac artery, and iliac bifurcation. The right common iliac artery along with the hypogastric artery and the external iliac artery is identified and mobilized (Fig. 15.2a). Care is taken to spare the right urether which crosses the common iliac artery before diving deep into the pelvis. A Rummel tourniquet is applied to control

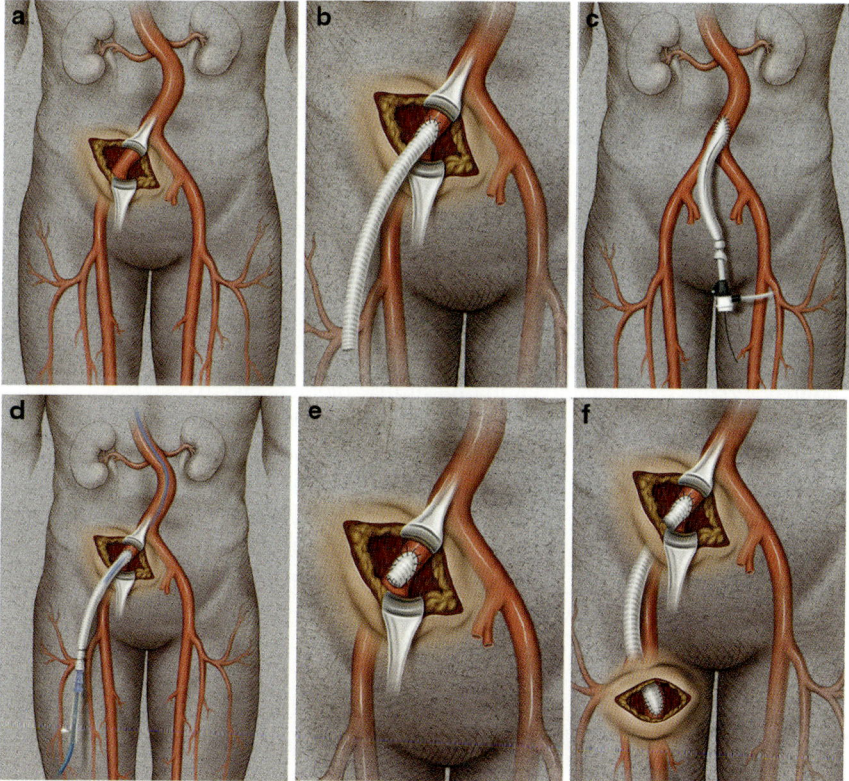

Fig. 15.2 (**a**) Retroperitoneal exposure; (**b**) 10 mm conduit sewn to iliac artery; (**c**) conduit brought out of incision with cannulation of conduit with an introducer sheath; (**d**) introducer sheath exchanged for a device sheath and advanced through the 10 mm conduit to the distal abdominal aorta; (**e**) ligation of 10 mm conduit; and (**f**) conduit tunneled and sewn to femoral artery as an ilio-femoral conduit

the proximal common iliac artery, the external iliac artery and origin of the hypogastric artery alternatively vascular clamps could be applied for control. Heparin is usually given to the patient prior to clamping the vessels. An arteriotomy is made on the common iliac artery with a #11 blade and extended with Pott's scissors close to the bifurcation of the hypogastric artery and the external iliac artery. A 10 mm conduit is then sewn in an end-to-side fashion using 5-0 prolene suture (Fig. 15.2b). The 10 mm graft is subsequently tunneled through the retroperitoneal space beneath the inguinal ligament and brought out through the groin incision used to expose the common femoral artery. The graft is subsequently flashed and clamped at the groin incision with the rummel tourniquets released from the common iliac artery, external iliac artery, and hypogastric artery. The 10 mm conduit is subsequently looped with a rummel tourniquet and ready to be punctured with an 18 G needle for access and introduction of a guidewire and an introducer sheath (Fig. 15.2c). The introducer sheath is subsequently exchanged for a device sheath which is advanced into the distal aorta (Fig. 15.2d). The endoluminal graft is then introduced into the delivery sheath and deployed to the target area. Wires and sheaths are removed from the 10 mm conduit and the conduit is clamped.

Either the conduit can be trimmed to the appropriate length and the conduit tied off as a stump (Fig. 15.2e) or the distal end of the conduit can be sewn to the more distal iliac system in an end-to-end fashion as an interposition graft or more commonly the conduit can brought out tunneled to the groin by tunneling the conduit under the inguinal ligament and performing either an end-to-end anastomosis or an ilio-femoral conduit. The ilio-femoral conduit is performed by making an arteriotomy on the adequately exposed common femoral artery after adequate proximal and distal control is achieved. An end-to-side anastomosis is constructed with a 5-0 prolene suture with adequate flushing maneuvers performed prior to completion of the anastomosis (Fig. 15.2f). The ilio-femoral conduit is the best for patients who may require further intervention for diffuse thoracic aneurismal disease as the conduit may be reused through a simple infra-inguinal incision in the future. The groin incision is approximated in layers. The right flank incision is irrigated, a 10 Fr Jackson-Pratt drain is placed in the retroperitoneal space and the incision closed in layers. The same technique can be applied to the infra-renal aorta and thoracic aorta. Similarly, end-to-side grafting of a conduit to the axillary artery as described elsewhere to facilitate deep hypothermic circulatory arrest also provides excellent access to the thoracic aorta via the innominate.[2]

15.3 Direct Iliac Artery Access via a Retroperitoneal Approach

A 15 cm semi-lunar right flank incision is made 4 finger breaths above the groin crease. Division of the external oblique, internal oblique and transversus abdominus muscle is performed. The peritoneum is identified and gently retracted medially with the help of a handheld retractor. The common iliac artery along with the hypogastric artery and the external iliac artery are identified and mobilized. Care

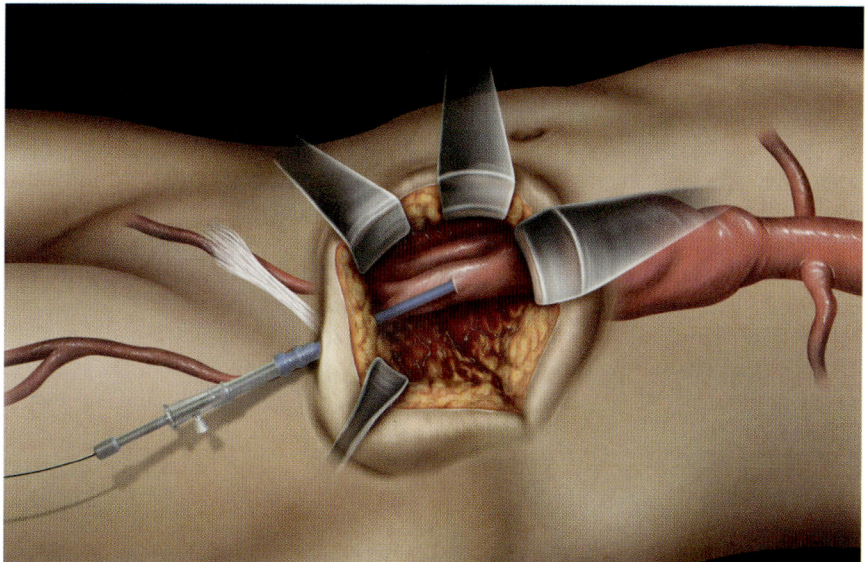

Fig. 15.3 Direct introduction of the device sheath through the common iliac artery through a retroperitoneal exposure

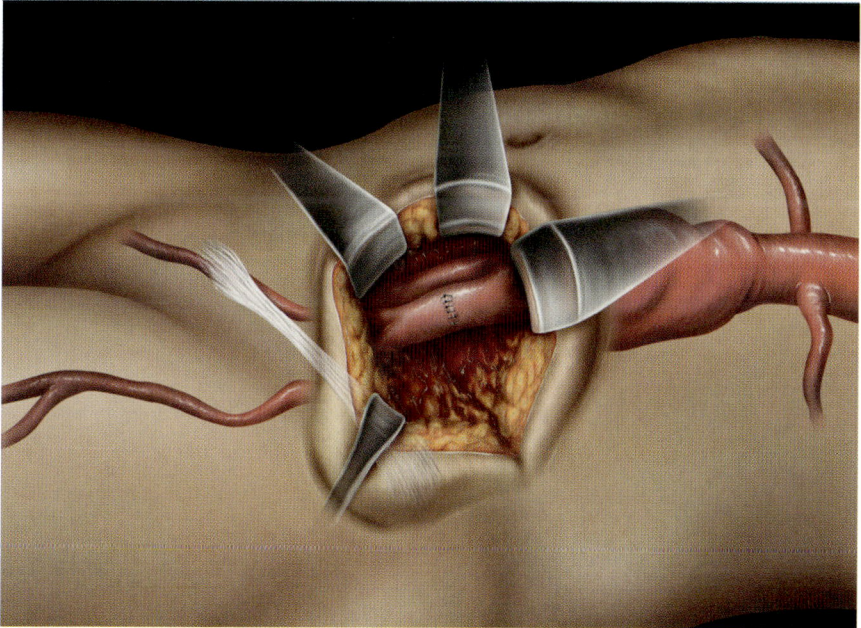

Fig 15.4 Direct repair of the iliac artery

is taken to spare the right urether which crosses the common iliac artery before diving deep into the pelvis. A Rummel tourniquet is applied to control the proximal common iliac artery, the external iliac artery and origin of the hypogastric artery alternatively vascular clamps could be applied for control. Heparin is usually given to the patient prior to clamping the vessels. Eighteen gauge needle is used to access the common iliac artery close to the hypogatric artery bifurcation and a guidewire and an introducer sheath are advanced. The introducer sheath is subsequently exchanged for a device sheath which is advanced into the distal aorta (Fig. 15.3). The endoluminal graft is then introduced into the delivery sheath and deployed to the target area. Wires and sheaths are removed and the arteriotomy repaired in a standard fashion (Fig. 15.4). The flank incision is irrigated, a 10 Fr Jackson-Pratt drain is placed in the retroperitoneal space, and the incision is closed in layers.

References

1. Abu-Ghaida AM, Clair DG, Greenberg RK, Srivastava S, O'Hara PJ, Ouriel K. Broadening the applicability of endovascular aneurysm repair: the use of iliac conduits. *J Vasc Surg.* 2002;36:111–117.
2. Diethrich EB, Ramaiah VG, Kpodonu J, Rodriguez JA. *Figures Courtesy of Endovascular and Hybrid Management of the Thoracic Aorta. A Case Based Approach.* 1st ed. West Sussex: Wiley Blackwell; 2008.

Chapter 16
Techniques for Constructing an Endoconduit

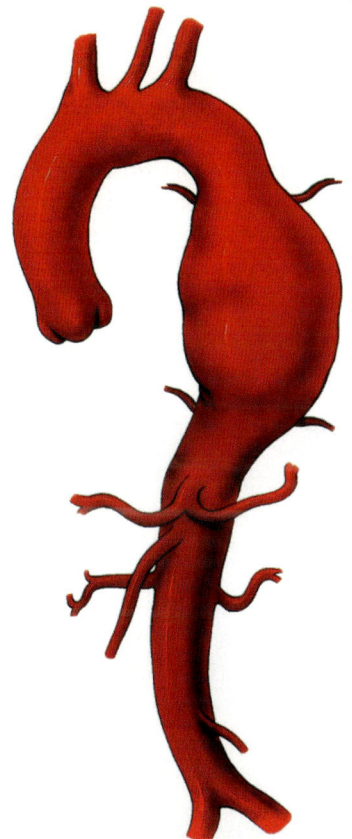

An endoconduit is an alternative percutaneous technique that can be used to deliver a thoracic endograft in a patient with a small, calcified, or tortuous vessel instead of the conventional ilio-femoral conduit. This technique can be applied in high-risk patients that have a relative contraindication to conventional open surgical techniques under general anesthesia. The endoluminal conduit technique allows

J. Kpodonu, *Manual of Thoracic Endoaortic Surgery*,
DOI 10.1007/978-1-84996-296-4_16, © Springer-Verlag London Limited 2010

aggressive balloon dilation of long segments of ilio-femoral stenosis without the risk of vessel rupture. The endoluminal graft conduit can be custom-assembled using grafts diameters of at least 8 mm and preferably 10 mm and can be back-loaded into a delivery sheath and deployed via a femoral arteriotomy into the common iliac artery covering the origin of the internal iliac artery.[1,2]

Retrograde percutaneous access of the common femoral artery is performed with an 18 G needle in the usual fashion and a 0.035 in. glide wire is advanced under fluoroscopic guidance into the distal thoracic aorta after heparin is administered. A 9 Fr sheath is then exchanged for the needle. A retrograde angiographic picture of the iliac vessels is performed noting the size, tortuosity, and calcification. The presence of a small or severely calcific or tortuous iliac vessel may preclude the introduction of a delivery sheath (Fig. 16.1). An attempt may be made to pass the delivery sheath and if any resistance is noted the patient would require a retroperitoneal conduit or an endoconduit. Using the existing 9 Fr sheath, balloon angioplasty can be performed to gently dilate the vessel; subsequently an endoluminal graft most commonly (Viahbahn W.L. Gore & Associates) endoluminal graft or an iCAST stent graft (Table 16.1) is deployed across the common iliac and external iliac artery covering the hypogastric vessels (Fig. 16.2). Post-deployment balloon angioplasty is subsequently performed with a balloon to expand the endoluminal graft; this technique has been referred to as cracking and paving. The 9 Fr sheath is subsequently exchanged to a 20–24 Fr delivery sheath that is required to deliver the thoracic endoluminal graft.

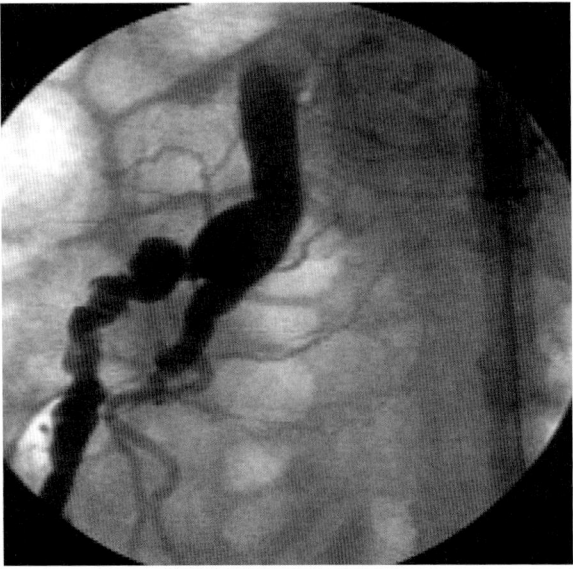

Fig. 16.1 Angiogram demonstrates a small, tortuous left iliac artery

Table 16.1 Commercially available covered stents used for peripheral indications

Fluency Plus	Bard	Tracheobronchial	Self-expanding
Jostent	Abbott	Coronary perforation	Balloon-expanded
Viabahn	Gore	SFA	Self-expanding
iCAST	Atrium	Tracheobronchial	Balloon-expanded

Fig. 16.2 Deployment of endoconduit

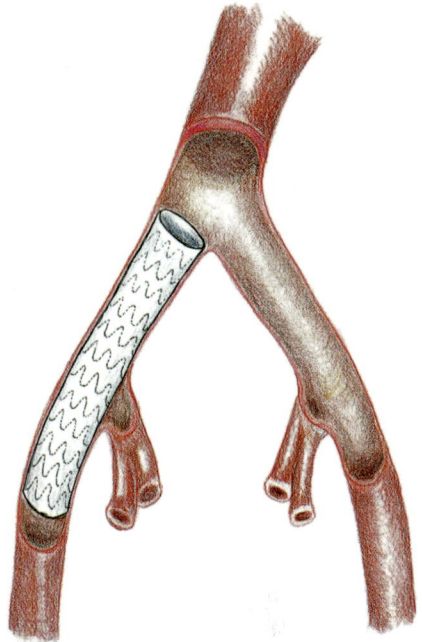

16.1 Case Scenario

An 80-year-old gentleman with previous coronary artery bypass graft surgery, hypertension, ilio-femoral vascular occlusive disease, and chronic obstructive pulmonary disease requiring home oxygen presented with increasing back pain.[2] His physical examination was notable for decreased femoral pulses and a decreased ankle brachial index. A CT scan of the chest and abdomen performed demonstrated a thoracic aortic aneurysm component measuring 7.0 cm and the infra-renal component measuring 3.0 cm (Fig. 16.3). The thoracic arch was very tortuous and the proximal neck diameter was measured at 29 mm with a short distal neck component measured at 31 mm. Due to his numerous co-morbidities he was felt not to be an open surgical candidate. He was offered the possibility of an endoluminal graft under local/sedation with a percutaneous approach.

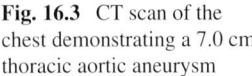

Fig. 16.3 CT scan of the
chest demonstrating a 7.0 cm
thoracic aortic aneurysm

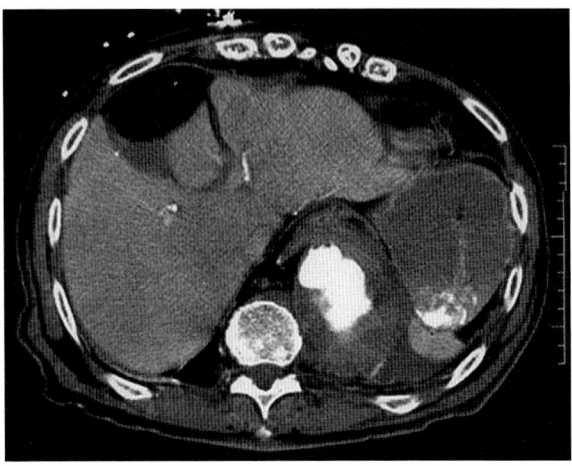

16.2 Endovascular Technique

Under local anesthesia with mild sedation, retrograde percutaneous cannulation of
both common femoral arteries was performed with an 18 G needle and a 0.035 in.
soft tip angled glide wire (Medi-tech/Boston Scientific) passed in the thoracic aorta
and exchanged for a 9 Fr sheath under fluoroscopic visualization. A retrograde iliac
angiogram performed demonstrated diffuse bilateral iliac disease (Fig. 16.4a). There
was a focal segment of disease in the left iliac artery that could be amenable to balloon angioplasty. Bilateral 9 Fr (sheath) was exchanged for a single, monorail, 10
Fr Prostar XL device (Perclose, an Abbott Laboratory Company, Redwood City,
CA). The two Perclose sutures (four suture ends) for each groin were left, untied,
to rest upon the patient in radial orientation until after the endograft deployment
had been completed. Five thousand units of heparin was given to keep activated
clotted time greater than 200 s. Wire access was regained through the monorail
side port on the shaft of the closure device and a 12 Fr groin sheath passed into
the aorta over a stiff wire and through the untied sutures. Balloon angioplasty of
the left common iliac artery was performed with an OPTA Pro 9 mm × 4 cm balloon with angiographic resolution of the focal area of stenosis as demonstrated by
a retrograde left iliac angiogram (Fig. 16.4b). A 5 Fr pigtail angiographic catheter
was advanced through the right groin sheath into the thoracic aorta and an oblique
thoracic arch aortogram was performed to visualize the orifices of the arch vessels and the descending thoracic aortic aneurysm. Intravascular ultrasound (IVUS)
was performed using a Volcano therapeutics 8.2-Fr probe to confirm the measurements on CT scan. A 34 mm × 15 cm TAG (W.L. Gore & Associates, Flagstaff,
AZ, USA) stent graft was selected to treat the aneurysm. An attempt to advance the
22 Fr delivery sheath was met with resistance and since the patient was not a candidate for a retroperitoneal conduit under general anesthesia and endoconduit was
planned. The 22 Fr sheath was exchanged for a 9 Fr sheath and a 13 mm × 10 cm

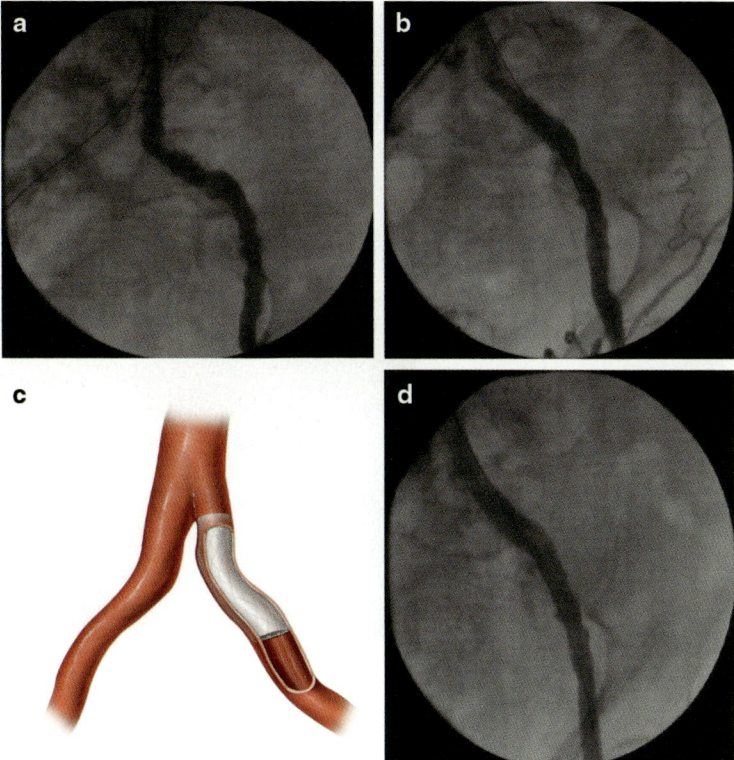

Fig. 16.4 (**a**) Left retrograde iliac angiogram demonstrating a diseased iliac vessel. (**b**) Retrograde left iliac angiogram after post-balloon angioplasty. (**c**) Illustration demonstrating a deployment of an endoluminal graft to the left common iliac and external iliac artery to be used as an endoconduit. (**d**) Retrograde left iliac angiogram after successful deployment of an endoconduit

Gore Viahbahn (W.L. Gore & Associates, Flagstaff, AZ, USA) endoluminal graft was deployed across the left common iliac and external iliac artery covering the hypogastric vessels (paving), with satisfactory angiographic picture (Fig. 16.4c, d). Post-deployment balloon angioplasty was performed with a Synergy 12 mm × 4 cm balloon to the left common iliac endoluminal graft to dilate the endoluminal graft with the possibility of rupturing the severely calcified and tortuous vessel (cracking). The 9 Fr sheath was subsequently exchanged for the delivery sheath that tracked smoothly up to the descending thoracic aorta. A 34 mm × 15 cm TAG stent graft device was advanced through the sheath and subsequently deployed over an extra stiff wire. Post-deployment balloon angioplasty was performed and a completion angiogram demonstrated satisfactory exclusion of aneurysm with no endoleak. Wires and sheaths were removed and the percutaneous closure device used to achieve hemostasis. Patient had bilateral palpable pulses at the end of the procedure and was transferred to recovery room and discharged on POD #2 in satisfactory condition. CT scan of the chest prior to discharge showed exclusion of the 7 cm aneurysm with no endoleak noted (Fig. 16.5).

Fig. 16.5 Post-operative CT scan demonstrating satisfactory exclusion of thoracic aortic aneurysm with no identifiable endoleak

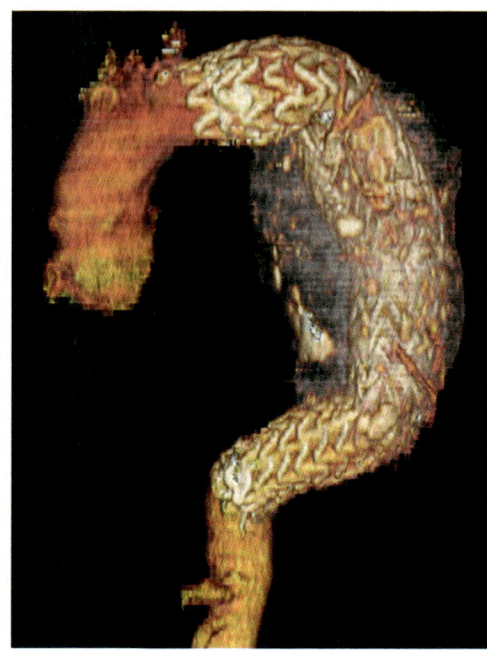

References

1. Diethrich EB, Ramaiah VG, Kpodonu J, Rodriguez JA. *Endovascular and Hybrid Management of the Thoracic Aorta. A Case Based Approach.* 1st ed. West Sussex: Wiley Blackwell; 2008.
2. Kpodonu J, Rodriguez JA, Ramaiah VG, Diethrich EB. Cracking and paving: a novel technique to deliver a thoracic endograft despite ilio-femoral occlusive disease. *J Card Surg.* 2009;24(2):188–190.

Part IV
Bolton Relay Thoracic Endovascular Stent Graft Device

Chapter 17
Bolton Relay Thoracic Stent Graft System

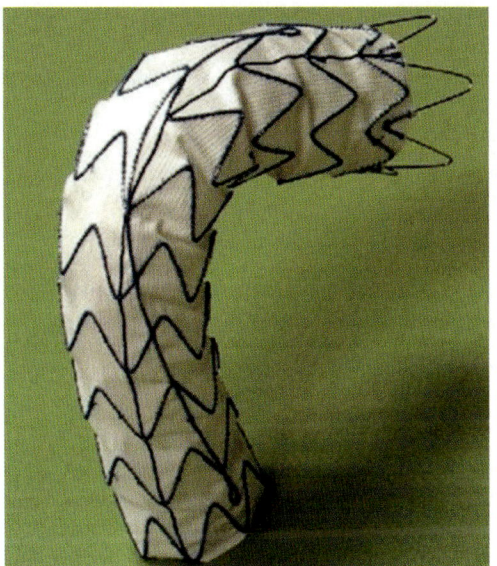

17.1 Device Description

The Relay Thoracic Stent Graft is a new endovascular device for the treatment of thoracic aortic pathologies. Clinical investigation is currently under way to assess its efficacy in the treatment of descending thoracic aneurysms. This device is composed of self-expanding nitinol stents that are sutured to a polyester fabric graft. The skeleton of the device is made up of a series of sinusoidal stents placed along the length of the graft fabric. To provide longitudinal support for this device, a curved nitinol wire is attached to the outer curve of the endograft fabric by a series of sutures. This design provides moderate column strength while maintaining desirable flexibility and torque response. A series of radiopaque markers, composed of platinum and iridium, are attached to the endograft in various locations to enhance fluoroscopic

J. Kpodonu, *Manual of Thoracic Endoaortic Surgery*,
DOI 10.1007/978-1-84996-296-4_17, © Springer-Verlag London Limited 2010

visualization. The Relay device is available in various sizes and configurations, both tapered and non-tapered. Graft lengths from 100 to 250 mm are available, with diameters from 22 to 46 mm (Fig. 17.1). The profile of the primary introducer sheath ranges from 22 to 26 Fr in size depending on graft diameter and length. The delivery system is a four-step controlled deployment for accuracy of positioning (Fig. 17.2).

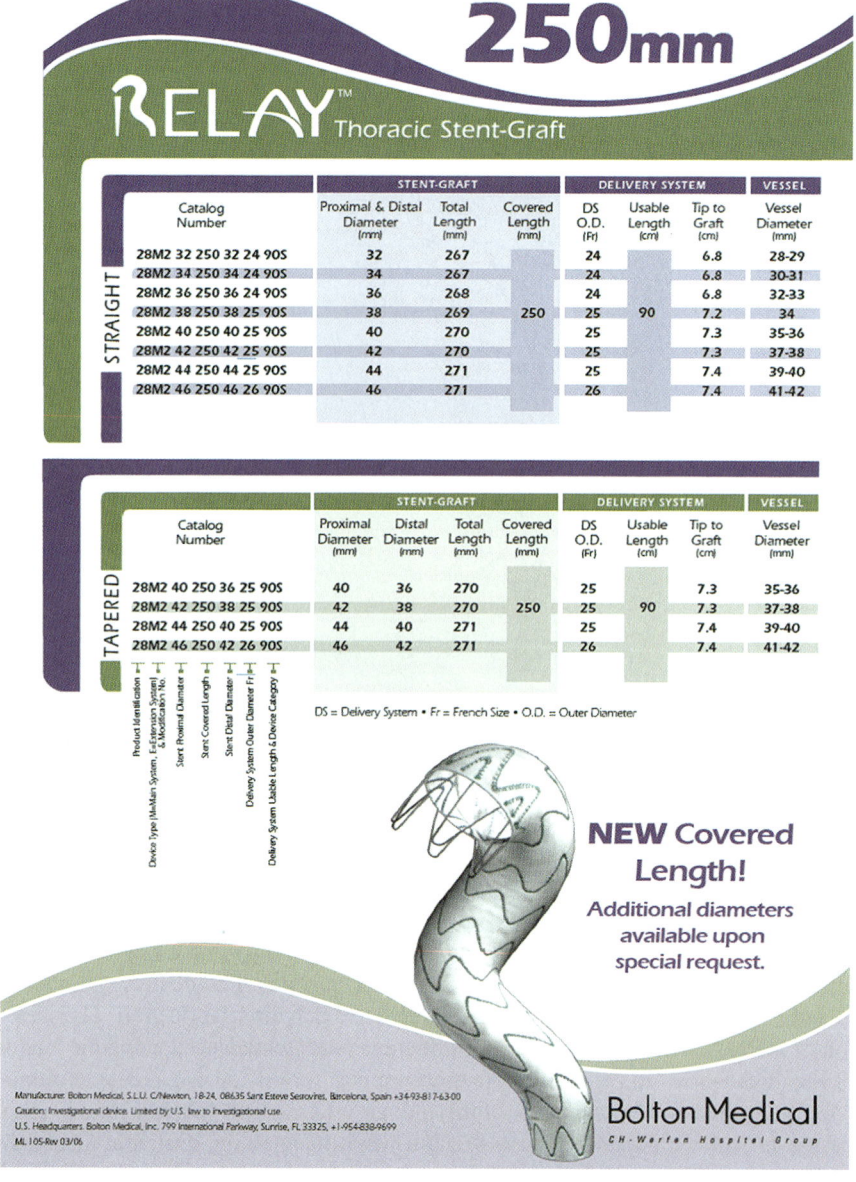

Fig. 17.1 Chart with various diameter sizes and lengths of the Bolton Relay Thoracic Stent Graft system

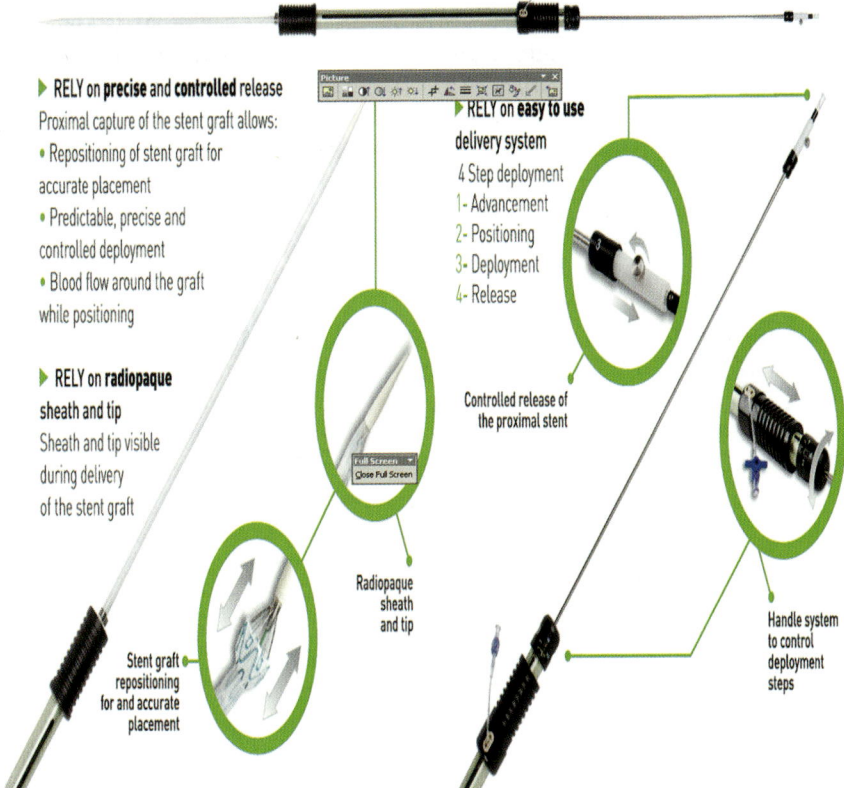

Fig. 17.2 RELAY Bolton Delivery system consists of four-step deployment system as depicted in Fig. 17.4

17.2 Brief Clinical Results

The feasibility or phase I study for the Relay Thoracic Stent Graft in the treatment of descending thoracic aortic aneurysms and penetrating ulcers was approved by the FDA in December 2004. This study was initially limited to 30 patients and 5 clinical sites. Regulatory approval to include two additional sites was granted in April 2005. Available information showed that more than 20 patients have been enrolled in the phase I study as of November 2005. Eighteen (90%) had thoracic aortic aneurysms and two (10%) had penetrating ulcers. Delivery and deployment of the device were deemed satisfactory in all instances except in three cases (15%), all involving a tendency toward distal device migration. This phenomenon occurred when the deployment sequence involved a "stop-and-go" maneuver with initial expansion of the first two to three stent segments before proceeding to full uncovering and expansion along its full length. These observations were similarly reproduced on bench testing, which led to a modification of the IFU involving the deployment technique. Since a modified deployment technique was instituted, no further occurrences relating to device migration were noted during the deployment process. Among all procedures that could be completed, there was a 100% technical success rate, with delivery and deployment of the device as intended and complete angiographic exclusion of the target lesion. There have been no 30-day mortalities. Two endoleaks have been reported on 6-month follow-up scans, although the precise cause remains undetermined. There have been no unanticipated device-related adverse events to date. Completion of the phase I study was achieved in 2006. An ongoing phase II trial is currently under way in the United States to evaluate 120 patients with the RELAY Stent Graft and compare them to 60 surgical controls. Expected completion of study is slated for 2010.

The Relay NBS^{TM} Thoracic Stent Graft has been designed to treat thoracic aortic pathologies (aneurysms, dissections, etc.). The proximal end of the Relay NBS design is an atraumatic design construction. The Relay NBS is similar in construction to the Relay device, with modification to the proximal end while maintaining proximal control during the delivery process. The Relay NBS is composed of self-expanding nitinol stents sutured to polyester vascular graft fabric. The skeleton of the device is a series of sinusoidal stents with different radial force according to the position along the length of the graft. The proximal end is covered by fabric and composed of a crown and proximal stent combination. The function of the crown stent is to support the edge of the fabric to optimize apposition of the proximal end of the graft and minimize the fabric enfolding. The crown stent presents a series of apexes that are connected by "flat sections." A curved nitinol wire provides longitudinal support for the stent graft. The curved wire is attached from the proximal to distal aspects of the graft with surgical suture. This design creates moderate column strength for the stent graft while at the same time provides flexibility and torque response. Additionally, radiopaque markers are also sewn in strategic places on the stent graft to aid in the visualization and accurate placement of the device. The distal end is a circumference of the terminating stent covered with fabric that is straight from the apexes of the stent. The Transport^{TM} delivery system is a two-stage delivery device consisting of a series of coaxially arranged sheaths and catheters (primary introduction sheath, secondary delivery sheath, through lumen), handle, and apex release mechanism. The stent graft is constrained within the secondary sheath, which is further constrained within the primary sheath. The radiopaque, polymeric primary sheath is tracked over a guidewire to facilitate introduction of the device through the femoral and iliac arteries. Once the system reaches the placement location, the proximal handle of the delivery system is advanced to advance the secondary sheath from the primary sheath in preparation for deployment. The secondary sheath, composed of thin wall, flexible fabric, enables the thoracic endograft to be more easily advanced and deployed in curved and tortuous portions of the anatomy than a polymeric sheath would allow. The secondary sheath, which is connected to the delivery catheter and the delivery handle, can be retracted to deploy the constrained stent graft in a controlled fashion. The apex release mechanism constrains the proximal end stent of the endograft. Sliding the outer control tube over the guidewire lumen after deployment from the secondary sheath controls this mechanism. This provides a controlled apposition of the proximal end of the stent to the vessel wall. The device diameter ranges from 22 to 46 mm and the device length 100 to 250 mm (Fig. 17.3).

Clinical experience: The Relay NBS Registry Relay NBS has commercial approval for CE market which was received in the summer of 2007 in Europe Dimensions and reference guides for RELAY NBS stent graft system are referenced in (Fig. 17.4).

Bolton Medical is introducing this device in select centers and is capturing this initial experience in a Registry. Relay NBS is not yet available in the United States as at the time of publishing this manual.

The Relay NBS Registry is a European Registry designed to capture multiple center results for the treatment of non-chronic pathologies. This data will include institutional procedure variation, acute technical results, clinician input on device performance, and acute and moderate clinical input. The study will include the support of five to seven Institutions throughout Europe. The goal would be to capture five procedures at each institution. Thus the study will capture a total of 25–35 patients. Regular follow-up will be conducted at 1, 6, and 12, 24-month intervals. Early experience was registered in 13 European centers involving 24 cases[1]: Policlinico (Bari): 1; Ospedale San Martino (Genoa): 3; Ospedale San Raffaele (Milano): 1; Ospedale Le Scotte (Siena): 2; Ospedale Pediátrico Apuano (Massa): 1; Hospital Clínico (Barcelona): 6; Umc (Utrecht): 3; Erasmus (Rotterdam): 1;

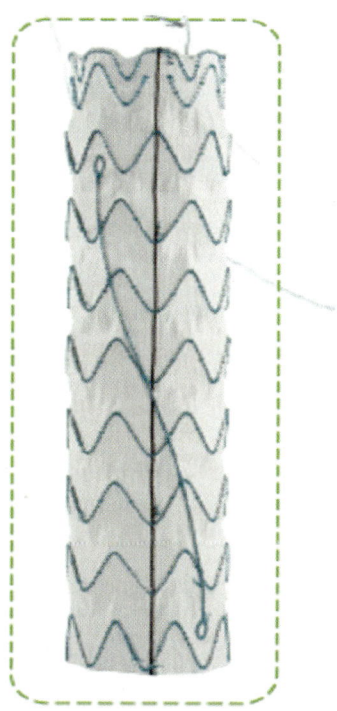

Fig. 17.3 The RELAY NBS endograft

a

STRAIGHT GRAFT	STENT GRAFT			DELIVERY SYSTEM			VESSEL
Catalog Number	Proximal/Distal Diameter (mm)	Length-Category (mm)	Covered Length (mm)	DS O.D. (Fr)	Usable Length (cm)	Tip to Graft (cm)	Vessel Diameter (mm)
28-N1 26 104 26 22 90S	26	100	104	22	90	4,9	22-23
28-N1 26 164 26 22 90S	26	150	164	22	90	4,9	22-23
28-N1 26 204 26 22 90S	26	200	204	22	90	4,9	22-23
28-N1 26 259 26 22 90S	26	250	259	22	90	4,9	22-23
28-N1 28 104 28 22 90S	28	100	104	22	90	4,9	24-25
28-N1 28 164 28 22 90S	28	150	164	22	90	4,9	24-25
28-N1 28 204 28 22 90S	28	200	204	22	90	4,9	24-25
28-N1 28 259 28 23 90S	28	250	259	23	90	5,1	24-25
28-N1 30 104 30 22 90S	30	100	104	22	90	4,9	26-27
28-N1 30 164 30 22 90S	30	150	164	22	90	4,9	26-27
28-N1 30 209 30 23 90S	30	200	209	23	90	5,1	26-27
28-N1 30 259 30 23 90S	30	250	259	23	90	5,1	26-27
28-N1 32 104 32 23 90S	32	100	104	23	90	5,1	28-29
28-N1 32 164 32 23 90S	32	150	164	23	90	5,1	28-29
28-N1 32 209 32 23 90S	32	200	209	23	90	5,1	28-29
28-N1 32 259 32 24 90S	32	250	259	24	90	5,3	28-29
28-N1 34 109 34 23 90S	34	100	109	23	90	5,1	30-31
28-N1 34 154 34 23 90S	34	150	154	23	90	5,1	30-31
28-N1 34 209 34 24 90S	34	200	209	24	90	5,3	30-31
28-N1 34 259 34 24 90S	34	250	259	24	90	5,3	30-31
28-N1 36 109 36 24 90S	36	100	109	24	90	5,3	32-33
28-N1 36 154 36 24 90S	36	150	154	24	90	5,3	32-33
28-N1 36 199 36 24 90S	36	200	199	24	90	5,3	32-33
28-N1 36 259 36 25 90S	36	250	259	25	90	5,5	32-33
28-N1 38 109 38 24 90S	38	100	109	24	90	5,3	34
28-N1 38 154 38 24 90S	38	150	154	24	90	5,3	34
28-N1 38 199 38 25 90S	38	200	199	25	90	5,5	34
28-N1 38 259 38 25 90S	38	250	259	25	90	5,5	34
28-N1 40 114 40 25 90S	40	100	114	25	90	5,5	35-36
28-N1 40 154 40 25 90S	40	150	154	25	90	5,5	35-36
28-N1 40 204 40 25 90S	40	200	204	25	90	5,5	35-36
28-N1 40 259 40 25 90S	40	250	259	25	90	5,5	35-36
28-N1 42 114 42 25 90S	42	100	114	25	90	5,5	37-38
28-N1 42 159 42 25 90S	42	150	159	25	90	5,5	37-38
28-N1 42 204 42 25 90S	42	200	204	25	90	5,5	37-38
28-N1 42 259 42 25 90S	42	250	259	25	90	5,5	37-38
28-N1 44 114 44 25 90S	44	100	114	25	90	5,5	39-40
28-N1 44 164 44 25 90S	44	150	164	25	90	5,5	39-40
28-N1 44 209 44 25 90S	44	200	209	25	90	5,5	39-40
28-N1 44 259 44 25 90S	44	250	259	25	90	5,5	39-40
28-N1 46 114 46 26 90S	46	100	114	26	90	5,5	41-42
28-N1 46 164 46 26 90S	46	150	164	26	90	5,5	41-42
28-N1 46 209 46 26 90S	46	200	209	26	90	5,5	41-42
28-N1 46 259 46 26 90S	46	250	259	26	90	5,5	41-42

Row groups by diameter: 26 mm, 28 mm, 30 mm, 32 mm, 34 mm, 36 mm, 38 mm, 40 mm, 42 mm, 44 mm, 46 mm Diameter

b

TAPERED/CONICAL GRAFT	STENT GRAFT			DELIVERY SYSTEM			VESSEL
Catalog Number	Proximal/Distal Diameter (mm)	Length Category (mm)	Covered Length (mm)	DS O.D. (Fr)	Usable Length (cm)	Tip to Graft (cm)	Vessel Diameter (mm)
28-N1 34 154 30 23 90S	34/30	150	154	23	90	5,1	30-31
28-N1 34 209 30 24 90S	34/30	200	209	24	90	5,3	30-31
28-N1 36 154 32 24 90S	36/32	150	154	24	90	5,3	32-33
28-N1 36 199 32 24 90S	36/32	200	199	24	90	5,3	32-33
28-N1 38 154 34 24 90S	38/34	150	154	24	90	5,3	34
28-N1 38 199 34 25 90S	38/34	200	199	25	90	5,5	34
28-N1 40 154 36 25 90S	40/36	150	154	25	90	5,5	35-36
28-N1 40 204 36 25 90S	40/36	200	204	25	90	5,5	35-36
28-N1 42 159 38 25 90S	42/38	150	159	25	90	5,5	37-38
28-N1 42 204 38 25 90S	42/38	200	204	25	90	5,5	37-38
28-N1 44 164 40 25 90S	44/40	150	164	25	90	5,5	39-40
28-N1 44 209 40 25 90S	44/40	200	209	25	90	5,5	39-40
28-N1 46 164 42 26 90S	46/42	150	164	26	90	5,5	41-42
28-N1 46 209 42 26 90S	46/42	200	209	26	90	5,5	41-42

Fig. 17.4 (**a**, **b**) Dimensions and reference guide for RELAY NBS stent graft system

Haukeland Universitets sykehus (Bergen) 2; Rikshospitalet (Oslo): 1; Linkopnig Univeristy Hospital (Linkopnig): 1; Inespital (Berna): 1 and CHU Jean Minjoz (Besancon): 1. Eleven thoracic aneurysms, nine acute and subacute type B dissections, and four leaks of previous TEVAR were attempted. Proximal landing segment involves zone 0 in two cases, zone 1 in 4, zone 2 in 4, zone 3 in 12, and zone 4 in 2. Successful repair was obtained in 23 cases (95.8%). Accuracy on deployment was classified by the implanters as excellent or good in all cases. No proximal extra stent grafts were necessary. In hospital morality was 4.2% (one case) non stent graft related. No clinical events were registered at 6 month follow-up. Long-term data are currently pending.

Reference

1. Riambau V, RESTORE collaborators. European experience with Relay: a new stent graft and delivery system for thoracic and arch lesions. *J Cardiovasc Surg (Torino).* 2008 Aug;49(4): 407–415.

Part V
Cook Zenith Thoracic Stent Graft Device

Chapter 18
Zenith TX2 Thoracic Endograft

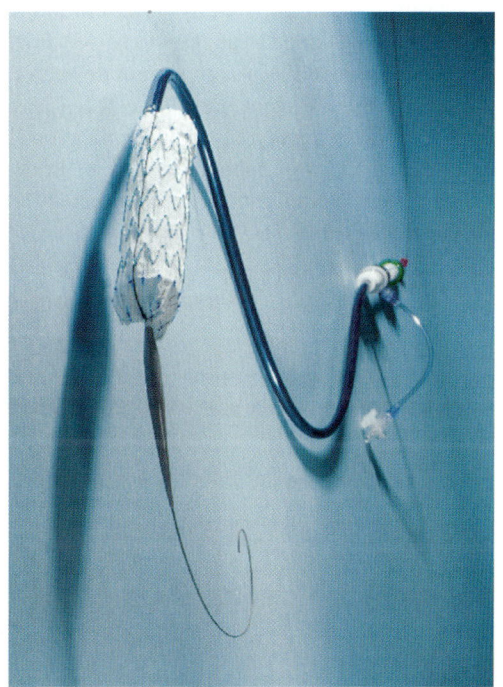

Case study courtesy Blackwell and Wiley to incorporate Case study including Figures 15–19 from Diethrich EB, Ramaiah VG, Kpodonu J, Rodriguez-Lopez JA. Endovascular and hybrid management of the thoracic aorta. A case based approach. Wiley Blackwell 2008.

J. Kpodonu, *Manual of Thoracic Endoaortic Surgery*, 169
DOI 10.1007/978-1-84996-296-4_18, © Springer-Verlag London Limited 2010

18.1 Zenith TX2 Stent Graft System

The Cook TX2 stent graft is designed as a two-piece system that incorporates hooks and barbs, distal fixation, and a proximal controlled deployment. Thoracic stent graft treatment of thoracic aortic pathologies, including thoracic aortic aneurysms, has been associated with migration of both proximal and distal fixation points,[1] erosion of uncovered proximal portion through the aortic arch,[2] and component separation with modular devices.[2,3] These problems have been described with most of the thoracic endoprosthesis implanted for thoracic aortic pathologies.[3–5] The ideal thoracic stent graft currently does not exist but would need to be flexible enough to accommodate the tortuosity of the arch, incorporate a fixation system that is secure both proximally and distally, seal within both straight and tortuous segments, be readily deliverable, and have favorable effects on the excluded region of the aorta. Additionally, delivery of the device would optimally not require the induction of hypotension or bradycardia even in the setting of extreme tortuousity. The Cook TX1 and TX2 device has been designed to attempt to solve some of these issues but currently at this time is not approved as a commercial device in the United States. The Zenith TX2 TAA Endovascular stent graft is designed as a two-piece modular endograft system for thoracic aneurysm repair application. Both the proximal and distal endograft components are a tubular stent graft in design. However, an additional uncovered bare stent configuration is incorporated in the lower segment of the distal endograft device (Fig. 18.1).

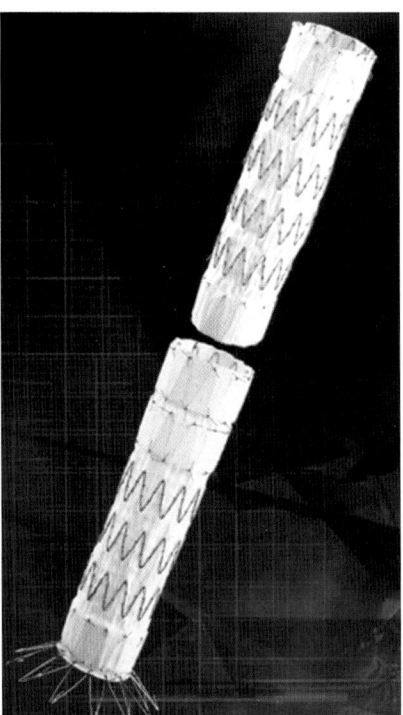

Fig. 18.1 Zenith TX2 two-piece thoracic endoluminal graft

The Zenith TX2 endograft is introduced through a preloaded catheter with triggers. The two stent grafts used for descending aortic repairs consist of a proximal stent with proximal engraved bare metal "V" wires with terminal barbs. After the first internal Z-stent, the remaining stents are external except for the last one of the proximal component. The second component has a proximal internal Z-stent, and the remaining intervening Z-stents are all external except the terminal one, which is internal and has external barbs attached to it.

The stents are attached to the fabric with large gaps (6, 8, or 10 mm, depending on device diameter) to provide flexibility of the device; diameter ranges from 22 to 42 mm. Unique to the Zenith system is that after introducing the proximal component to the site of choice, it is released out of the delivery catheter; however, the bare metal barbs are not released until positioning is certain, at which point a trigger allows for release of the barbed component. Before triggering the barbs, positioning can be adjusted, but this should be avoided. The second component is then seated in the first. If components are correctly chosen, balloon fixation is usually not required. Because the proximal barbs and stent are released by a trigger, hypotension and bradycardia are not needed for seating the stent graft.

Several design variations exist, and the justification for each component is as follows:

1. *Proximal fixation system:* Barbs were added to mimic a surgical anastomosis and discourage migration. Uncovered proximal stents are not used because of concern about unequal proximal stent apposition with subsequent erosion of the aortic wall or potential for creating retrograde proximal dissection.
2. *Distal fixation systems:* Two distal fixation systems exist. For large fusiform aneurysms, a desire to incorporate barbs intended to prevent proximal migration of the distal stent prompted the addition of an uncovered distal stent with cranially oriented barbs. Such a design is not intended for use with dissections or in the setting of marked distal tortuosity. Therefore, the option to have a distal component without an uncovered stent or barbs exists and is used in those circumstances.

18.1.1 Device Description

The Zenith TX2 TAA Endovascular stent graft is designed as a two-piece modular system, although implantation of a single device may be sufficient for focal thoracic aortic lesions (see Fig. 18.8). The Zenith TX2 endograft is constructed of Dacron fabric covered by stainless steel Z-stents. In this device, the proximal end is covered and has stainless steel barbs protruding through the graft fabric (Fig. 18.10), which anchor the graft directly to the aortic wall. This also protects against distal stent graft migration during high-velocity systolic blood flow. The device uses an active fixation mechanism with external barbs oriented in opposing directions and designed to engage the aortic wall to decrease the risk of proximal and distal migration. Full deployment of the proximal stent is released by pulling a trigger wire once the optimal graft position is confirmed. The stents are modified Gianturco

Z-stents, with small gaps left between each stent to allow some flexibility. Each end of the graft is held within a cap; inadvertent release during positioning within the aorta is prevented by a safety catch. The full length of the graft material is stent supported to prevent graft torsion or compression. The placement of the stents relative to the fabric is varied along the length of the device. At the ends of the endograft, the stents are sewn inside the fabric, whereas in its midportion, they are outside the fabric. The intent of this design was to optimize fabric apposition to the aortic lumen and fabric–fabric interstent junctions. The Zenith TX2 proximal component (Fig. 18.2) is available in diameters ranging from 28 to 42 mm and lengths from 12.0 to 21.6 cm. The Z-Trak delivery systems for the Zenith TX2 device have profiles between 20 and 22 Fr. Device deployment is achieved by withdrawing an external sheath.

The Zenith TX2 distal component (Fig. 18.3) differs slightly in design configuration compared with the proximal component. The distal end of the device

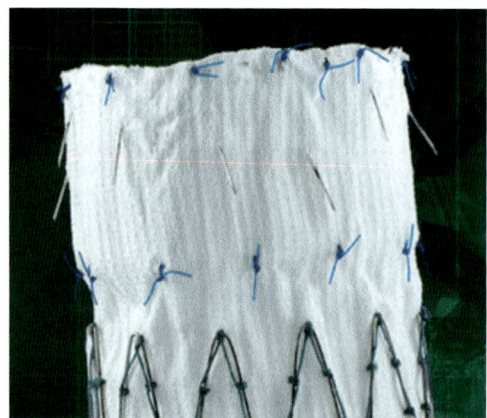

Fig. 18.2 Close-up view of the proximal end of the TX2 proximal component. Note the hooks protruding from the fabric

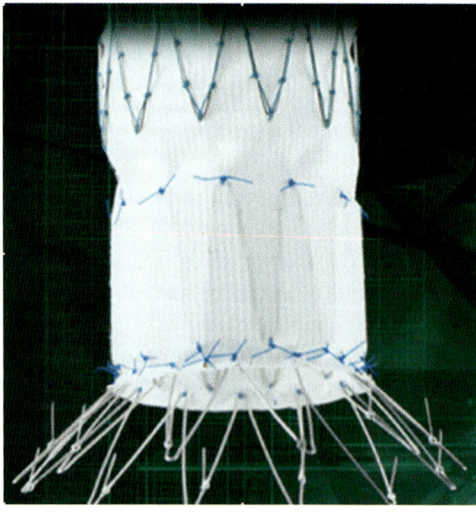

Fig. 18.3 Close-up view of the distal end of the TX2 distal component. Note the bare stent with the retrograde-oriented hooks

has an uncovered bare metal stent similar to the proximal end of the Zenith Abdominal Aortic Endovascular Graft for AAA. The barbs are on this bare stent and are oriented in a retrograde manner opposite to the direction of the proximal hooks (Fig. 18.11). This bare stent configuration allows fixation of the device over

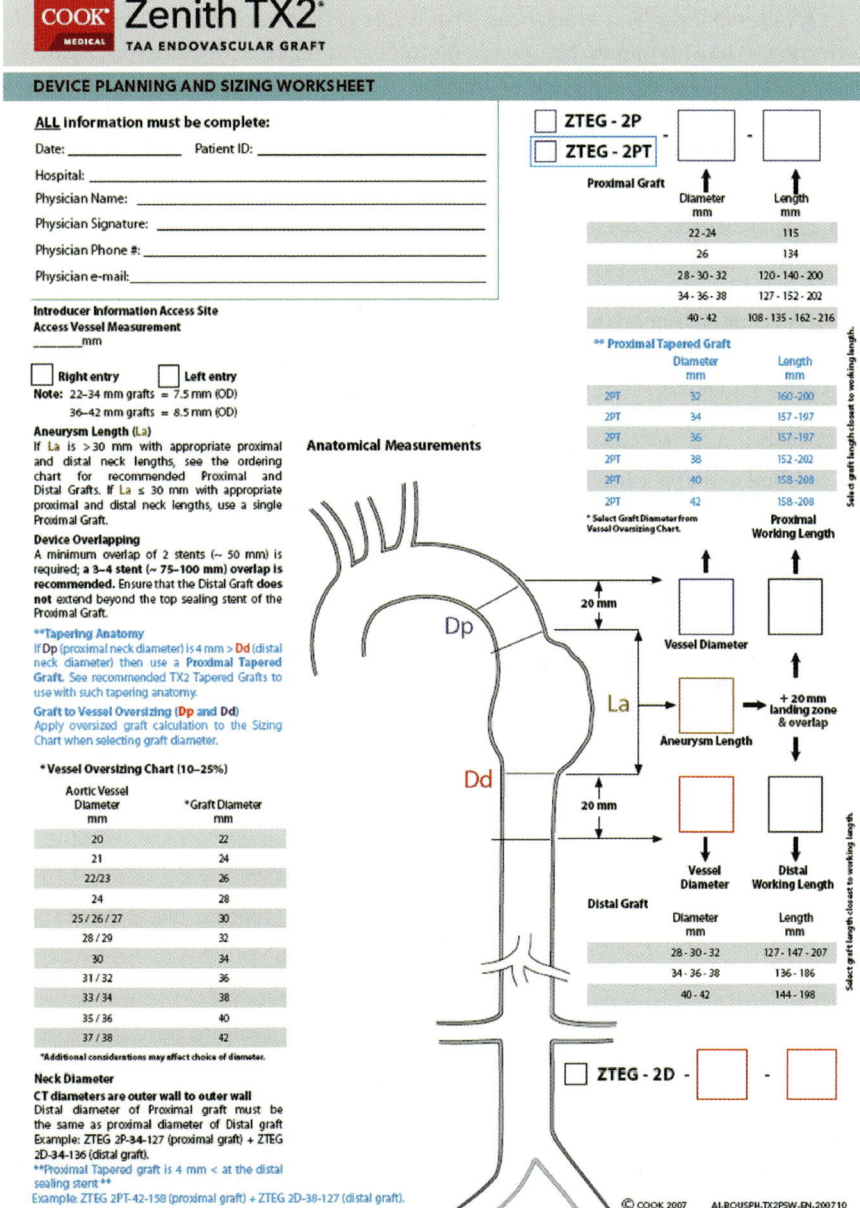

Fig. 18.4 Device planning and worksheet

the origins of the visceral vessels, where it may be relatively less diseased, and the covered portion to extend right to the origin of the celiac artery. Similar to the proximal component, the TX2 proximal component device diameters range from 28 to 42 mm and lengths from 120 to 207 mm. The deployment method similarly involves first unsheathing the stent graft and, after precisely positioning the distal end, releasing trigger wires to deploy the distal bare metal stents.

Device planning and worksheet (Fig. 18.4) permits accurate planning for the selection of an appropriate endoluminal graft based on a pre-operative CT scan.

18.2 Deployment of TX2 Cook Endoluminal Graft

18.2.1 General Cautions

- Exercise extreme caution when manipulating interventional and angiographic devices in the region of the barbs.
- Do not advance the wire guide or delivery system if resistance is felt. Exercise particular care in areas of stenosis, thrombus, calcification, or tortuosity.
- With the exception of the left subclavian, do not cover arch or mesenteric arteries with the graft. If covering the subclavian, be aware of possible compromise to cerebral and upper limb perfusion.
- Use caution during manipulation of catheters, wires, and sheaths within the aneurysm, as thrombus dislodgement and embolization may occur.
- Do not attempt to re-sheath the graft after partial or complete deployment.
- Avoid damaging the graft or disturbing graft positioning if reinstrumentation is necessary.
- Anatomy and graft position can change with sheath removal, constantly monitor graft position, using angiography as necessary.

18.2.2 Deployment Overview

18.2.2.1 Position Stiff Lunderquist Wire in Aortic Arch

Through the radiopaque banded pigtail flush catheter, replace the standard wire guide with a stiff 0.035 in. 260 cm Lunderquist wire guide. Advance the wire guide up to the level of the aortic arch and remove the pigtail flush catheter (Fig. 18.5).

18.2.2.2 Position Proximal Component

Introduce the delivery system for the proximal component over the stiff Lunderquist wire guide and advance until the desired graft position is reached (Fig. 18.6).

Caution: To avoid twisting the graft, never rotate the delivery system. Do not advance the sheath while the graft is still within; doing so may cause the barbs to perforate the sheath.

Fig. 18.5 Lunderquist wire is
advanced into the aortic arch

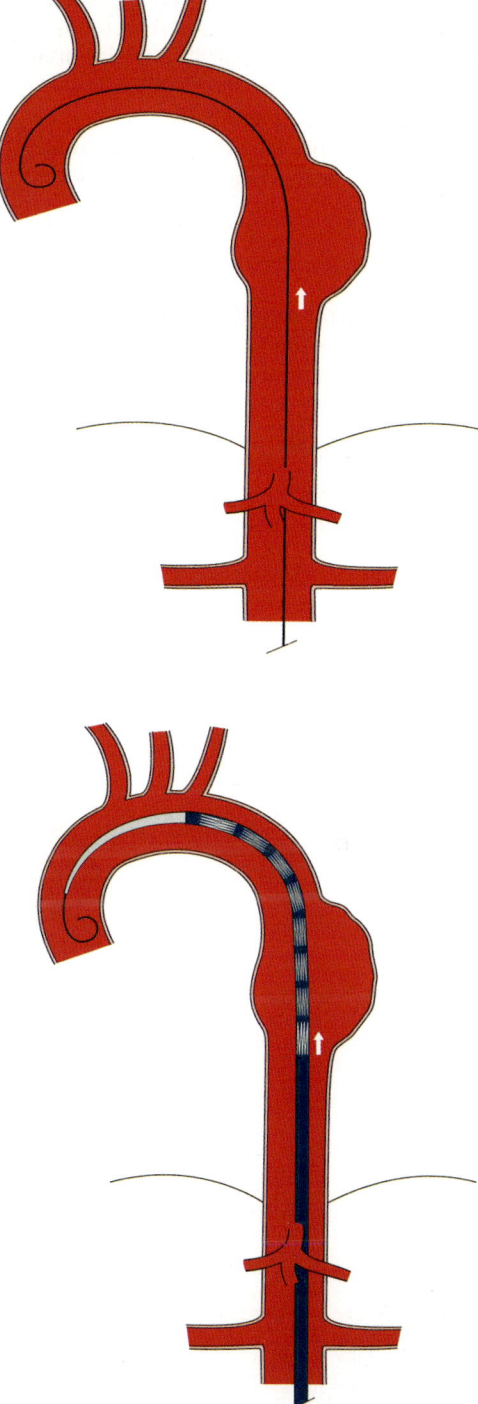

Fig. 18.6 Delivery system
advanced into the aortic arch

18.2.2.3 Unsheath Proximal Component

While constantly monitoring graft position, withdraw the sheath until the graft is fully expanded. Continue sheath withdrawal until the valve assembly docks with the control handle (Fig. 18.7).

Caution: Barbs are now exposed; limited forward advancement is possible, but retracting the device may damage the aorta.

18.2.2.4 Release Proximal Component Trigger Wires

Unscrew and remove the safety lock from the green trigger-wire release mechanism. Withdraw the trigger wire slowly until the proximal end of the graft opens (Fig. 18.8). Withdraw the trigger wire completely to release the distal attachment to the introducer. Make sure that all trigger wires are removed prior to withdrawal of the delivery system.

18.2.2.5 Remove Introducer Sheath for Proximal Component

Remove the delivery system entirely, leaving the wire guide positioned in the graft (Fig. 18.9).

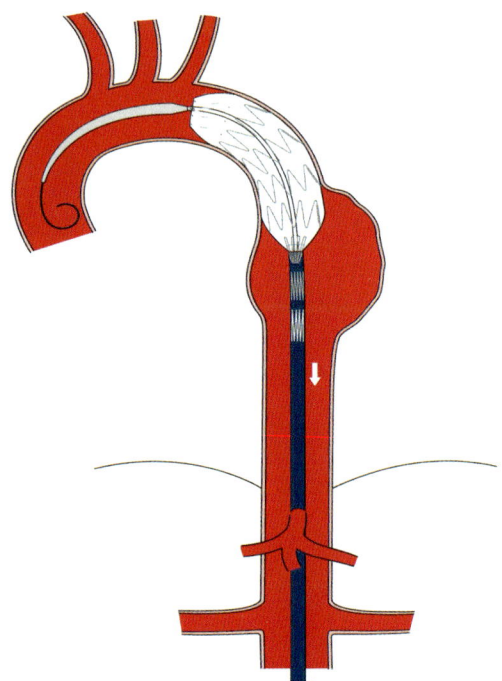

Fig. 18.7 Outer sheath is withdrawn to fully expand TX2 endoluminal graft

Fig. 18.8 Removal of trigger wire by unscrewing green cap to release proximal and distal end of TX2 endoluminal graft

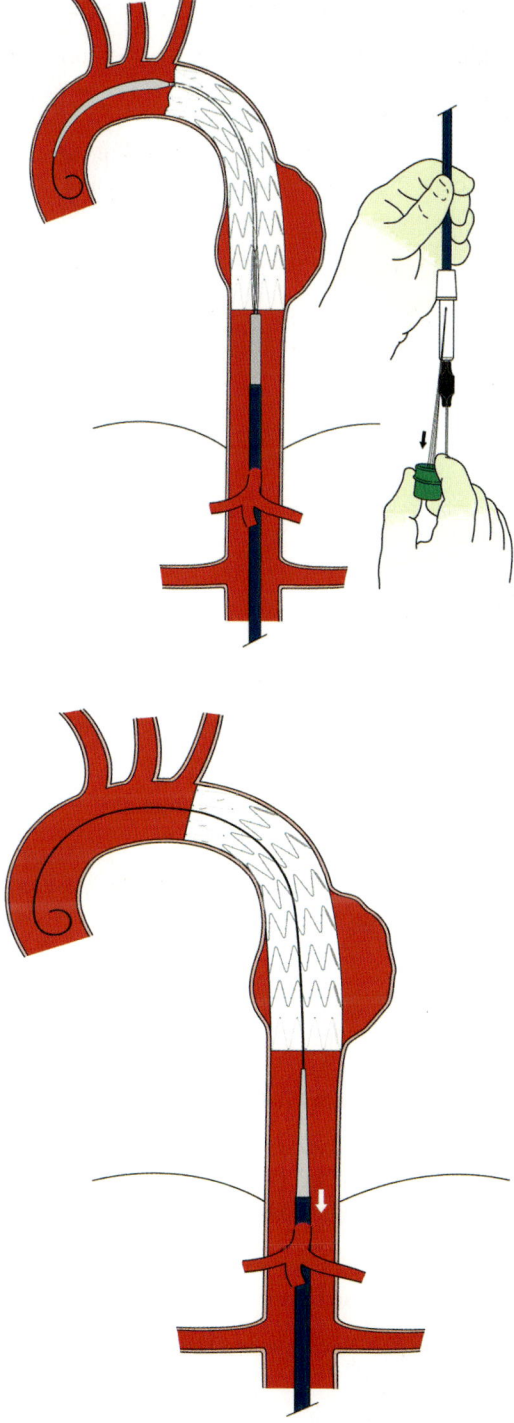

Fig. 18.9 Removal of introducer sheath of proximal component of endoluminal graft

Fig. 18.10 Delivery system
of distal component advanced
and positioned in the
deployed proximal
component with 3–4 stent
overlap

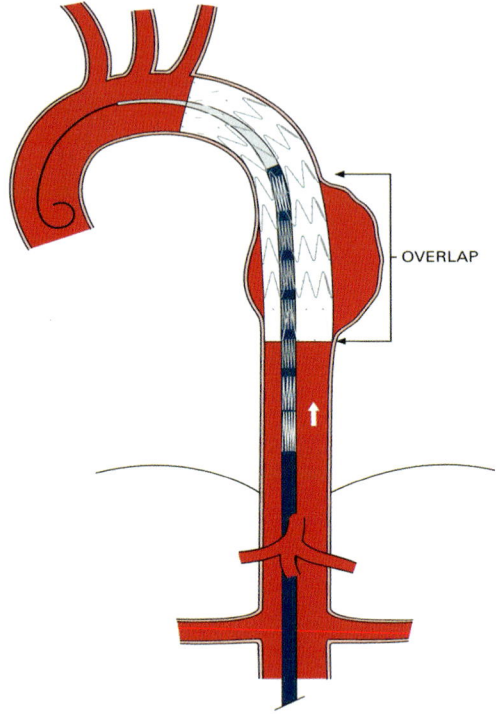

18.2.2.6 Position Distal Component

Introduce the delivery system for the distal component over the stiff Lunderquist
wire guide and advance until the desired position inside of the proximal component
is reached (Fig. 18.10). Advance the delivery system of the distal component until
the collapsed stent graft inside is in its intended location, with a recommended 3–4
stent overlap (75–100 mm) with the proximal component.

Note: The stainless steel stent bodies are easily visualized under fluoroscopy.

18.2.2.7 Unsheath Distal Component

While constantly monitoring graft position, withdraw the sheath until the graft is
fully expanded (Fig. 18.11). Continue sheath withdrawal until the valve assembly
docks with the control handle.

18.2.2.8 Release Distal Component Trigger Wires

Using the 1-2-3 deployment sequence

Fig. 18.11 Outer sheath withdrawn to fully expose distal component of TX2 endoluminal graft

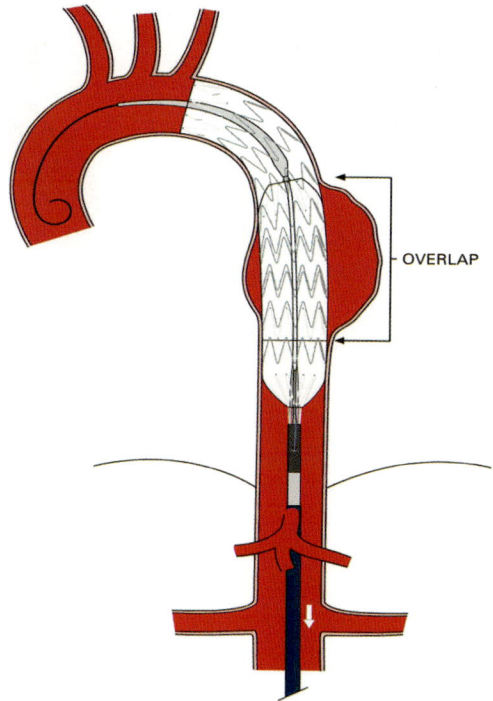

OVERLAP

- Unscrew and remove the trigger-wire safety lock; then withdraw and remove the white trigger-wire release mechanism labeled #1.
- Unscrew and remove the safety lock on the telescoping handle labeled #2. Stabilize the delivery system and slide the telescoping handle together with the gray tube and outer sheath in a distal direction until it locks into position with a click.
- Unscrew and remove the safety lock from the green trigger-wire release mechanism labeled #3. Withdraw the release wires slowly until the proximal end of the graft opens, continuing withdrawal until the graft is fully opened and released (Fig. 18.12).

18.2.2.9 Optional: Molding Balloon

Position molding balloon and utilizing diluted contrast media (as directed by manufacturer), expand it in areas of the proximal covered stent, proximal component/distal component overlap, and distal fixation site, starting proximally and working in a distal direction (Fig. 18.13). Confirm complete deflation of balloon prior to repositioning.

Warning: Do not inflate the balloon in aorta outside confines of the graft.

Fig. 18.12 Unscrew and removal of safety locks labeled 1, 2, and 3 to fully open and deploy distal component of TX2 endoluminal graft

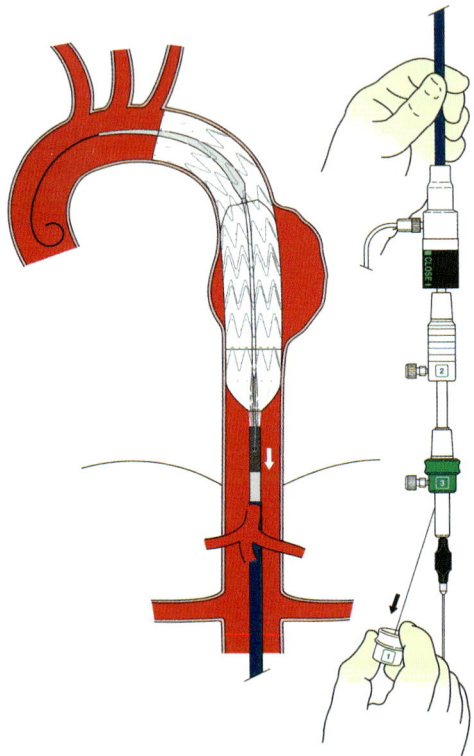

18.2.2.10 Perform Final Flush Aortogram

Position angiographic pigtail flush catheter just above the level of the deployed endovascular graft and perform angiography to verify: correct graft position, patency of arch vessels and celiac plexus, that there are no endoleaks or kinks at position of proximal and distal gold radiopaque markers (Fig. 18.14). Withdraw introducer sheath for distal component, catheters, and wires. Repair vessels and close in standard surgical fashion.

Warning: To avoid impaling any in situ catheters, rotate the delivery system during withdrawal. Overlap balloon expansion/graft sealing sites.

18.3 Case Study

An 80-year-old man with a 40 pack year smoking history with a past medical history of open abdominal aortic aneurysm repair, coronary artery disease with recent coronary artery bypass graft surgery, chronic obstructive lung disease with steroid and oxygen dependency, hypertension and left ventricular dysfunction was found to have a thoracic aortic aneurysm of the mid and descending thoracic aorta after evaluation on a routine CXR.[6] A CT scan of the chest

Fig. 18.13 Balloon
angioplasty of proximal and
distal fixation sites and areas
of component overlap for
adequate fixation of TX2
endoluminal graft to aortic
wall

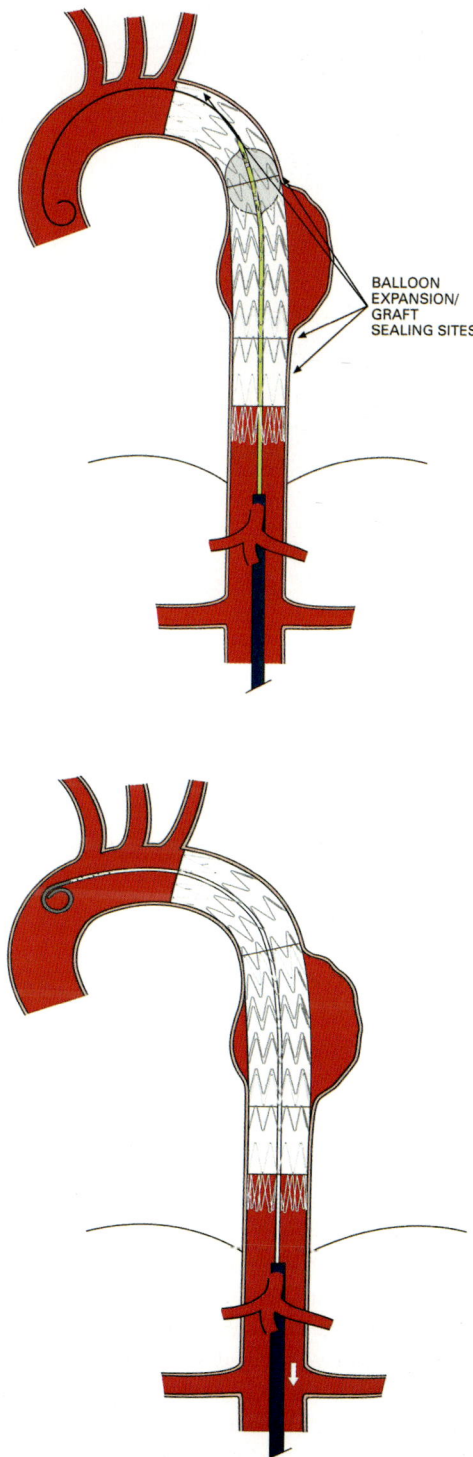

BALLOON
EXPANSION/
GRAFT
SEALING SITES

Fig. 18.14 Completion
angiogram is performed after
introduction of a flush
catheter in the aortic arch to
confirm exclusion of thoracic
aneurysm and absence of
endoleak

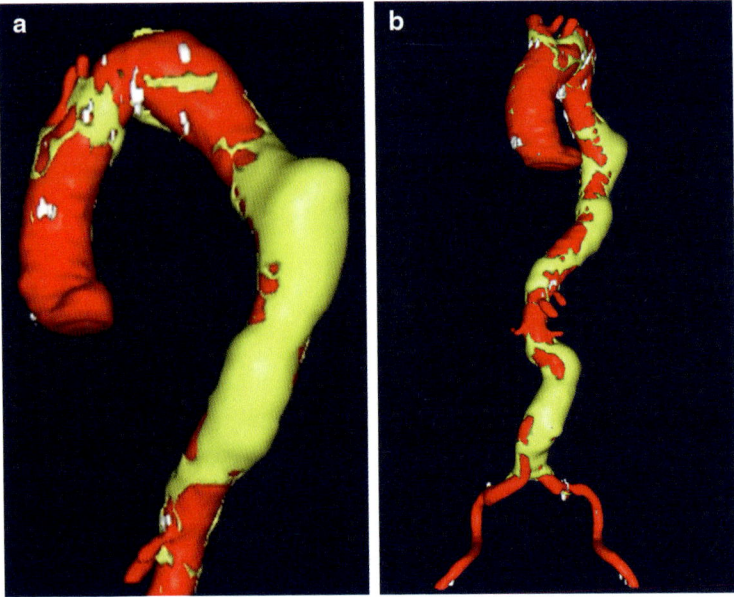

Fig. 18.15 (**a**, **b**) Reconstructed CT scan of the chest demonstrating a thoracic aortic aneurysm measuring 6.0 cm in diameter with adequate-sized iliac vessels with minimal tortuosity and calcium

performed demonstrated a 6.0 cm thoracic aortic aneurysm with mural thrombus (Fig. 18.15a, b). Due to the extensive co-morbidities he was felt to be a high-risk candidate for open surgical repair and enrolled in the multicenter TX2 trial.

18.4 Endovascular Procedure

The right common femoral artery was exposed through a small oblique incision and cannulated with a 9 Fr sheath. Percutaneous access of the left common femoral artery was performed and a 5 Fr sheath was introduced. Oblique thoracic aortogram was performed through the left groin sheath via a 5 Fr pigtail angiographic catheter to delineate the arch and the descending thoracic aorta aneurysm (Fig. 18.16a). Intravascular ultrasound was performed using a (Volcano Therapeutics, Inc.) 8.2 Fr probe through the right groin sheath to confirm the size of aneurysm, presence or absence of thrombus, proximal neck diameter and length, and distal neck diameter and length. The proximal neck and distal neck diameters were measured at 30 mm. Based on the measurements, a 36 mm Cook Zenith TX2 thoracic endoluminal graft was chosen for exclusion of the thoracic aortic aneurysm. An extra stiff Lunderquist wire (Cook Bloomington, IN, USA) was exchanged through the IVUS catheter. The right 9 Fr sheath was exchanged for a Cook Zenith TX2 device

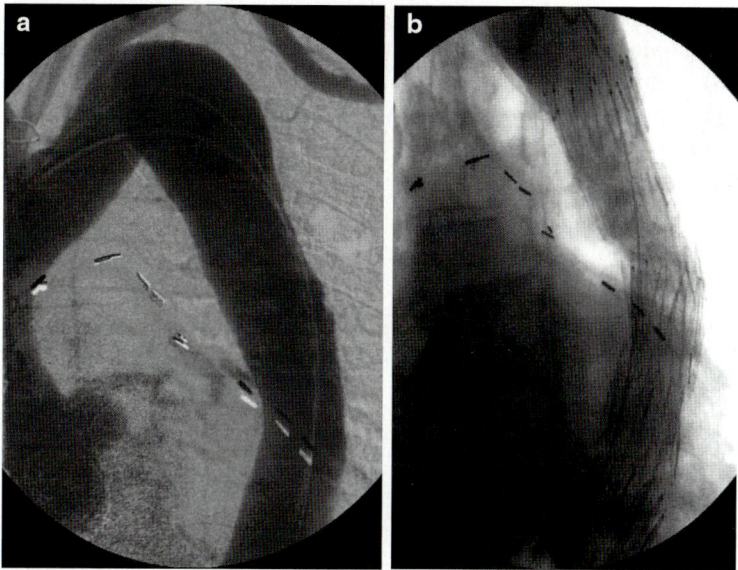

Fig. 18.16 (**a**, **b**) A pre- and post-thoracic aortogram demonstrating an angulated and tortuous arch and exclusion of the aneurysm

(Bloomington, IN) measuring 36 mm × 152 mm and deployed 2 cm distal to the left subclavian artery with at least a 3 cm proximal neck. A second Cook Zenith device 36 mm × 136 mm was deployed distally with adequate overlap between grafts to a level just above the celiac trunk. A completion angiogram demonstrated satisfactory exclusion of the thoracic aortic aneurysm with no endoleak (Fig. 18.16b). All

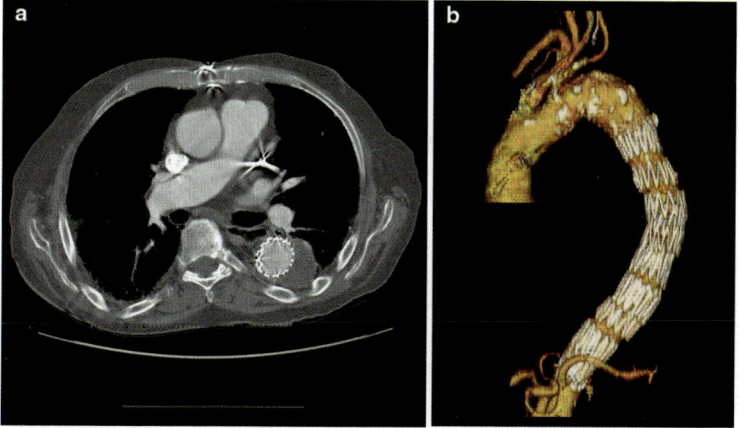

Fig. 18.17 (**a**, **b**) Post-operative CT scan of the chest demonstrating satisfactory exclusion of aneurysm

wires and sheaths were removed. The right common femoral artery was closed in a transverse fashion with restoration of flow. A vascular closure device was deployed to the left common femoral artery with satisfactory bilateral palpable pulses of the feet at the end of the procedure. The patient was subsequently extubated and transferred to recovery room. A post-operative CT scan demonstrated adequate exclusion of thoracic aortic aneurysm with no endoleak (Fig. 18.17a, b).

References

1. Greenberg R, Resch T, Nyman U, et al. Endovascular repair of descending thoracic aortic aneurysms (an early experience with intermediate-term follow-up). *J Vasc Surg.* 2000;31(1):147–156.
2. Malina M, Brunkwall J, Ivancev K, et al. Late aortic arch perforation by graft-anchoring stent (complication of endovascular thoracic aneurysm exclusion). *J Endovasc Surg.* 1998;5(3):274–277.
3. Criado FJ, Clarke NS, Barnaton M. Stent-graft repair in the aortic arch and descending thoracic aorta (a 4-year experience). *J Vasc Surg.* 2002;36:1121–1128.
4. White RA, Donayre CE, Walot L, Kopchok G, Woody J. Endovascular exclusion of descending thoracic aortic aneurysms and chronic dissections (initial clinical results with the AneuRx device). *J Vasc Surg.* 2001;33:927–934.
5. Dake MD, Miller DC, Mitchell RS. The first generation of endovascular stent grafts for patients with descending thoracic aortic aneurysms. *J Thorac Cardiovasc Surg.* 1998;116:689–704.
6. Diethrich EB, Ramaiah VG, Kpodonu J, Rodriguez-Lopez JA. *Endovascular and Hybrid Management of the Thoracic Aorta. A Case Based Approach.* West Sussex: Wiley Blackwell; 2008.

Chapter 19
Cook Zenith Dissection Endovascular Stent

The recently introduced Zenith Dissection Endovascular Stent component is designed to be used in conjunction with the Zenith TX2 covered stent in the setting of aortic dissection. This bare stent component is constructed of stacked Z-stents joined by polypropylene sutures, which can be deployed through a 16 Fr sheath and inserted through the existing Zenith TX2 proximal component sheath. A single stent diameter accommodates aortic luminal diameters ranging from 24 to 38 mm and is available in 82, 123, and 164 mm lengths (Fig. 19.1). The Z-stents exert minimal radial force, which allows gradual opposition of the dissection septum and re-expansion of the true lumen. The large open strut architecture allows maintenance of branch vessel perfusion so that the stent can be safely deployed across the origins of the intercostal, visceral, and renal arteries. In the scenario of persistent malperfusion owing to a dissection flap into or a re-entry tear near a vessel origin, the bare Z-stent component provides structural scaffolding for placement of a bare or covered peripheral stent from the true lumen into the branch vessel bridging across the false lumen (Fig. 19.2). A device planning sheet (Fig. 19.3) is helpful in choosing the appropriate diameter and length of graft required to treat each individual patient based on a pre-operative CT scan.

19.1 Cook Zenith Dissection Endovascular System Deployment Overview

19.1.1 General Precautions

1. Exercise extreme caution when manipulating interventional and angiographic devices in the region of the (stent graft) barbs.
2. Do not advance the wire guide or delivery system if resistance is felt. Exercise particular care in areas of stenosis, thrombus, calcification, or tortuosity.

Permission granted by Blackwell and Wiley to incorporate Case study including Figures 13–18 in chapter from Endovascular and hybrid management of the thoracic aorta (Wiley-Blackwell 2008). Diethrich EB, Ramaiah VG, Kpodonu J, Rodriguez-Lopez JA.

3. With the exception of the left subclavian, do not cover arch or mesenteric arteries with the stint graft. If covering the subclavian, be aware of possible compromise to cerebral and upper limb perfusion.
4. Use caution when manipulating catheters, wires, and sheaths within an aneurysm or dissection. Significant disturbances may induce further injury or dislodge fragments of thrombus, which can cause distal or cerebral embolization.
5. Avoid twisting or rotating the gray positioner against the introducer sheath assembly. Doing so may cause the loaded stent to become entangled and to deploy in a twisted state, or not to release from the delivery system.

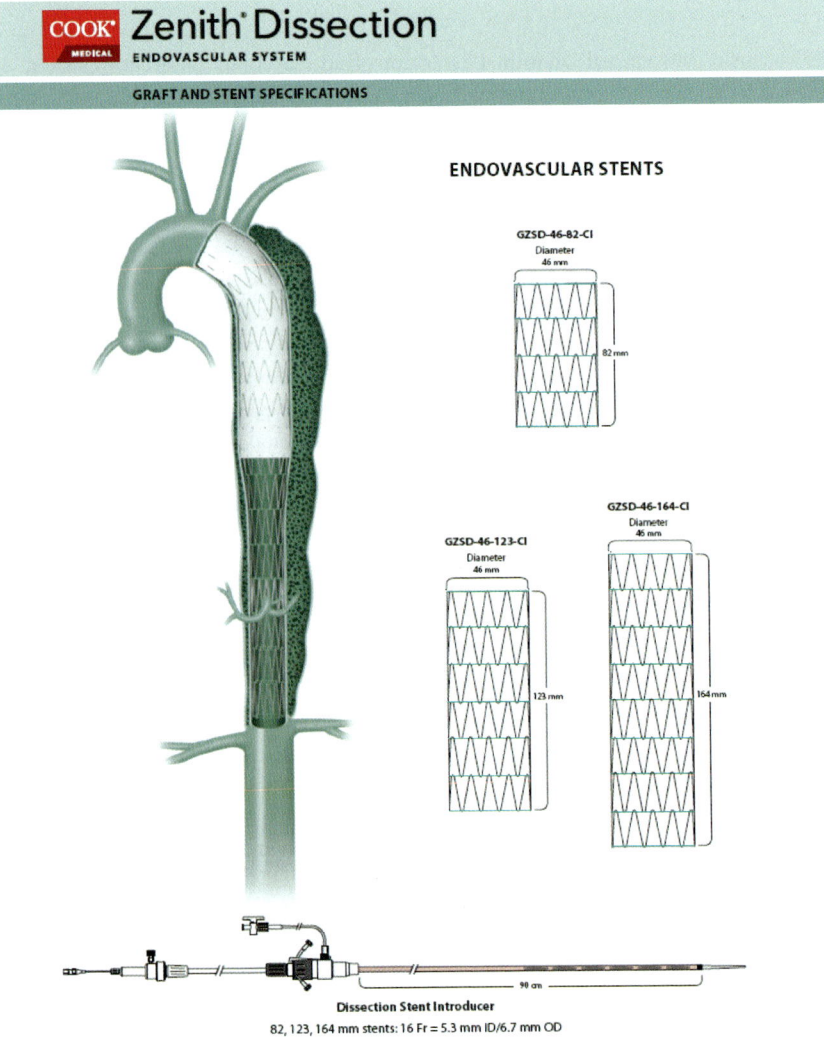

Fig. 19.1 Zenith dissecting endovascular system with graft and stent specifications

PROXIMAL COMPONENTS

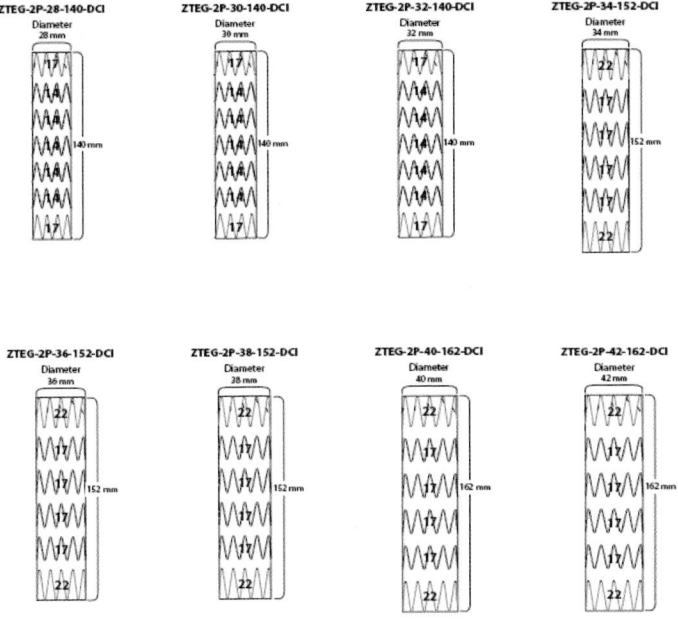

Note: Numbers on stents indicate stent lengths in millimeters (mm).

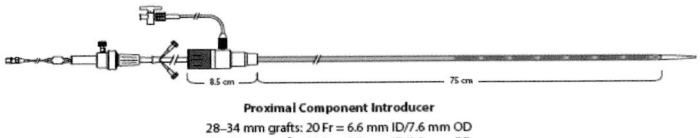

Proximal Component Introducer
28–34 mm grafts: 20 Fr = 6.6 mm ID/7.6 mm OD
36–42 mm grafts: 22 Fr = 7.3 mm ID/8.3 mm OD

Investigational device, limited by federal (U.S.A.) law to investigational use.

Fig. 19.1   (continued)

PROXIMAL TAPERED COMPONENTS

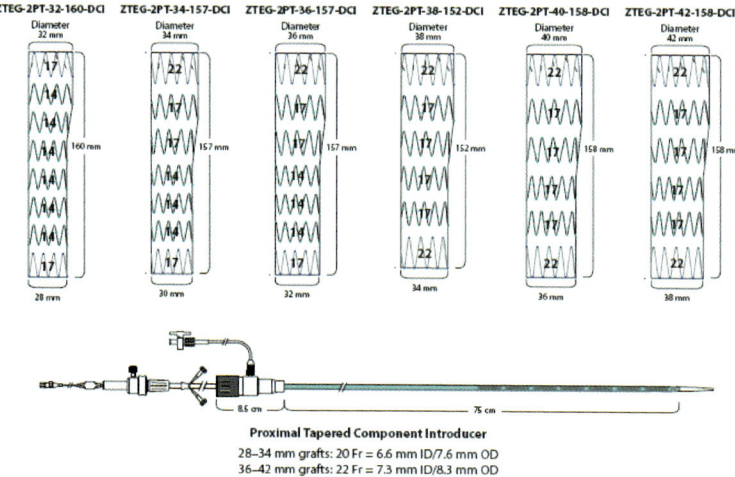

Proximal Tapered Component Introducer
28–34 mm grafts: 20 Fr = 6.6 mm ID/7.6 mm OD
36–42 mm grafts: 22 Fr = 7.3 mm ID/8.3 mm OD

PROXIMAL EXTENSIONS

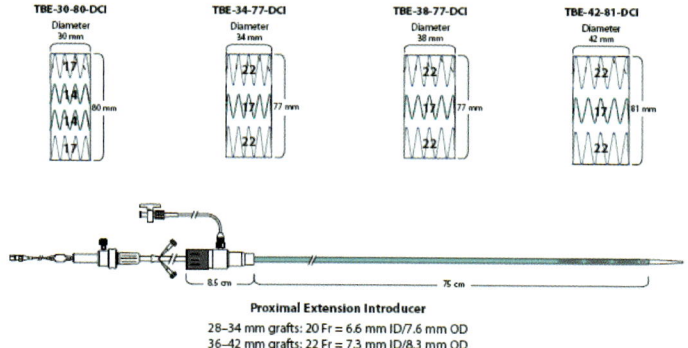

Proximal Extension Introducer
28–34 mm grafts: 20 Fr = 6.6 mm ID/7.6 mm OD
36–42 mm grafts: 22 Fr = 7.3 mm ID/8.3 mm OD

Investigational device, limited by federal (U.S.A.) law to investigational use.

Fig. 19.1 (continued)

DISTAL EXTENSIONS

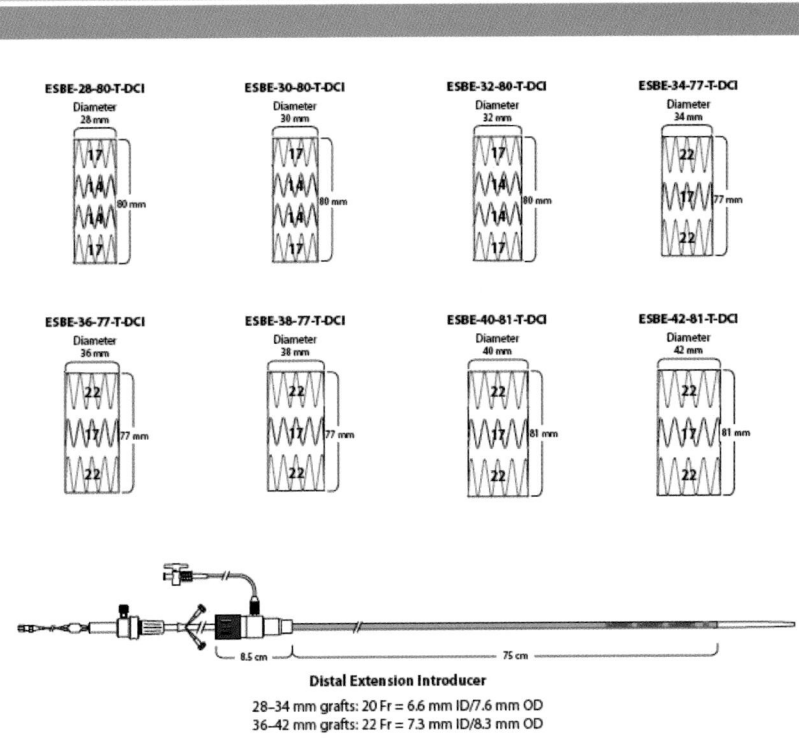

Distal Extension Introducer

28–34 mm grafts: 20 Fr = 6.6 mm ID/7.6 mm OD
36–42 mm grafts: 22 Fr = 7.3 mm ID/8.3 mm OD

Investigational device, limited by federal (U.S.A.) law to investigational use.

Fig. 19.1 (continued)

6. To avoid twisting the stent graft, never rotate the delivery system during the procedure. Allow the stent to conform naturally to the curves and tortuosity of the vessels.

19.1.2 Position Extra Stiff Lunderquist^TM Wire Guide in Aortic Arch

Through the radiopaque-banded pigtail flush catheter, replace the standard wire guide with a stiff 0.035 in. 260 cm LES-DC wire guide (Fig. 19.4). Advance the wire guide up to the level of the aortic arch and remove the pigtail flush catheter.

Fig. 19.2 A model depicting the treatment strategy using the TX2 proximal component with the distal bare stent component. Note how the bare stent can be deployed over the abdominal visceral vessels in the setting of aortic dissection or malperfusion syndrome

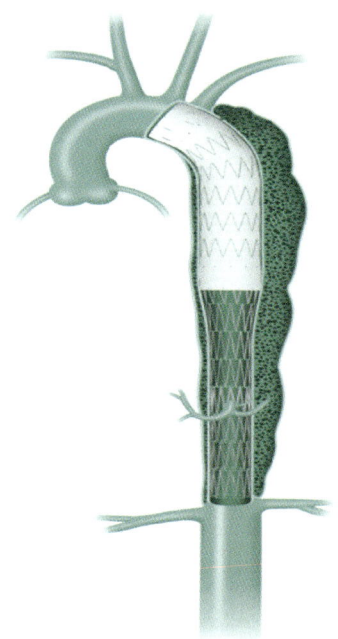

19.1.3 Position Proximal Component to Cover Entry Tear

Introduce the delivery system for the TX2 proximal component over the stiff Lunderquist wire guide and advance until the desired graft position is reached (Fig. 19.5).

Caution: To avoid twisting the stent graft, never rotate the delivery system. Do not advance the sheath while the graft is still within; doing so may cause the barbs to perforate the sheath.

Caution: If a left subclavian artery is to be covered with the device in order to achieve an adequate proximal landing zone, the clinician should be aware of potential compromise to cerebral and upper limb circulation.

19.1.4 Unsheath Proximal Component

While constantly monitoring graft position, withdraw the sheath until the graft is fully expanded. Continue sheath withdrawal until the valve assembly docks with the control handle (Fig. 19.6).

Caution: The barbs are now exposed; limited forward advancement is possible, but retracting the device may damage the aorta.

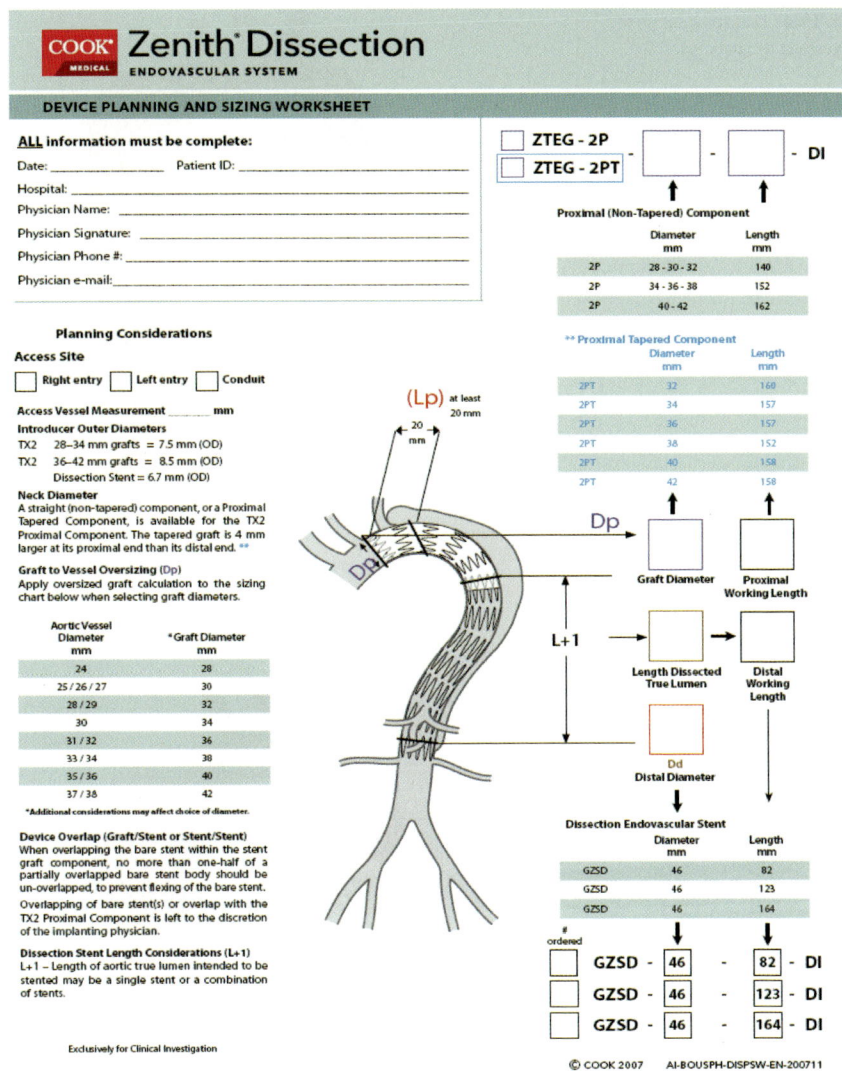

Fig. 19.3 Device planning sheet

19.1.5 *Release Proximal Component Trigger Wires*

Unscrew and remove the safety lock from the green trigger-wire release mechanism. Withdraw the trigger wire slowly until the proximal end of the graft opens. Withdraw the trigger wire completely to release the distal attachment to the introducer. Make sure that all trigger wires are removed prior to withdrawal of the delivery system (Fig. 19.7).

Fig. 19.4 Lunderquist wire
advanced to aortic arch

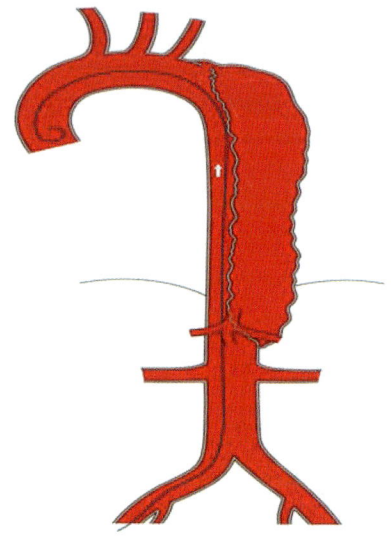

Fig. 19.5 Delivery system
advanced over the stiff
Lunderquist wire

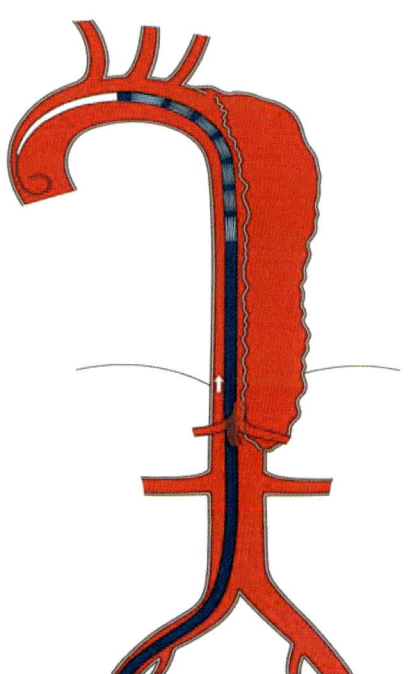

Fig. 19.6 Sheath is withdrawn to fully expand graft

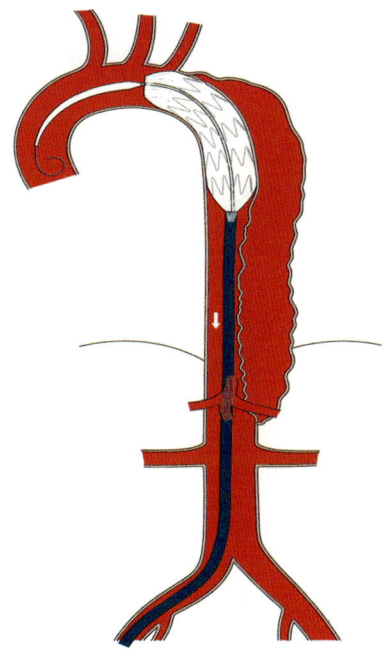

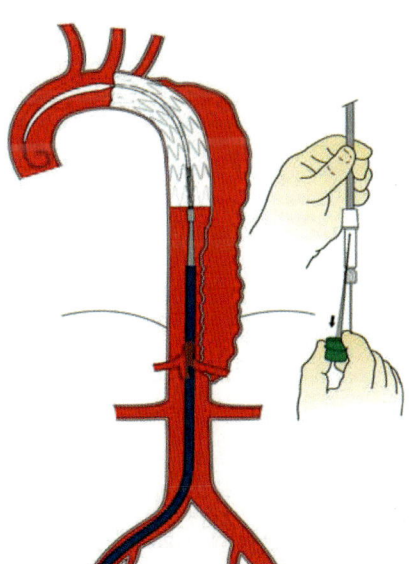

Fig. 19.7 Proximal and distal attachments of grafts are released by withdrawing the proximal and distal trigger wires

19.1.6 Remove Gray Positioner from Proximal Component
Introducer Sheath

Note: The TX2 proximal component sheath is left in place if the intent is to use a dissection stent.

The gray positioner is removed from the introducer sheath and the wire is left in place across the valve (Fig. 19.8). Tighten the Captor® Hemostatic Valve with gentle pressure around the wire guide by turning it clockwise.

19.1.7 Position Dissection Endovascular Stent(s)

Introduce (coaxially) the delivery system for the Dissection Endovascular Stent over the stiff Lunderquist wire guide and advance until the desired position is reached (Fig. 19.9).

Caution: When overlapping the bare stent within the stent component, no more than one-half of a partially overlapped bare stent body should be un-overlapped, so as to prevent flaring of the bare stent.

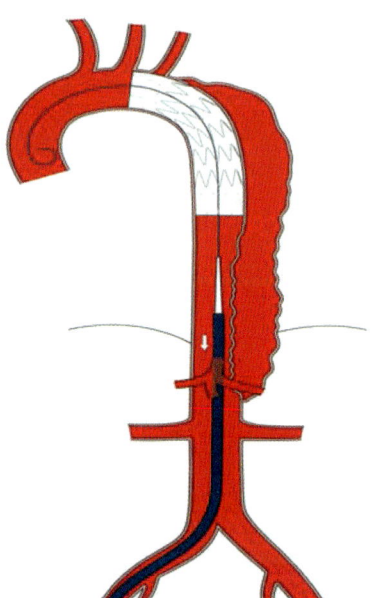

Fig. 19.8 Introducer system
is removed leaving the wire in
position

Fig. 19.9 Introduction of dissection endovascular stent graft system into desired position

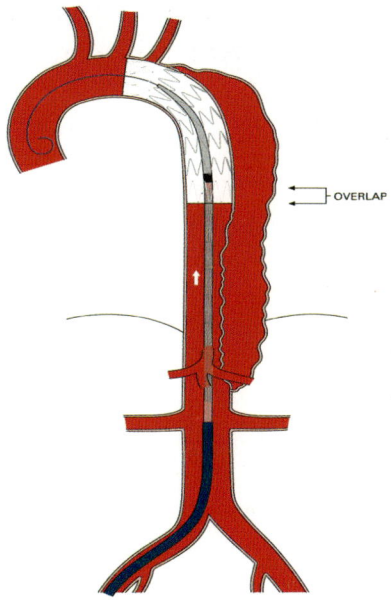

OVERLAP

19.1.8 Unsheath Dissection Endovascular Stent

Just before withdrawing the sheath to deploy the stent, unlock the black cap on the anti-torque device by rotating it counterclockwise. The anti-torque device is now released from the gray dilator and fixed only to the captor hemostatic valve. Stabilize the gray positioner (introduction system shaft) and begin withdrawing the sheath until the stent is fully expanded and the valve assembly docks with the control handle (Fig. 19.10).

19.1.9 Release Dissection Endovascular Stent Trigger Wires

Loosen the safety lock from the green trigger-wire release mechanism. Withdraw the trigger wire slowly until the proximal end of the stent opens. The distal end of the stent is still fixed. Continue to withdraw the trigger wire slowly until the distal end opens. Withdraw the trigger wire completely. Remove the introduction system, leaving the wire guide in the graft (Fig. 19.11).

Note: If deployment of multiple bare Dissection Endovascular Stents is anticipated, their introducer sheath(s) may be inserted coaxially through the in situ (TX2 proximal component) sheath.

Fig. 19.10 Dissecting
endovascular stent graft is
unsheathed from the
introduction system shaft

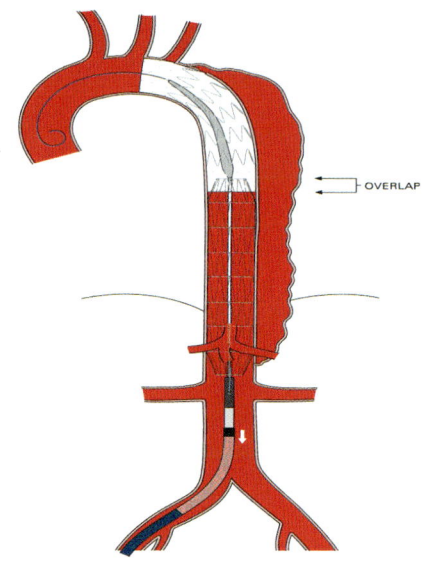

Fig. 19.11 Introduction
system is removed with wire
left in place

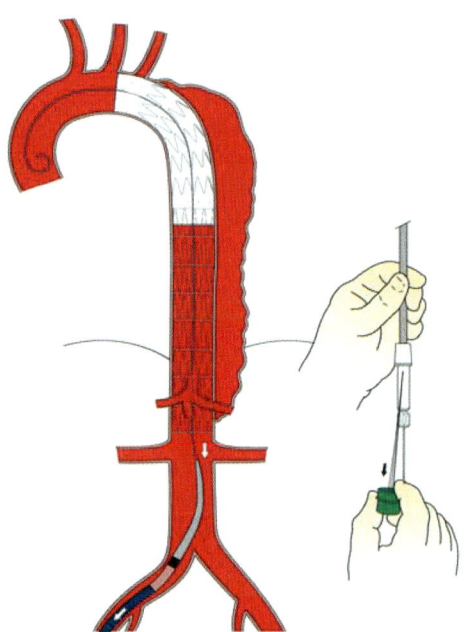

19.2 Final Angiogram

Position angiographic catheter just above the level of the endovascular graft and stent (Fig. 19.12). Perform angiography to verify correct graft and/or stent position, patency of arch vessels, there are no endoleaks or kinks, and patency of vessels inside the stented area. *Caution*: Use of a molding balloon inside a section of aorta treated with the Zenith Dissection Endovascular Stent is not recommended.

Fig. 19.12 Angiographic catheter is advanced to arch for a completion angiogram

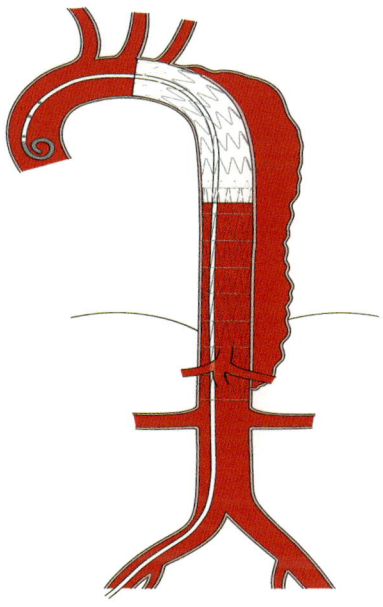

Aortic dissection is a catastrophic cardiovascular disease associated with high morbidity and mortality, affecting approximately 10 per 100,000 of the population per year.[1] Deaths due to aortic dissection exceed those due to ruptured abdominal aortic aneurysm (AAA) and 35% are not diagnosed before death.[2] Covered stent grafts have recently been advocated to treat the primary entry tear in type B dissections and in some centers have become the treatment of choice. Such treatment consists of placing a stent graft across the primary entry tear with the aim of depressurizing the false lumen and inducing proximal false lumen thrombosis. However, due to re-entry tears or intimal fenestrations related to branch vessels, false lumen flow often persists in the lower thoracic and abdominal aorta. This flow acts to prevent complete thrombosis of the false lumen. Repair is therefore incomplete and the dissection persists, leaving the potential for aneurysmal change, rupture, or redissection.[3-6] This case study describes a novel treatment of a dissection using a stent graft with bare stents below it for a more holistic repair of the dissected aorta.[7,8]

19.3 Case Study

A 40-year-old man with a history of poorly controlled hypertension presented to his local hospital with sudden onset chest and back pain.[9] Two years prior, he had been diagnosed with an uncomplicated type B aortic dissection. He was then managed conservatively, with antihypertensive therapy using Candesartan (an angiotensin II receptor antagonist) and atenolol (a beta-blocker), in conjunction with twice-yearly surveillance CT scanning. During the initial 18 months post-diagnosis, the patient's CT scans demonstrated progressive dilatation of the proximal descending thoracic aorta from 4.5 to 5.5 cm in diameter. Six months later, the patient deteriorated clinically, with the recurrence of severe back and chest pain, suggestive of redissection. Multi-slice CT imaging confirmed marked aneurysmal change, with a maximum proximal descending thoracic aortic diameter of 6.5 cm (Fig. 19.13). In addition, dynamic obstruction of the infra-renal aortic true lumen was evident, along with hypoperfusion of the renal arteries and downstream aorta (Fig. 19.14). Emergent surgical reconstruction of the aorta was considered; however, it was felt that this approach carried an unacceptably high risk of mortality, given the patient's unstable condition with organ malperfusion. Endovascular aortic reconstruction was, therefore, selected with the goal of endograft placement over the primary entry tear aimed at preventing rupture and providing expansion of the true lumen and

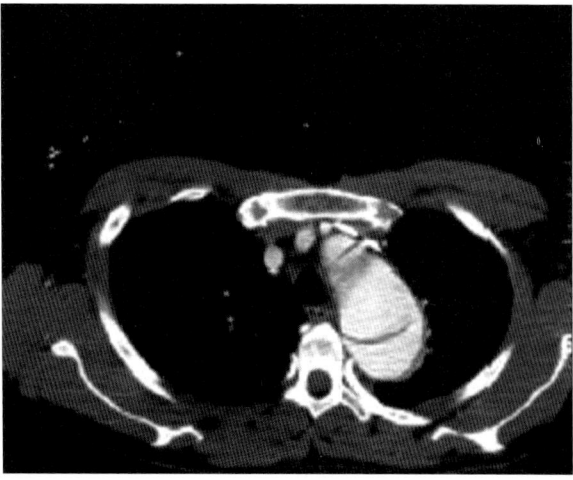

Fig. 19.13 Axial CT scan image demonstrates aneurysmal changes of the proximal descending thoracic aorta with a diameter of 6.5 cm

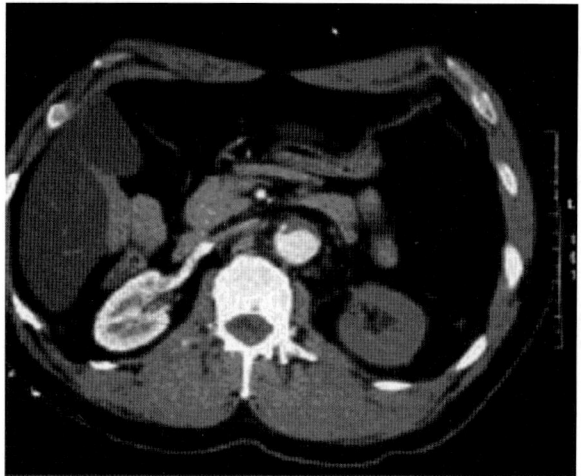

Fig. 19.14 Axial CT scan of the abdominal aorta demonstrates dynamic obstruction of the infra-renal true lumen with hypoperfusion of the renal arteries

reperfusion of the renal and infra-renal aortic segments. Angiographic evaluation revealed a high-flow primary entry tear just distal to the left subclavian artery, with severely compromised abdominal aortic and renal artery perfusion (Fig. 19.15). Near-static renal perfusion was noted immediately following endograft implantation (Fig. 19.16).

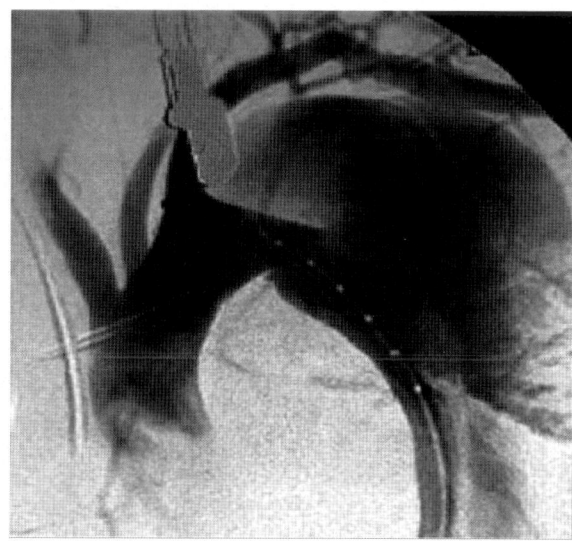

Fig. 19.15 Angiogram demonstrates a high-flow proximal entry tear distal to the left subclavaian artery with compressed true lumen flow

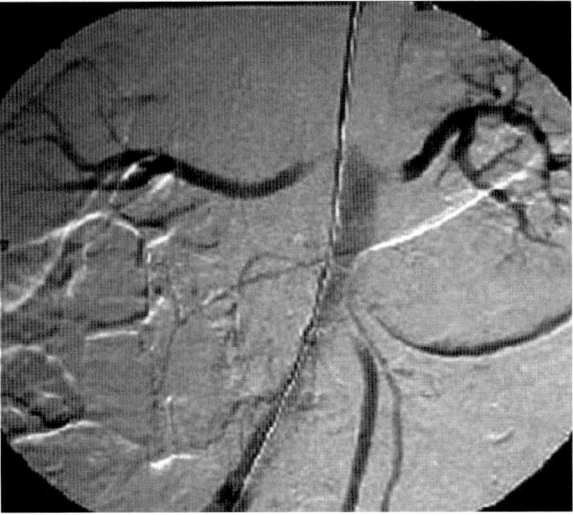

Fig. 19.16 Angiogram demonstrates severely compromised abdominal and renal perfusion with near-static renal flow

19.3.1 Zenith® Dissection™ Case Study

The first stage of the endovascular repair involved implantation of the proximal component of a 34 mm diameter Zenith® TX2™ TAA Endovascular Graft[†] Proximal Component under transesophageal echocardiography and angiographic guidance. This stent graft covered the origin of the subclavian artery and the primary entry tear, thereby eliminating inflow into the proximal thoracic false lumen. As part of the same procedure, stenting of the statically obstructed left renal ostium was performed to enable re-establishment of left renal artery inflow. The patient made a satisfactory recovery after the procedure, in terms of both dramatically reduced pain levels and successful reperfusion of the kidneys and lower limbs. Urine output was re-established and renal function normalized after 4 days. Follow-up CT scan at 1 week showed thrombosis of the upper thoracic false lumen. However, there was persistent false lumen perfusion distally with reduced true lumen caliber. To address this, bare Z-stents (Zenith® Dissection™ Endovascular Stents) were deployed in the aortic true lumen just distal to the stent graft to

---

[†] Investigational device, limited by federal (U.S.A.) law to investigational use.

Fig. 19.17 Glass model of a
Cook Zenith dissection
endovascular stent graft
system

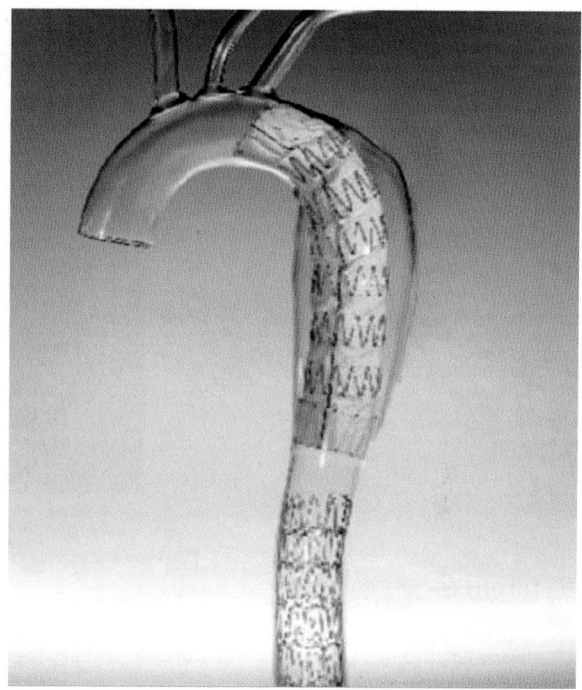

promote true lumen remodeling and distal flow (Fig. 19.17). Follow-up CT examination at one month demonstrated thrombosis of the thoracic aortic false lumen;
however, the abdominal aortic false lumen remained patent because of re-entry
tears in the abdominal aorta and the left common iliac artery. A third procedure,
consisting of stent graft implantation and coil embolization, successfully obliter-
ated these re-entry tears and subsequently induced thrombosis of the abdominal
false lumen. One year later, the patient remained well and asymptomatic. Total
false lumen thrombosis was maintained, and significant remodeling of the aortic
true lumen had occurred (Fig. 19.18). Currently, the patient remains under close
follow-up CT surveillance and is receiving aggressive hypertensive therapy. The
classic endovascular approach to type B dissection has previously demonstrated
advantages over medical treatment.[8] However, it does not address the problem of
continued false lumen patency, which in turn promotes remote-phase complications such as progressive aneurysmal change. To address this problem, the more
holistic staged endovascular repair of both the thoracic aorta and abdominal aorta
can be carried out. This approach permits remodeling to restore normal aortic
morphology and is an exciting future direction for endovascular repair of aortic
dissection.[9]

Fig. 19.18 Sixty-four slice
CT image at 1 year follow-up
with complete thrombosis of
the false lumen and
remodeling of the aortic true
lumen

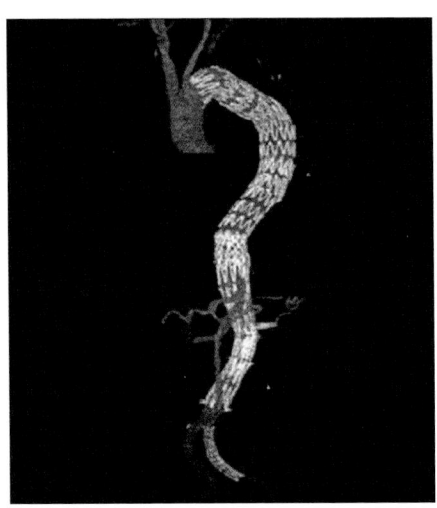

References

1. Svensson L. Aortic dissection and aortic aneurysm surgery: clinical observations, experimental investigations, and statistical analyses. Part II. *Curr Probl Surg.* 1992;29:915–1057.
2. Svensson L. Chapter 3. *Degenerative Aortic Aneurysms, Cardiovascular and Vascular Disease of the Aorta.* Philadelphia, PA: W.B. Saunders Co.; 1997:29–41.
3. Lissin LW, Vangelos R. Acute aortic syndrome: a case presentation and review of the literature. *Vasc Med.* 2002;7:281–287.
4. Umana JP, Miller DC, Mitchell RS. What is the best treatment for patients with acute type B aortic dissection-medical, surgical, or endovascular stent grafting? *Ann Thorac Surg.* 2002;74:S1840–S1843.
5. Onitsuka S, Akashi H, Tayama K, et al.: Long term outcome and prognostic predictors of medically treated acute type B aortic dissections. *Ann Thorac Surg.* 2004;78:1268–1273.
6. Sueyoshi E, Sakamoto I, Hayashi K, Yamaguchi T, Imada T. Growth rate of aortic diameter in patients with type B aortic dissection during the chronic phase. *Circulation.* 2004;110(11 Suppl. 1):S11256–S11261.
7. Mossop P. Staged endovascular treatment for type B aortic dissection. *NCP Cardiovasc Med.* 2005;2(6):316–321.
8. Dake MD, Kato N, Mitchell RS, et al. Endovascular stent-graft placement for the treatment of acute aortic dissection. *N Engl J Med.* 1999;340:1546–1552.
9. Diethrich EB, Ramaiah VG, Kpodonu J, Rodriguez-Lopez JA. *Endovascular and Hybrid Management of the Thoracic Aorta.* West Sussex: Wiley-Blackwell; 2008.

Chapter 20
COOK Medical Accessories Used for Deployment of the TX2 COOK Stent Graft

20.1 Wire Guides

Wire guides navigate tortuous anatomy while offering support to the aorta and iliac vessels during the deployment and advancement of endovascular grafts and accessories used in endovascular aortic repair (EVAR).

20.2 Lunderquist Wire

This device is intended for complex diagnostic and interventional procedures where increased body, flexibility, and low surface friction of the wire guide are needed. There are three different types of Lunderquist wires: the straight exchange Lunderquist, the curved exchange Lunderquist, and the double-curve Lunderquist wire. They have increased body, flexibility, and low surface friction intended for complex diagnostic and interventional procedures. They are packaged as five wire guides in a box in the United States (Fig. 20.1a–c).

Ultra-stiff wire guides are used for interventional cardiovascular procedures, interventional biliary drainage, abscess drainage, uroradiology procedures and catheter exchanges (Fig. 20.2).

Rosen wire is commonly used for angioplasty catheter exchange (Fig. 20.3).

Nimble and firm wire guides are used for complex diagnostic and interventional procedures (Fig. 20.4).

Hydrophilic wire guides are used to facilitate the placement of devices during diagnostic and interventional procedures (Fig. 20.5).

Introducers facilitate endovascular graft placement by providing continual vessel access while maintaining hemostasis (Fig. 20.6).

Introducers with high-Flex dilator, hydrophilic coating, and a radiopaque band are used to introduce balloon, closed and non-tapered end catheters, and other devices for intervention (Fig. 20.7).

J. Kpodonu, *Manual of Thoracic Endoaortic Surgery*,
DOI 10.1007/978-1-84996-296-4_20, © Springer-Verlag London Limited 2010

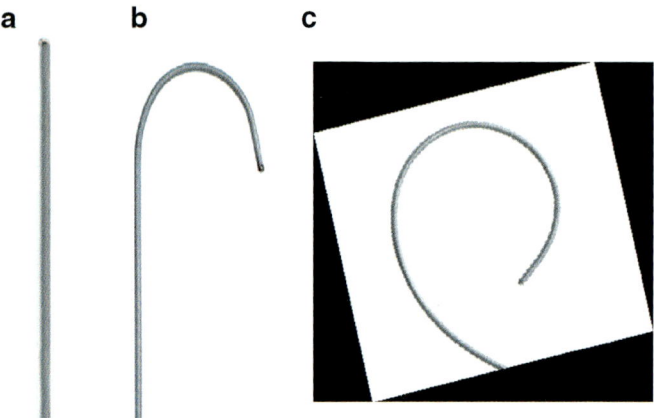

Fig. 20.1 (**a**) Straight Lunderquist. (**b**) Curved Lunderquist. (**c**) Double-curve Lunderquist

Fig. 20.2 Amplatz wire

Fig. 20.3 Rosen wire

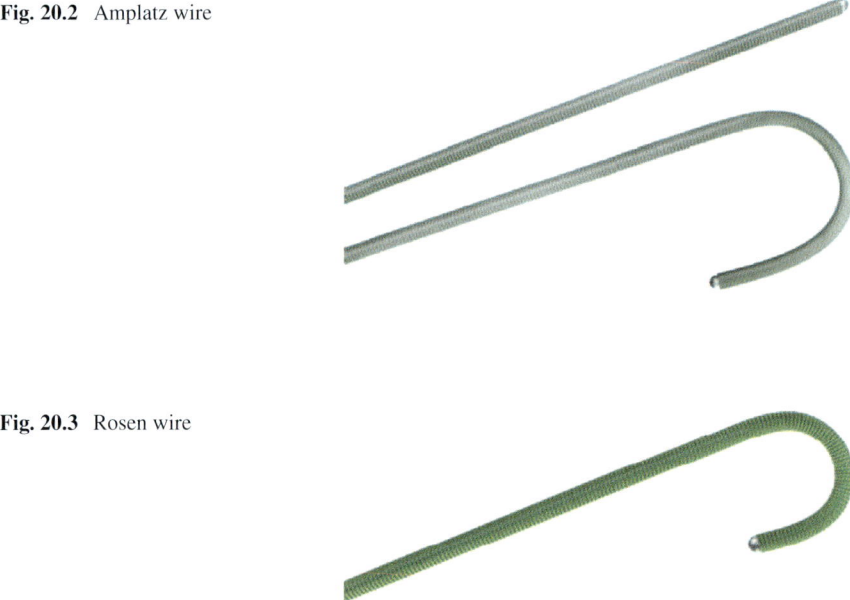

Introducers with radiopaque band are used to introduce balloon, closed and non-tapered end catheters, and other devices for intervention (Fig. 20.8).

Extra large Check-Flo introducers are used to introduce large devices for vascular intervention (Fig. 20.9).

Fig. 20.4 Roadrunner PC wire

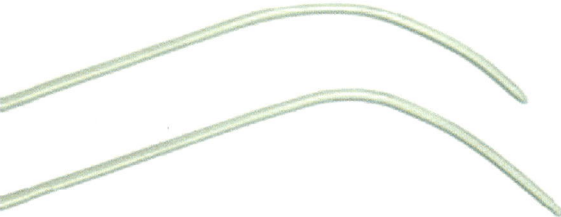

Fig. 20.5 HiWire

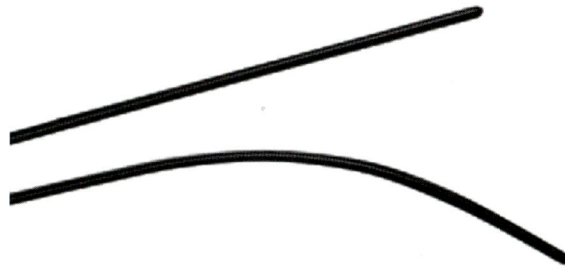

Fig. 20.6 Introducers

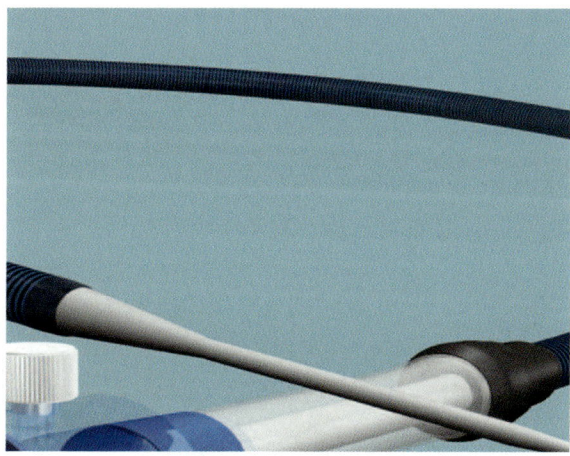

Introducer sets are used to introduce balloon, electrode, closed or non-tapered end, and other catheters (Fig. 20.10).

Introducers with AQ Hydrophylic and a radiopaque band are used to introduce balloon, closed and non-tapered end catheters, and other devices (Fig. 20.11).

Fig. 20.7 Flexor Check-Flo
introducers

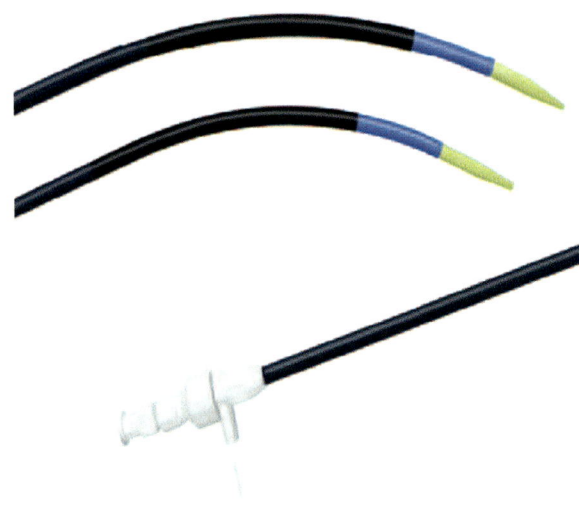

Fig. 20.8 Large Check-Flo
introducers

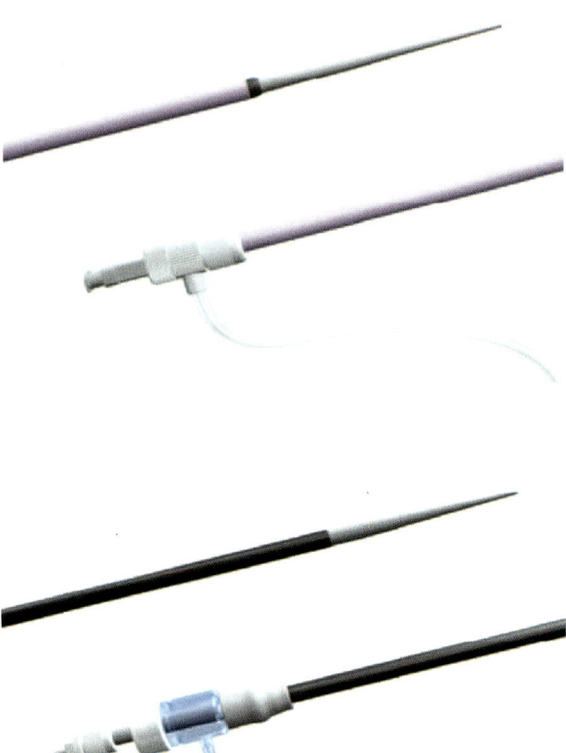

Fig. 20.9 Extra large
Check-Flo introducers

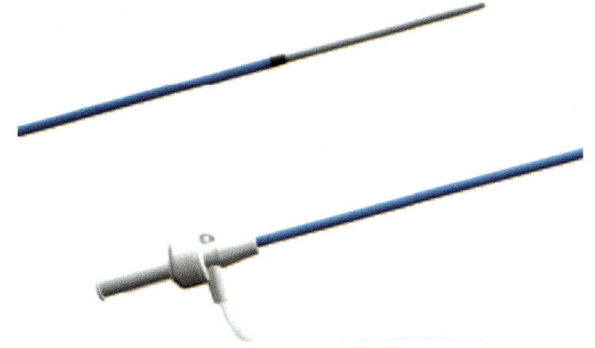

Fig. 20.10 Check-Flo performer introducer

Fig. 20.11 Flexor
Keller-Timmermans
introducers

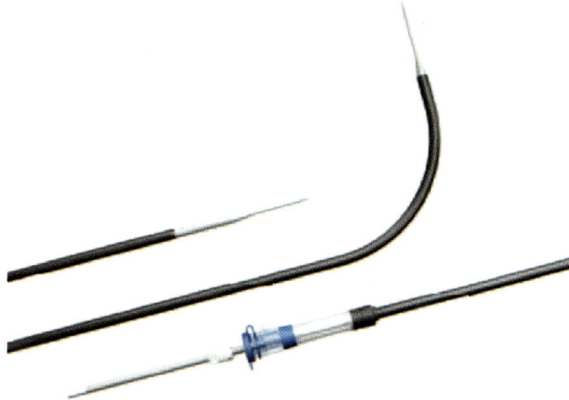

20.3 Catheters

Diagnostic catheters determine anatomical measurements, locate and select specific vessels, advance and precisely position endovascular devices, and cannulate limbs of endovascular grafts (Fig. 20.12).

AURUS centimeter sizing catheters are used to determine accurate sizing of vessel lumen prior to aortic graft surgery, angioplasty, embolization, and other interventional procedures.

Beacon Tip Van Schie seeking catheters are used for catheterization of bifurcated endoluminal AAA stent grafts (Fig. 20.13).

Catheters are used for intra-procedural angiography (Fig. 20.14).

Beacon Tip Royal Flush Plus High-Flow Angiographic Flush catheters are used for high flow rate applications (Fig. 20.15a).

Catheters are used for high flow rate applications (Fig. 20.15b).

Fig. 20.12 AURUS
centimeter sizing catheter

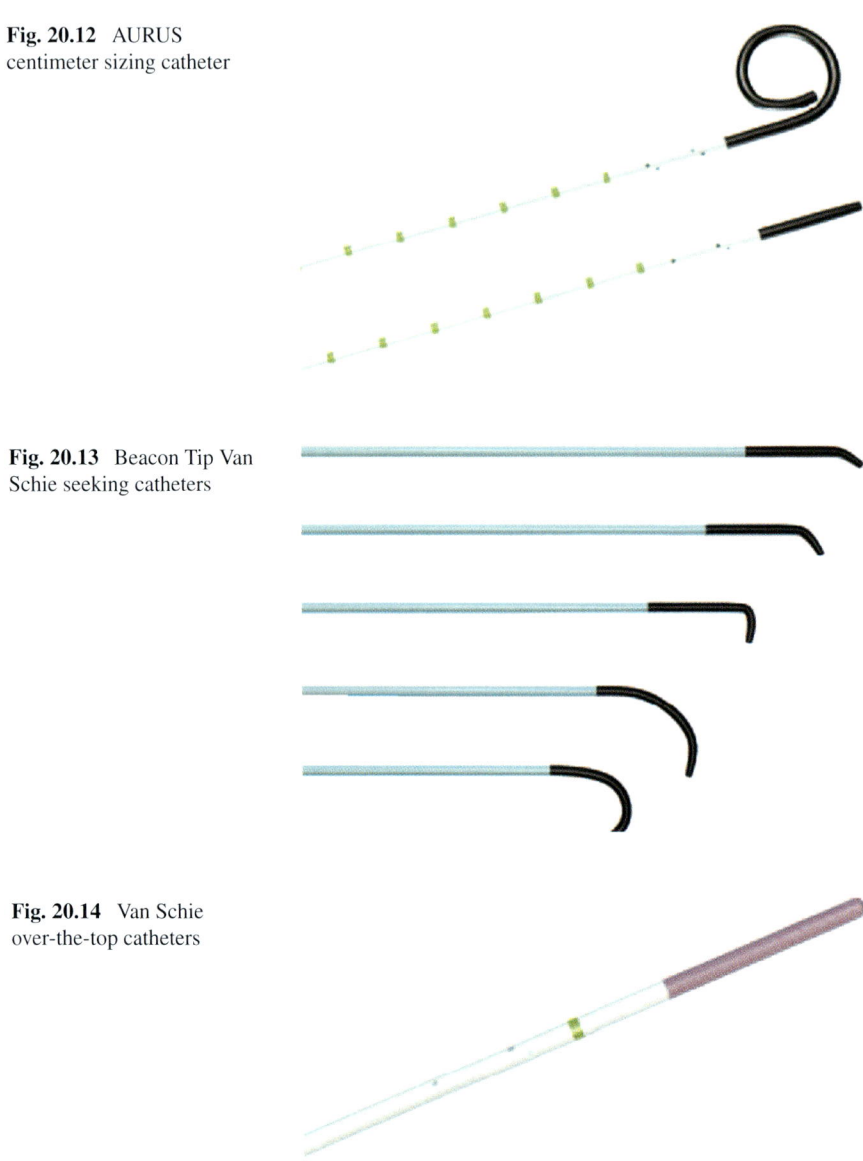

Fig. 20.13 Beacon Tip Van
Schie seeking catheters

Fig. 20.14 Van Schie
over-the-top catheters

20.4 Embolization

Embolization coils occlude vessels that commonly contribute to type II endoleaks. Occlusion balloon catheters temporarily close off large vessels or expand vascular prostheses (Fig. 20.16).

Fig. 20.15 (**a**) Beacon Tip
Royal Flush Plus High-Flow
Angiographic Flush catheters.
(**b**) Beacon Tip angiographic
catheters

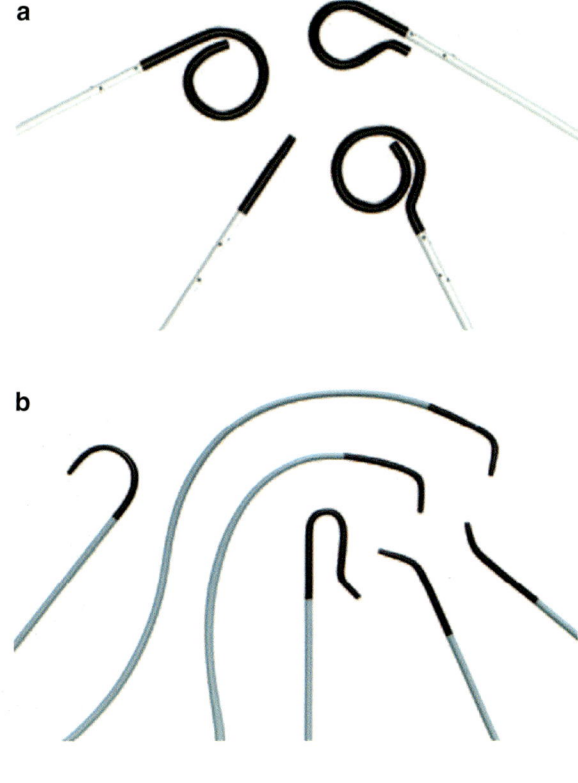

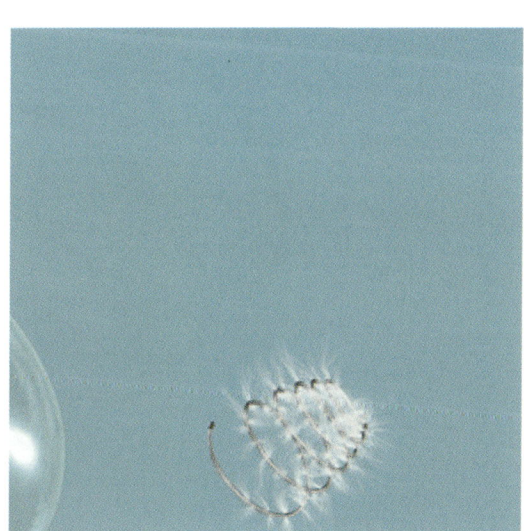

Fig. 20.16 Embolization
coils

Nester embolization coils are used for arterial and venous embolization (Fig. 20.17).

Tornado embolization coils are used for embolization of selective vessel supply to arteriovenous malformations and other vascular lesions (Fig. 20.18).

Compliant balloons are used for temporary occlusion of large vessels or to expand vascular prostheses (Fig. 20.19).

Used for fascial tissue tract and vessel dilation prior to catheter introduction. Dilators are used to pre-dilate tortuous iliac arteries, which must be surpassed in order to deliver and deploy endovascular devices. The dilators that comprise the

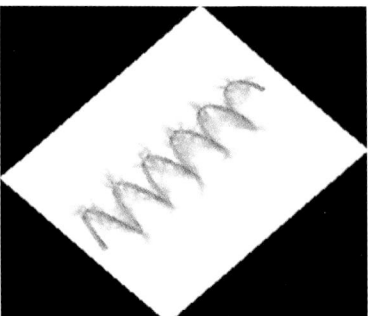

Fig. 20.17 Nester embolization coils – platinum

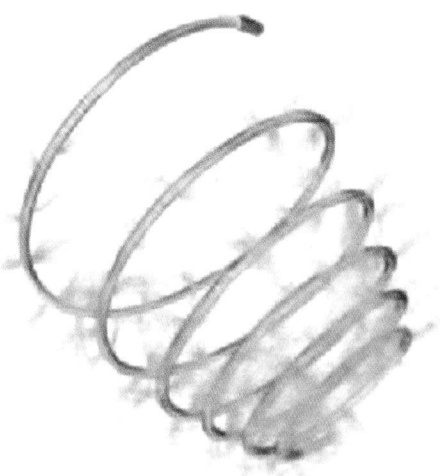

Fig. 20.18 Tornado embolization coils – platinum

Fig. 20.19 Coda balloon
catheters

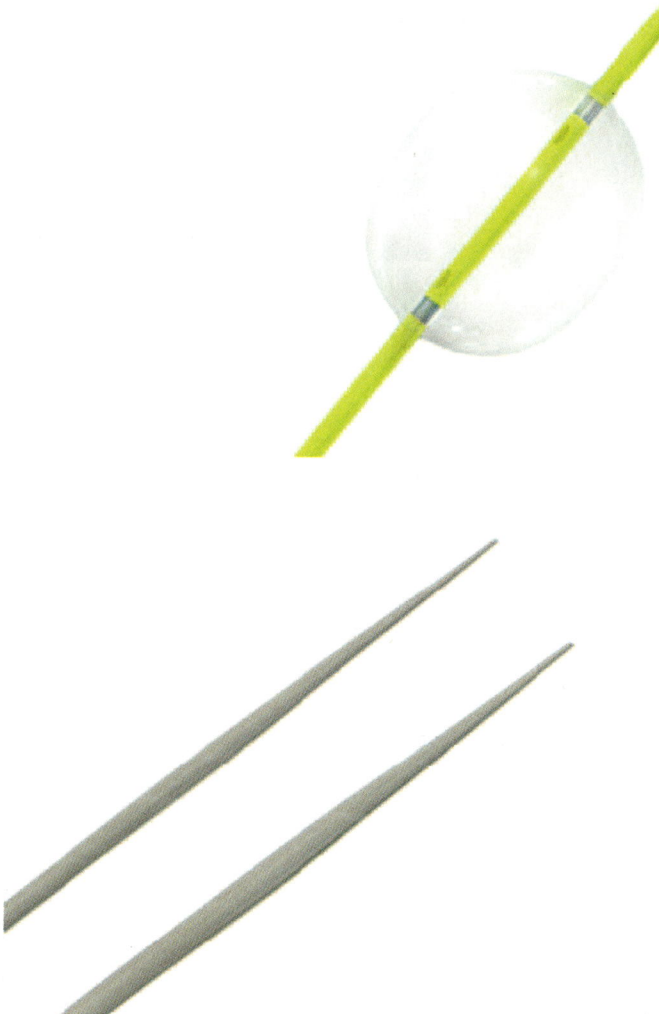

Fig. 20.20 Endovascular dilator set

endovascular dilator set (Fig. 20.20) are designed with hydrophilic-coated, long tapered dilator tips that provide excellent over-the-wire tractability.

20.5   Access Needle

Needle accesses arteries during endovascular aortic repair (Fig. 20.21).

Fig. 20.21 Percutaneous
entry thin wall needle

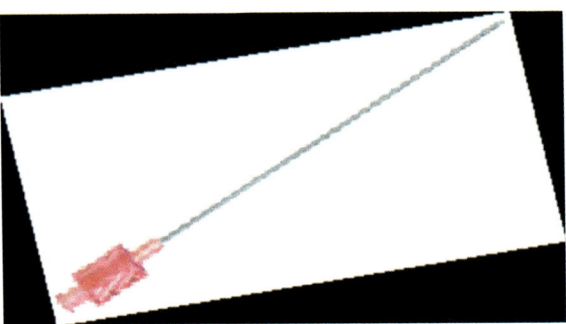

Reference

1. Cook Aortic Physician Reference Manual.

Chapter 21
Clinical Data Using the Zenith TX2 Thoracic Graft

21.1 The STARZ Trial

The STARZ-TX2 trial (Study of Thoracic Aortic Aneurysm Repair with the Zenith TX2 TAA Endovascular Graft) is a North American multicenter, nonrandomized, prospective clinical trial. It is seeking to enroll 270 patients at 35 sites in the United States and Canada. It includes a control group consisting of patients with concurrent and recent historical open surgical procedures. Subject selections are based on the inclusion and exclusion criteria listed in Tables 21.1 and 21.2. Control subjects are those who do not meet the anatomic inclusion criteria for the endovascular treatment group but otherwise fit the study criteria.

The primary safety hypothesis is that the subjects treated with the Zenith device will have 30-day survival rates equivalent to those of the surgical control group. The secondary hypothesis under investigation is that patients treated with the TX2 stent graft will have equivalent or fewer complications compared with the surgical arm up to 30 days after the procedure. Other outcome measures include 12-month survival, aneurysm-related survival, incidence of rupture and conversion, aneurysm size reduction, rates of major adverse effects, device-related events, and secondary intervention rates.

The screening process includes a thorough history and physical, an ankle/brachial index, and a pre-operative Short Form-36 quality-of-life questionnaire, as well as a pre-operative angiography or a contrast-enhanced CT scan. Follow-up physical examination, Short Form-36 quality of life, ankle/brachial index, chest radiograph, and a CT scan of the chest are obtained before discharge at 1, 6, and 12 months after implantation with annual follow-up thereafter up to 5 years. The study started enrolling patients in March 2004 and has completed its enrollment targets at this time. Results of this multicenter trial are currently not available to make any meaningful conclusion. It is hoped that within mid-2008 the Federal Drug Administration will grant approval of the Cook Zenith TX1 and TX2 device approval for use in the United States to treat thoracic aortic aneurysm.

Table 21.1 Inclusion criteria

Criterion	Cook TX2
Age (years)	>18
Women	Negative pregnancy test 7 days before treatment
Open surgical candidate	Yes
Neck length	Minimal 3 cm proximal and distal
Aneurysm	Fusiform DTA at least twice the size of normal thoracic aorta
Penetrating ulcer	No
Proximal landing zone location	30 mm distal to left CCA
Distal landing zone location	20 mm proximal to celiac axis
Landing zone diameter (mm)	24–38

CCA, common carotid artery; *DTA*, descending thoracic aortic aneurysm

Table 21.2 Exclusion criteria

Criterion	Cook TX2
Creatinine (mg/dl)	
Unstable rupture	Yes
Mycotic aneurysm	Yes
Connective tissue disease	Yes
Significant landing zone thrombus	Yes
Previous descending aortic surgery or endovascular repair of DTA or AAA	Yes
Aortic dissection	Yes
Coagulopathy	Yes
MI/CVA	<3 months
Major operation within 30 days	Yes
Participation in another investigational study	<30 days

DTA, descending thoracic aortic aneurysm; *AAA*, abdominal aortic aneurysm; *MI*, myocardial infarction; *CVA*, cerebrovascular accident; *N/A*, not applicable

21.2 International Controlled Clinical Trial of Thoracic Endovascular Aneurysm Repair with the Zenith TX2 Endovascular Graft: 1-Year Results

21.2.1 Trial Design

The study was a nonrandomized, controlled, multicenter, international trial designed to evaluate the safety and effectiveness of the TX2, a contemporary thoracic aortic endograft, in patients with descending thoracic aneurysms ≥5 cm, rapid growth ≥5 mm/year, or ulcers ≥10 mm in depth and 20 mm in diameter. Type I thoracoabdominal aneurysms were eligible if the placement of endograft fabric was planned to be above the visceral vessels or if there was no planned mesenteric revascularization with open repair. The primary end points were 30-day survival and 30-day rupture-free survival. Secondary end points included 30-day morbidity and clinical utility.

Fifty-seven prespecified events were considered in calculating a composite morbidity score (Table 21.3). Because all 57 events were weighted equally when calculating the composite score, but not of the same clinical severity, a subset of severe morbid events (Table 21.4) were identified in part from reporting standards for endovascular aneurysm repair. These were considered in calculating a severe morbidity composite index that would be more clinically relevant when endovascular and open aortic repair operations were compared.

Table 21.3 All events comprising the composite morbidity score

Category	Event type
Cardiovascular	1. Q-wave myocardial infarction 2. Non-Q-wave myocardial infarction 3. Congestive heart failure 4. Arrhythmia requiring intervention or new treatment 5. Cardiac ischemia requiring intervention 6. Inotropic support 7. Refractory hypertension (systolic blood pressure ≥ 160 despite receiving medication) 8. Cardiac event involving arrest, resuscitation, or balloon pump
Pulmonary	9. Ventilation >24 h 10. Reintubation 11. Pneumonia requiring antibiotics 12. Supplemental oxygen at time of discharge 13. Chronic obstructive pulmonary disease 14. Pleural effusion requiring treatment 15. Pulmonary edema requiring treatment 16. Pneumothorax 17. Hemothorax 18. Pulmonary event requiring tracheostomy or chest tube
Renal	19. Urinary tract infection requiring antibiotic treatment 20. Renal failure requiring dialysis 21. Serum creatinine rise >30% from baseline resulting in a persistent value >2.0 mg/dl 22. Permanent dialysis, hemofiltration, or kidney transplant
Gastrointestinal	23. Bowel ischemia 24. Gastrointestinal infection requiring treatment 25. Gastrointestinal bleeding requiring treatment 26. Paralytic ileus >4 days 27. Bowel resection

Table 21.3   (continued)

Category	Event type
Neurologic	28. Stroke
	29. Transient ischemic attack/reversible ischemic neurologic deficit
	30. Carotid artery embolization/occlusion
	31. Paraparesis
	32. Paraplegia
Vascular	33. Pulmonary embolism
	34. Pulmonary embolism involving hemodynamic instability or surgery
	35. Vascular injury
	36. Aneurysm leak/rupture
	37. Aneurysm or vessel leak requiring reoperation
	38. Pseudoaneurysm requiring surgical repair
	39. Increase in aneurysm size >0.5 cm relative to first post-procedure measurement
	40. Aorto-esophageal fistula
	41. Aorto-bronchial fistula
	42. Aortoenteric fistula
	43. Arterial thrombosis
	44. Embolization resulting in tissue loss or requiring intervention
	45. Amputation involving more than the toes
	46. Deep vein thrombosis
	47. Deep vein thrombosis requiring surgical or lytic therapy
	48. Hematoma requiring surgical repair
	49. Hematoma requiring receipt of blood products
	50. Coagulopathy requiring surgery
	51. Post-procedure transfusion
Wound	52. Wound infection requiring antibiotic treatment
	53. Incisional hernia
	54. Lymph fistula
	55. Wound breakdown requiring debridement
	56. Seroma requiring treatment
	57. Wound complication requiring return to the operating room

21.2.2 Follow-Up

Device integrity was assessed using chest radiograph and 3D reformatted CT imaging.

21.2.2.1 Repair Techniques

The endovascular and open surgical aneurysm/ulcer repair techniques consisted of institutional standard of care executed within the limits of the study protocol.

Table 21.4 Events comprising the severe morbidity composite index

Organ system	Event
Cardiovascular	1. Q-wave myocardial infarction 2. Cardiac event involving arrest, resuscitation, or balloon pump
Pulmonary	3. Ventilation >72 h or reintubation 4. Pulmonary event requiring tracheostomy or chest tube
Renal	5. Permanent dialysis, hemofiltration, or kidney transplant
Gastrointestinal	6. Bowel resection
Neurologic	7. Stroke or severe impairment (paraplegia)
Vascular	8. Amputation involving more than the toes 9. Aneurysm or vessel leak requiring reoperation 10. Deep vein thrombosis requiring surgical or lytic therapy 11. Pulmonary embolism involving hemodynamic instability 12. Coagulopathy requiring surgery
Wound	13. Wound complication requiring return to the operating room

21.2.3 Results

Enrollment began on March 30, 2004, and was completed on July 6, 2006. The results reported here reflect data received as of September 12, 2007. A total of 160 patients for endovascular repair and 70 patients for open surgical repair were enrolled at 42 institutions. Enrollment for 51 of 70 open patients (73%) was retrospective, but the treatment groups were reasonably concurrent, with 81% of open patients treated within the period of TEVAR enrollment.

21.2.4 Patient Characteristics

Evaluation of pre-existing conditions or risk factors showed similar pre-operative demographic, medical, and laboratory characteristics in the TEVAR and open study groups, with a few exceptions. As summarized in Table 21.5, patients in the TEVAR group were older ($P < 0.01$), weighed more ($P = 0.02$), had a larger body mass index ($P = 0.03$), and had more previous access site surgery ($P = 0.02$), whereas patients in the open group had a higher incidence of prior thoracic surgery or trauma ($P < 0.01$). The preprocedure hemoglobin (g/dl) was higher in the TEVAR patients than in the open patients (13.5 ± 1.6 versus 13.0 ± 1.6, $P = 0.03$); however,

Table 21.5 Patient demographics, medical history, and risk assessment

Item	TEVAR	Open	P
Sex, male	72 (115/160)	60 (42/70)	0.09
Age (years)	72±9.6 (160)	68±12 (70)	<0.01
Weight (kg)	80.5±16 (158)	75.9±15 (70)	0.02
Body mass index	27.2±4.9 (153)	25.9±3.7 (69)	0.03
Cardiovascular			
Myocardial infarction	22 (35/158)	25 (17/68)	0.73
Congestive heart failure	13 (20/160)	12 (8/69)	>0.99
Coronary artery disease	44 (69/158)	42 (29/69)	0.88
Arrhythmia	30 (48/159)	19 (13/69)	0.1
Vascular			
Thromboembolic event	10 (16/159)	8.7 (6/69)	>0.99
Peripheral vascular disease	24 (39/160)	26 (18/69)	0.86
Family history of aneurysm	17 (24/140)	20 (11/54)	0.67
Hypertension	89 (143/160)	83 (58/70)	0.19
Thoracic surgery/trauma	10 (16/160)	26 (18/70)	<0.01
Diagnosed AAA	31 (50/160)	23 (16/70)	0.2
Repaired AAA	19 (31/160)	14 (10/70)	0.47
COPD	45 (71/159)	43 (30/70)	0.88
Renal failure requiring dialysis	3.1 (5/160)	2.9 (2/70)	>0.99
Diabetes mellitus	19 (30/160)	14 (10/70)	0.45
Sepsis	1.9 (3/156)	1.5 (1/68)	>0.99
Neurologic			
Cerebrovascular accident	15 (24/160)	15 (10/68)	>0.99
Carotid endarterectomy	5.7 (9/159)	2.9 (2/70)	0.51
Gastrointestinal disease	41 (64/158)	30 (21/70)	0.14
Liver disease	6.3 (10/160)	4.3 (3/70)	0.75
Cancer	25 (40/159)	16 (11/70)	0.12
Excessive alcohol use	3.2 (5/157)	0.0 (0/67)	0.32
Tobacco use			0.19
Current smoker	22 (35/156)	18 (12/68)	
Quit smoking	66 (103/156)	62 (42/68)	
Never smoked	12 (18/156)	21 (14/68)	
Access site			
Previous surgery	10 (16/159)	1.4 (1/69)	0.02
Previous radiation	0.0 (0/159)	0.0 (0/69)	NA
Allergies	44 (70/160)	40 (28/70)	0.66
ASA classification			<0.01
Healthy patient: 1	8.8 (14/160)	7.1 (5/70)	
Mild systemic disease: 2	50 (80/160)	41 (29/70)	
Severe systemic disease: 3	37 (59/160)	29 (20/70)	
Incapacitating systemic disease: 4	4.4 (7/160)	23 (16/70)	
Moribund patient: 5	0 (0/160)	0 (0/70)	
Total SVS/ISCVS risk score	6.4±3.0 (159)	5.4±3.5 (68)	0.03

AAA, abdominal aortic aneurysm; *ASA*, American Society of Anesthesiologists; *NA*, not applicable; *TEVAR*, thoracic endovascular aneurysm repair; SVS/ISCVS, Society for Vascular Surgery/International Society for Cardiovascular Surgery

Categoric data are presented as percentages (no.) and continuous data as mean ± standard deviation (no.)

both values were within the normal range for hemoglobin measurements. The TEVAR patients had a lower ASA classification ($P < 0.01$) and higher Society for Vascular Surgery/International Society for Cardiovascular Surgery risk score ($P = 0.03$).

21.2.5 Aneurysm/Ulcer Characteristics

Both the endovascular treatment group and open surgical control group had patients with aneurysms (86 and 90%) and patients with ulcers (14 and 10%), with the distribution in morphology being similar in the two groups ($P = 0.40$). As summarized in Table 21.6, the distribution in primary location (proximal, middle, or distal) of the aneurysm or ulcer was different between groups ($P = 0.02$). Specifically, the percentage of patients with a proximal location was lower in the TEVAR group compared with the open group (22.5 versus 36.9%). The major axis diameter of the aneurysm was not different between the two groups ($P = 0.20$; Table 21.6), but the ulcer depth was smaller for the TEVAR group than the open group (14 ± 4.7 versus 21 ± 7.8 mm, $P = 0.01$). Protocol-driven anatomic differences included smaller mean neck diameters, such as at 30 mm distal to the left common carotid artery ($P < 0.01$) and 30 mm proximal to the celiac axis artery ($P < 0.01$), in the TEVAR group compared with the open group.

Table 21.6   Core laboratory analysis of preprocedure anatomy

Item	TEVAR[a]	Open[a]	P
Morphology type			0.4
Aneurysm	86 (137/160)	90 (63/70)	
Ulcer	14 (23/160)	10 (7/70)	
Morphology location			0.02
Proximal	23 (36/160)	37 (24/65)	
Middle	55 (88/160)	52 (34/65)	
Distal	23 (36/160)	11 (7/65)	
Dimensions (mm)			
Aneurysm major axis	60.8 ± 10.7 (137)	63.0 ± 10.8 (53)	0.2
Ulcer depth	14.4 ± 4.7 (22)	20.7 ± 7.8 (7)	0.01
Proximal neck[b]	35.5 ± 7.8 (158)	41.2 ± 9.9 (55)	<0.01
Distal neck[c]	32.3 ± 5.0 (157)	41.5 ± 13.5 (56)	<0.01

TEVAR, thoracic endovascular aneurysm repair
[a]Categoric data are presented as percentages (no.) and continuous data as mean $\pm$ standard deviation (no.)
[b]Major axis at 30 mm distal to left common carotid artery
[c]Major axis at 30 mm proximal to celiac axis artery

21.2.6 Mortality

The 30-day survival estimate from all-cause mortality was noninferior ($P < 0.01$) in the endovascular treatment group compared with the open surgical control group

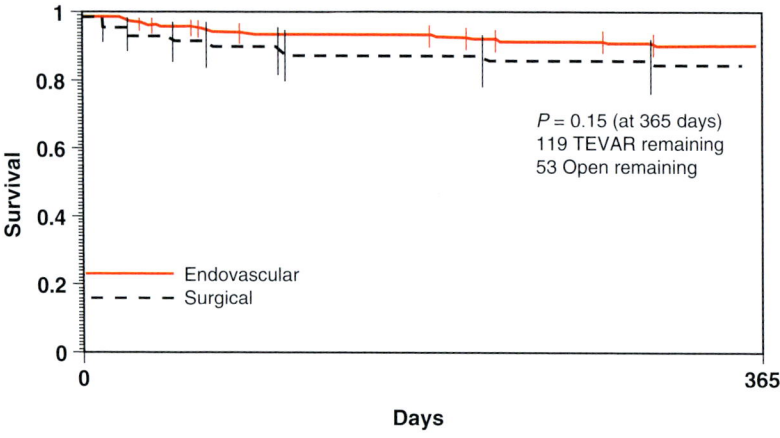

Fig. 21.1   All-cause mortality survival curves

(98.1 versus 94.3%). Propensity score analysis confirmed noninferior 30-day survival for the endovascular treatment group. The 365-day survival estimate from
all-cause mortality was 91.6% in the endovascular group and 85.5% in the open
surgical group, as illustrated in Fig. 21.1 (log-rank = 0.15). The 365-day survival
estimate from aneurysm-related mortality was 94.2% in the endovascular group and
88.2% in the open surgical group, as illustrated in Fig 21.2 (log-rank = 0.12). All
aneurysm-related deaths were considered procedure-related by the clinical events
committee, and no deaths were considered device-related.

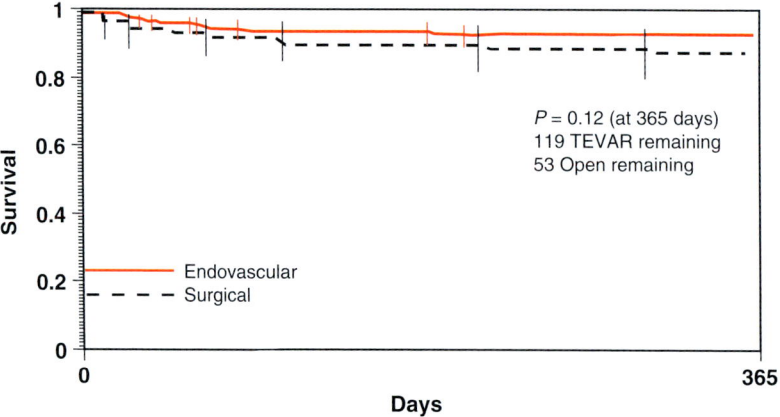

Fig. 21.2   Aneurysm-related mortality survival curves

21.2.7 All Morbidity

Cardiovascular ($P < 0.01$), pulmonary ($P < 0.01$), and vascular ($P = 0.01$) categories of morbid events were lower in the endovascular treatment group compared with the open surgical control group (Table 21.7). The composite 30-day morbidity score (mean number of events per patient) was lower with TEVAR compared with open repair (1.3 ± 3.0 versus 2.9 ± 3.6; $P < 0.01$). Propensity score analysis confirmed lower 30-day morbidity for the endovascular treatment group. The percentage of patients experiencing at least one morbid event was also lower with TEVAR compared with open (41.9 versus 68.6%, $P < 0.01$).

Table 21.7   Morbid events (by category) occurring ≤ 30 days

Category	TEVAR, % (no.)	Open, % (no.)	P
Cardiovascular	15.6 (25/160)	44.3 (31/70)	<0.01
Pulmonary	15.6 (25/160)	44.3 (31/70)	<0.01
Renal	8.8 (14/160)	14.3 (10/70)	0.24
Gastrointestinal	6.9 (11/160)	7.1 (5/70)	>0.99
Neurologic	8.1 (13/160)	14.3 (10/70)	0.15
Vascular	22.5 (36/160)	40 (28/70)	0.01
Wound	6.3 (10/160)	4.3 (3/70)	0.75

TEVAR, thoracic endovascular aneurysm repair

21.2.8 Neurologic Morbidity

An assessment of neurologic morbidity consisted of evaluating five prespecified events: carotid artery embolization/occlusion, stroke, transient ischemic attack (TIA)/reversible ischemic neurological deficit (RIND), paraplegia, and paraparesis (lower extremity weakness but still able to walk). Table 21.8 reviews the percentage of patients experiencing each of these categories of neurologic events ≤ 30 days.

Table 21.8   Neurologic events occurring ≤ 30 days

Event	TEVAR, % (no.)	Open, % (no.)	P
Carotid artery embolization/occlusion	0 (0/160)	0 (0/70)	–
Stroke	2.5 (4/160)	8.6 (6/70)	0.07
TIA/RIND	0.6 (1/160)	1.4 (1/70)	0.51
Paraplegia	1.3 (2/160)	5.7 (4/70)	0.07
Paraparesis	4.4 (7/160)	0 (0/70)	0.10

TEVAR, thoracic endovascular aneurysm repair

21.2.9 Stroke

Stroke occurred in four TEVAR patients; all had general cardiovascular risk factors, none had history of TIA or carotid endarterectomy, all had proximal location of the graft distal to the left subclavian artery, one had a brain biopsy 11 days after TEVAR, and three of the patients died.

21.2.10 Paraplegia

Two TEVAR patients experienced paraplegia after treatment of the aneurysm. The aneurysms in both patients were in the mid-descending thoracic aorta, there was no history of abdominal aneurysm repair, the proximal aspect of the grafts was deployed distal to the left subclavian artery, and no spinal drains were used. In the first patient, approximately 70% of the descending aorta was covered by the graft and paraplegia developed on post-operative day 0; in the second patient (who also had a stroke), approximately 100% of the descending aorta was covered by the graft and paraplegia developed on post-operative day 3. Both patients died.

21.2.11 Paraparesis

Seven patients in the TEVAR group were diagnosed with paraparesis ≤ 30 days. Four had a history of AAA repair, three had a spinal drain placed, and two had a proximal graft location that was proximal to the left subclavian artery (one did and one did not have subclavian revascularization). One patient died without resolution of the paraparesis at post-operative day 37 of septicemia complicated by respiratory failure. Paraparesis resolved in the other six patients.

21.2.12 Rupture

There were no early or late ruptures with either TEVAR or open through 365 days.

21.2.12.1 Secondary Interventions

The percentage of patients requiring reintervention through 12 months was similar ($P = 0.74$) for endovascular repair (4.4%, 7 of 158) and open surgical repair (5.7%, 4 of 70) and included three endovascular patients and three open surgical patients requiring secondary intervention ≤ 7 days of the initial aneurysm repair. In the TEVAR group, seven patients underwent secondary interventions, including one patient who underwent two secondary interventions for treatment of a distal type I endoleak (bare stent placement and stent placement/coil embolization/distal extension placement). The other six endovascular patients had reintervention for proximal type I endoleak (proximal main body extension placement), distal type I endoleak (molding balloon angioplasty and distal extension placement), type III endoleak (angiogram to rule out endoleak), iliac artery occlusion (femorofemoral bypass), aneurysm growth but no detectable endoleak (distal extension placement in overlap and distal end of in situ graft), and a proximal aortic pseudoaneurysm (proximal extension placement). There were no open conversions in the TEVAR group through 365 days. Three open surgical control patients underwent re-exploration for bleeding, and one underwent custom endograft placement for an aorto-esophageal fistula.

21.2.13 Change in Aneurysm or Ulcer Size

At 12 months, aneurysm/ulcer size decreased for 48% (54 of 112) of the patients and remained unchanged for 45% (50 of 112). Aneurysm growth was identified in 7.1% (8 of 112) at 12 months. Two of these patients have had follow-up at 24 months and do not have sac growth compared with baseline, one has been re-treated for distal type I endoleak, one has been re-treated for growth, and four have not had further follow-up. In the latter four patients, there is no detectable endoleak at 12 months or evidence of graft infection, but the aortic neck diameter at the actual graft placement does not meet the recommended oversizing of at least 10%. Each of these four patients also has an inverted funnel-shaped proximal aortic neck or a funnel-shaped distal neck.

21.2.14 Endoleak

Endoleak rates at predischarge, 30 days, 6 months, and 12 months were 13, 4.8, 2.6, and 3.9% (Table 21.9). Several patients had reintervention in the first year such that no patients were identified with type I or IV endoleak at 12 months. One patient with a one-piece system has a type III endoleak at 12 months (unknown type per site assessment) that was not associated with aneurysm growth and has not had subsequent imaging or reintervention.

21.2.15 Migration

Proximal or distal graft migration of >10 mm was noted in 2.8% (3 of 107) through 12 months, consisting of two cases of caudal migration of the proximal graft and one case of cranial migration of the distal graft. None have been associated with endoleak or increase in aneurysm size, and none have had secondary intervention. All three patients have aortic neck diameter at the actual graft placement that does not meet the recommended oversizing of at least 10%. All three also have placement of the pertinent barbed stent in a neck that is either an acutely angled segment or in an area of thrombus.

Table 21.9 Percentage of patients with endoleak at each follow-up time point based on core lab analysis

Type	Time point, % (no.)			
	Predischarge	30 days	6 months	12 months
Any	12.6 (17/135)	4.8 (6/126)	2.6 (3/114)	3.9 (4/103)
Multiple	0 (0/135)	0 (0/126)	0 (0/114)	0 (0/103)
Proximal type I	0 (0/135)	0 (0/126)	0 (0/114)	0 (0/103)
Distal type I	0.7 (1/135)	0.8 (1/126)	0.9 (1/114)	0 (0/103)
Type IIa	1.5 (2/135)	0.8 (1/126)	0 (0/114)	0 (0/103)
Type IIb	5.9 (8/135)	2.4 (3/126)	1.8 (2/114)	1.9 (2/103)
Type III	1.5 (2/135)	0.8 (1/126)	0 (0/114)	1.0 (1/103)
Type IV	1.5 (2/135)	0 (0/126)	0 (0/114)	0 (0/103)
Unknown	1.5 (2/135)	0 (0/126)	0 (0/114)	1.0 (1/103)

21.2.16 Device Integrity

Device integrity was assessed at each examination period through 12 months. None of the patients have had stent fracture, barb separation, stent-to-graft separation, or component separation. One patient (0.8%) has distal bare stent strut entanglement from predischarge through 12 months, which is not associated with migration, endoleak, or the need for secondary intervention. It is unclear whether the entanglement is related to a device failure, barb entanglement during loading, movement during deployment, or very tortuous anatomy.

21.2.17 Device Patency

No patients have had loss of patency through 12 months. A kink was noted in 1.6% (2 of 123) of patients at 12 months and compression was noted in 0.9% (1 of 108), but none of these three patients have adverse clinical sequelae or required a secondary intervention. The compression is a concentric constriction of one mid-body stent of the device not associated with tortuosity or flow limitation with expansion of the stents above and below the compressed segment. This should be distinguished from the phenomena of endovascular graft collapse described in the literature.

21.3 Conclusion

The most recent version of The Cook Zenith Tx2 device for the treatment of thoracic aortic aneurysms has just undergone a US phase II multicenter trial and is commercially available in Europe, Australia, and Canada.

Greenberg et al.[1] studied 100 patients (42% women) under a single site device exemption protocol to assess the technical success and outcomes of patients with thoracic aortic pathology at high risk for conventional therapy using the Cook Zenith TX1 and TX2 thoracic stent graft between 2001 and 2004. The study population consisted of patients at high risk for conventional surgical therapy presenting with chronic aortic dissections, thoracic aneurysms, and aorto-bronchial or aorto-esophageal fistulas. Follow-up studies included radiographic evaluation before discharge and at 1, 6, 12, and 24 months. Most patients (55%) included in the study had undergone prior aortic aneurysm repair. The pathology treated included 81 aneurysms, 15 aortic dissections (with aneurysms), 2 patients with fistulous connections (1 aorto-bronchial and 1 aorto-esophageal), 1 subclavian artery aneurysm, and 1 aortic rupture. Mean aneurysm size was 62 mm and patients had a 14 month mean follow-up. Hybrid interventions were necessary to create adequate implantation sites in 29% patients, including 14 elephant trunk/arch reconstructions, 18 carotid-subclavian bypasses, and 4 visceral vessel bypasses. Iliac conduits were required in 19 patients. Overall mortality in this cohort group was 17%, and aneurysm-related mortality was 14% at 1 year. Sac regression (>5 mm maximum diameter decrease) was observed in 52 and 56% at 12 and 24 months. Growth was noted in one patient (1.6%) at 12 months. Endoleaks were detected in eight patients (8.5%) at 30 days and three patients (6%) at 12 months. Secondary interventions were required in 15 patients. Migration (>10 mm) of the proximal or distal stent was noted in three patients (6%) (two proximal and one distal), none of which required treatment or resulted in an adverse event. The authors concluded that acceptable intermediate-term outcomes have been achieved in the treatment of high-risk patients in the setting of both favorable and challenging anatomic situations with these devices.

A 1-year result of this recent international TX2 trial trial[2] demonstrates similar overall and aneurysm-related survival with TEVAR using the TX2 compared with open repair. Significant reductions in severe and major adverse events contributed to improved clinical utility with TEVAR compared with open surgical repair. There were no ruptures or conversions in the endovascular treatment group, and reintervention rates were similar in both groups. Radiographic findings of sac enlargement, endoleak, migration, and other device issues were infrequent but underscore the value of careful procedure planning and regular follow-up with imaging before and after TEVAR. These 1-year results provide reasonable assurance that the TX2 is a safer and effective alternative to open surgical repair. Patient follow-up beyond 1-year remains ongoing and is essential for assessing long-term performance and the durability of these early benefits.

References

1. Greenberg RK, O'Neill S, Walker E, et al. Endovascular repair of thoracic aortic lesions with the Zenith TX1 and TX2 thoracic grafts (intermediate-term results). *J Vasc Surg.* 2005;41:589–596.
2. Matsumura JS, Cambria RP, Dake MD, Moore RD, Svensson LG, Snyder S; TX2 Clinical Trial Investigators. International controlled clinical trial of thoracic endovascular aneurysm repair with the Zenith TX2 endovascular graft: 1-year results. *J Vasc Surg.* 2008;47(2):247–257; Discussion 257.

Part VI
W.L. Gore TAG Thoracic Endovascular Stent Graft Device

Chapter 22
The Gore TAG Endoprosthesis

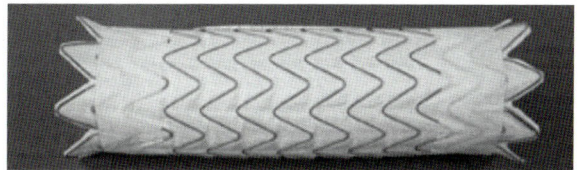

The Gore TAG endoprosthesis is composed of a symmetric expanded polytetrafluo-roethylene (ePTFE) tube externally reinforced with a layer of ePTFE and fluorinated ethylene propylene (FEP) (Fig. 22.1). An exoskeleton consisting of nitinol stents is attached to the entire external surface of the graft with ePTFE-FEP bonding tape. Both the proximal and distal segments of the endograft have scalloped flares, which are to facilitate endograft conformity in a tortuous thoracic aorta. Two radiopaque gold bands are attached to the base of the flares, serving as a guide during deployment and in graft surveillance. A polytetrafluoroethylene sealing cuff, which is affixed to the base of the flares, is attached on one end with FEP, whereas the other end is allowed to remain free. This is designed to enhance the device attachment to the aortic wall and potentially reduce type 1 endoleaks.

The Gore TAG endoprosthesis contains a unique deployment mechanism in which the endograft is constrained by an ePTFE-FEP sleeve connected to a deployment knob located at the control end of the delivery catheter (Fig. 22.2).

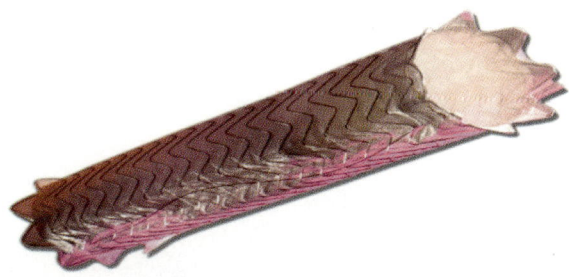

Fig. 22.1 Gore TAG endoprosthesis

J. Kpodonu, *Manual of Thoracic Endoaortic Surgery*,
DOI 10.1007/978-1-84996-296-4_22, © Springer-Verlag London Limited 2010

Fig. 22.2 Deployment of the
Gore TAG endoprosthesis. (**a**)
Initial deployment involves
turning and pulling the
deployment knob. (**b**) The
endoprosthesis is fully
constrained on the delivery
catheter. (**c**) The stent graft is
deployed from the middle
segment, expanding outward.
(**d**) Fully deployed thoracic
device

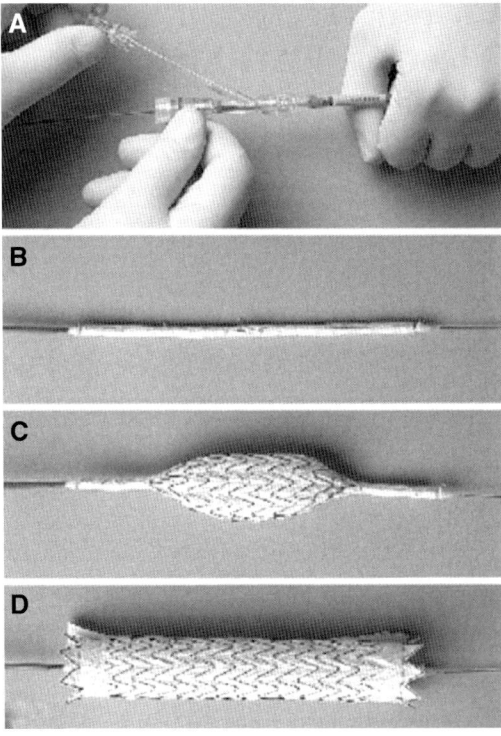

Release of the endograft begins in the midgraft region to reduce distal displacement
via a "windsock" effect. Following device deployment, a unique tri-lobed balloon,
which permits continuous antegrade aortic blood flow during balloon inflation, is
used to ensure full device attachment to the aortic wall (Fig. 22.3).

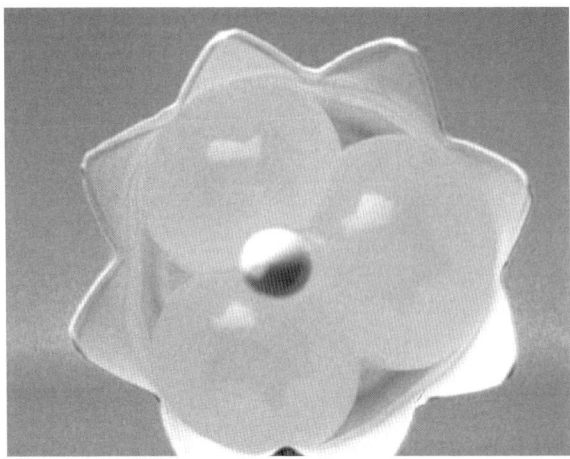

Fig. 22.3 A tri-lobed balloon
is used to inflate the aortic
stent graft while allowing
continuous antegrade blood
flow during balloon inflation

22.1 Gore TAG Delivery System

Gore TAG Delivery system consists of a flexible delivery catheter of a low-profile design which facilitates passage through tortuous iliac anatomy and the aortic arch. The delivery sheath has a 100 cm long working length and has a 20, 22, and 24 Fr delivery sheath. A radiopaque olive is present at both ends for enhanced visualization which helps in precise placement. The Gore deployment system is flexible and allows device to conform to tortuous anatomy. The sheathless deployment system results in low deployment forces with a unique middle to end deployment which results in an accurate and rapid placement. The endoprosthesis has lengths ranging from 10 to 20 cm and diameters from 26–40 mm (Table 22.1). The construction is with a low-permeable and abrasion-resistant PTFE material which conforms to the contours of the aorta without kinking. The graft is supported by external self-expanding nitinol stents which provide radial force and MRI safe. Sealing cuffs at both ends are made to prevent endoleaks.

Table 22.1   Gore device sizing table

US catalogue number	Outside US catalogue number	Endoprosthesis diameter (mm)	Endoprosthesis length (cm)	Aortic treatment, range (mm)	Sheath size (Fr)	Balloon inflation volume (cc)
TG2610	TAG2610	26.0	10.0	23–24	20	7
TG2810	TAG2810	28.0	10.0	24–26	20	9
TG2815	TAG2815	28.0	15.0	24–26	20	9
TG3110	TAG3110	31.0	10.0	26–29	22	12
TG3115	TAG3115	31.0	15.0	26–29	22	12
TG3410	TAG3410	34.0	10.0	29–32	22	15
TG3415	TAG3415	34.0	15.0	29–32	22	15
TG3420	TAG3420	34.0	20.0	29–32	22	15
TG3710	TAG3710	37.0	10.0	32–34	24	18
TG3715	TAG3715	37.0	15.0	32–34	24	18
TG3720	TAG3720	37.0	20.0	32–34	24	18
TG4010	TAG4010	40.0	10.0	34–37	24	21
TG4015	TAG4015	40.0	15.0	34–37	24	21
TG4020	TAG4020	40.0	20.0	34–37	24	21
TG4510*	TAG4510	45.0	10.0	37–42	24	30
TG4515*	TAG4515	45.0	15.0	37–42	24	30
TG4520*	TAG4520	45.0	20.0	37–42	24	30

22.2 Patient Selection

As outlined in the indication for use manual (IFU), critical factors for successful clinical outcomes include te appropriate patient selection, including patients who meet the indications for use:

Adequate iliac/femoral access must be determined on pre-operative CT scan (Figs. 22.4 and 22.5). Aortic inner diameter in the range of 23–37 mm in the United

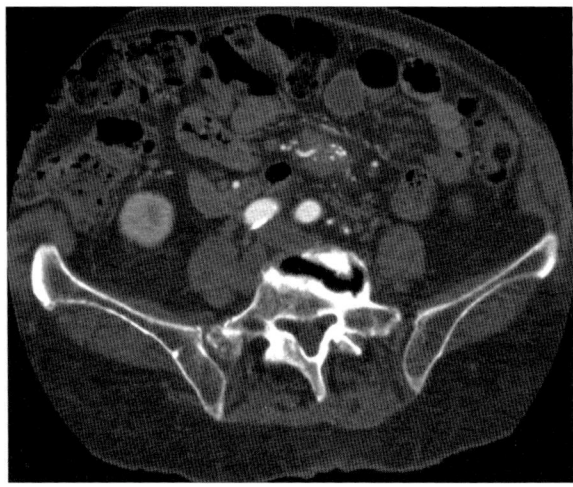

Fig. 22.4 An axial CT image demonstrating adequate-sized iliac arteries for access with mild calcification in the posterior wall of right iliac artery

Size (Fr)	ID (mm)	OD (mm)
20	6.7	7.6
22	7.3	8.3
24	8.1	9.1

Fig. 22.5 Recommended iliac diameter for the introduction of Gore delivery sheaths. ID, inner diameter; OD, outer diameter

Device diameter(mm)	Vessel diameter(mm)	Oversizing %
26	23-24	8-14
28	24-26	8-17
31	26-29	7-19
34	29-32	9-16
37	32-34	9-16
40	34-37	9-18

Fig. 22.6 Gore TAG sizing chart as recommended by IFU

States (23–42 mm outside the United States[1]) as well as the presence of ≥2 cm non-aneurysmal aorta proximal and distal to the aneurysm is required for successful endovascular treatment of thoracic aneurysms. Device selection and deployment must be in accordance with the IFU (Fig. 22.6). Appropriate and timely patient follow-up is required when a patient is managed with a thoracic endoprosthesis.

22.3 Pre-procedural Planning and Imaging

Key anatomic elements that may affect successful exclusion of thoracic aneurysm include severe proximal neck angulation, short proximal aortic neck and significant aortic neck thrombus (Fig. 22.7a), and/or calcium (Fig. 22.7b) at the arterial implantation sites, specifically the proximal aortic neck and distal iliac artery interface. In the presence of anatomical limitations, a longer neck length may be required to obtain adequate sealing and fixation. The US clinical studies quantify significant thrombus as thrombus ≥2 mm in thickness and/or ≥25% of the vessel circumference in the intended seal zone of the aortic neck. Irregular calcium and/or plaque may compromise the fixation and sealing of the implantation sites. Sizing of aortic neck diameters should be measured from axial CTA films and should consist only of the flow lumen and not the aortic wall. When determining the diameter of the proximal and distal necks for thoracic endografting (Fig. 22.8a), it is recommended that the thrombus be included in the aortic wall diameter (Fig. 22.8). When calcium is present in the aortic wall it is recommended to measure around the calcium and not the circumference. For deployment of the Gore TAG thoracic endograft aortic neck diameters should range from 23 to 37 mm in the United States (23–42 mm outside the United States). Three diameter measurements at least 1 cm apart are required for both the proximal (A–C) and distal (E–G) necks (Fig. 22.9). Diameter measurements along the entire aortic neck must be within one intended aortic inner diameter range. Measurements of all lengths should be along greater curve of flow lumen. Proximal (I) and distal (J) neck lengths should be a minimum of 20 mm.

Maximum aneurysm diameter (D) and length of aneurysm (H) are taken for characterization and follow-up purposes. Total treatment length (K) is the minimum length of aorta that needs to be treated. Iliac and femoral diameters need to accommodate the appropriate size sheath or a conduit may be necessary: a screening planning (Fig. 22.10) and case planning form (Fig. 22.11) are helpful in preplanning for endovascular management of the thoracic aorta using a Gore TAG endoprosthesis. C-arm imaging angles can be determined pre-operatively on CT scan imaging by drawing a line bisecting patient and another line perpendicular to the flow lumen at the proximal landing site. For optimal visualization, the C-arm is positioned so that it is perpendicular to the flow lumen at the target landing zone. For proximal landing zones in the arch, the C-arm is angulated 45–75° left anterior oblique (LAO). For steeper LAO projections placement of a left shoulder roll or cushion may be helpful. For distal landing zones, the C-arm angulation of 90° lateral typically positions the C-arm perpendicular to the flow lumen as well as the origin of the celiac artery.

22.4 Thrombus in Proximal Neck

22.5 Calcium in Proximal Neck

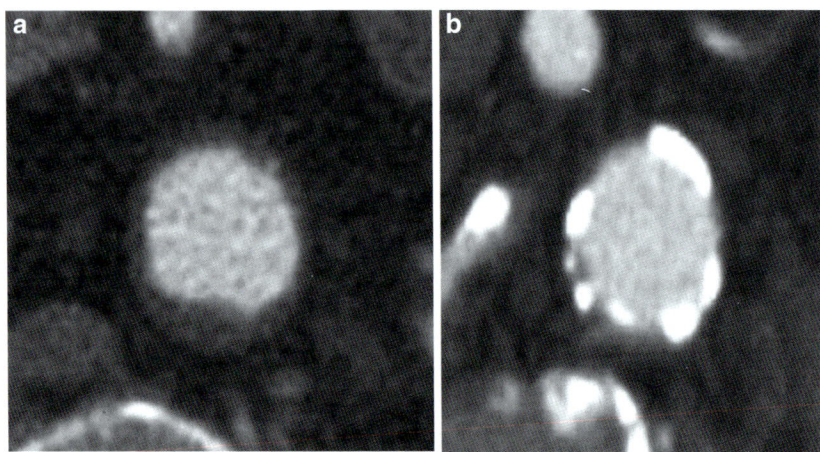

Fig. 22.7 (**a**) Axial CT image demonstrating thrombus in aortic wall. Include thrombus in diameter measurements (**b**) Axial CT image of the thoracic aorta with calcium in the neck. Measurement is made around focal calcium and circumferential calcium is excluded from diameter measurements

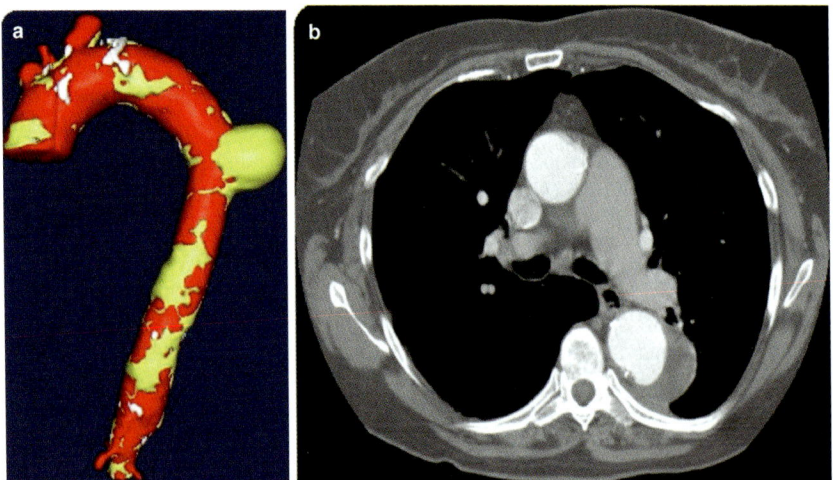

Fig. 22.8 (**a**) Three-dimensional reconstruction demonstrates the patient's thoracic aortic anatomy and of the proximal and distal landing zones. (**b**) Axial CT scan of the chest with IV contrast demonstrating a descending thoracic aneurysm with mural thrombus[2]

Fig. 22.9 A pre-operative worksheet for the Gore TAG endograft to evaluate the candidacy for stent graft placement. A, proximal implantation site; B, 1 cm proximal to implantation site; C, 2 cm from implantation site; D, aneurysm diameter; E, secondary aneurysm – N/A; F, 2 cm distal to implantation site; G, 1 cm from distal implantation site; H, distal implantation site; M, aneurysm length; N, distal neck, distance from aneurysm to celiac axis; O, total treatment length

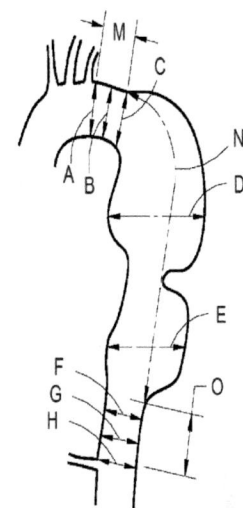

22.6 Deployment Optimization Techniques

Fluoroscopic C-arm angulation must be appropriately positioned to adequately visualize target landing zones.

The GORE TAG® Device is advanced past the target location and pulled back to release any stored energy prior to initiating deployment. The guidewire is advanced and the delivery catheter manipulated prior to deployment to ensure that the device is positioned along the outer curve of the flow lumen to allow any confirmed stored energy to be released from the deployment system. Using a two-person deployment technique ensures that sheath and delivery catheter are stabilized during deployment.

The deployment knob is then pulled with one steady rapid motion.

22.7 Procedural Steps for Deployment of Gore Device

The patient is placed in a supine position. Both groins and the entire abdomen are prepped and draped. If the right radial/brachial artery needs to be accessed, the right arm is prepped and draped. TEVAR may be performed under general, regional, or local anesthesia. Cerebrospinal fluid drainage is recommended for patients with previous abdominal aortic aneurysm repair, in whom iliac conduit or coverage of subclavian artery is planned. Patients with underlying thoracic aortic aneurysm requiring extensive stent graft coverage may require a prophylactic placement of the cerebrospinal fluid drainage catheter. The femoral artery is the access site most commonly used in (80% of the time); in 15% of times a 10 mm conduit is sewn to the common iliac artery (Fig. 22.12) and in 5% of times the ascending aorta and

PATIENT SCREENING FORM

Patient ID:		Calibration Factor:		NOTES
Institution:		CT Date:		
		Angio Date:		

Type of Aneurysm: ☐ FUSIFORM   ☐ SACULAR

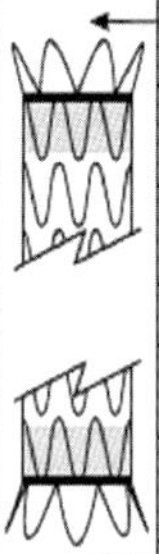

	LOCATION	MEASUREMENT List single value used to select devices	RANGE List range of measurements taken	CT TABLE POSITION / ANGIO Specify CT frame # or specify angio
DIAMETER				
A	Proximal implantation site	mm	mm	
B	1 cm from proximal implantation site	mm	mm	
C	2 cm from proximal implantation site	mm	mm	
D	Aneurysm	mm	mm	
E	2 cm from distal implantation site	mm	mm	
F	1 cm from distal implantation site	mm	mm	
G	Distal implantation site	mm	mm	
H	R common iliac	mm	mm	
I	L common iliac	mm	mm	
J	R ext. iliac/femoral	mm	mm	
K	L ext. iliac/femoral	mm	mm	
LENGTH				
L	Proximal neck Distance from aneurysm to L subclavian or L carotid	cm	cm	
M	Aneurysm			

Fig. 22.10 Screening form

distal abdominal aorta is the access site of choice. The right brachial/radial artery is accessed when planning on excluding any brachiocephalic vessels with the covered stent graft (zone 0–2 deployment in the aortic arch).[3–5] The details of iliac access have been discussed elsewhere within the access chapter.[2,5]

A femoral artery cut down is performed on the device access site. The patient is heparinized for a target activated clotting time ≥300 s. This level of anticoagulation is maintained throughout the procedure, until the femoral artery cut down is repaired and distal pulses are verified. A 12 Fr sheath is used for femoral access to potentially accommodate a large diameter occlusion balloon if acute rupture occurs. An angled soft tip guidewire is used to access the abdominal aorta, and then advanced under fluoroscopic guidance into the ascending aorta. The soft tip of the guidewire should reflect off the aortic valve, back into ascending aorta. It is important to keep this

T A G

TMORGICEXDOPROSTHESIS GORE **CASE PLANNING FORM**

Institution: _____ Patient ID: _____

Reviewer: _____ Anticipated Procedure Date: _____

| Intended Prosthesis Introduction Site | ☐ Right | ☐ Iliac | ☐ Infra-renal Aorta |
| | ☐ Left | ☐ Femoral | |

TREATMENT OPTION 1

Devices listed as implanted (proximal to distal)	Order of implantation (#1, #2, etc.)		Intended Aortic Diameters (mm)	Recommended Prosthesis Diameter (mm)	Prosthesis Lengths (cm)
			23-24	26	10
			24-26	28	10, 15
			26-29	31	10, 15
			29-32	34	10, 15, 20
			32-34	37	10, 15, 20
			34-37	40	10, 15, 20

TREATMENT OPTION 2

Devices listed as implanted (proximal to distal)	Order of implantation (#1, #2, etc.)		Additional Procedural Notes

Fig. 22.11 Case planning form

guidewire in place during the entire endovascular procedure. The anesthesiologist should be forewarned about these guidewires and watch for any arrhythmias they may cause.

The angled catheter is exchanged for an intravascular ultrasound (IVUS). The IVUS and guidewire are advanced together, under direct IVUS imaging and fluoroscopy, into the ascending aorta. This is to keep the wire out of the contained perforation site or to keep the guidewire in the true lumen (in case of aortic dissection), respectively.

The guidewire is then exchanged through the IVUS catheter for a stiff (soft tip) guidewire and the thoracic aorta interrogated with IVUS. The use of IVUS for thoracic procedures allows the surgeon to interrogate the thoracic arch and potentially map out (on the fluoroscopic screen) the arch vessels without the use of contrast. Vessel diameter and detailed pathology of the thoracic aorta including neck length, neck diameter, and aneurysm size can accurately be determined with the use of IVUS. The device can be advanced and positioned in the arch and then the first

Fig. 22.12 Ilio-femoral
conduit performed for a
retroperitoneal approach to
deployment of an endograft

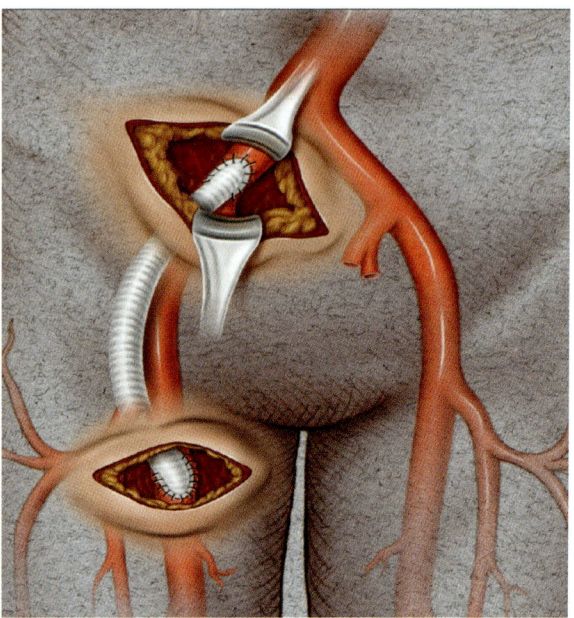

angiogram performed to confirm branch vessel location, which may have changed
with the device in place. IVUS is also invaluable in dissections to assure the device
is in the true lumen along the length.

A percutaneous 5 Fr sheath is placed in the contralateral femoral artery and a
second guidewire positioned in the ascending aorta. If the endoluminal device will
be deployed distal to the subclavian artery (landing zones 3 and 4), a 6 Fr pigtail
catheter will be positioned in the ascending aorta. (If the left subclavian artery is
going to be excluded with the covered device (landing zone 2), this guidewire will
serve as a "bailout" access guidewire. If the device is deployed inadvertently over
the left carotid artery, an 8 mm × 8 cm balloon will quickly be advanced over this
guidewire and inflated across the proximal end of the device, to allow perfusion to
the carotid artery orifice.)

A percutaneous 5 Fr sheath and subsequent pigtail catheter are placed in the
right brachial artery when the left subclavian artery is planned to be excluded or
when tortuous thoracic aorta and arch are present and the body floss maneuver is
planned. The pigtail catheter is positioned in the ascending aorta in these scenarios.

When dealing with a very tortuous aorta or an arch with a small radius, the body
floss maneuver may be helpful in advancing the device through the arch. This is
accomplished by advancing a 0.035 × 450 cm hydrophilic guidewire from the right
brachial artery to the femoral artery. The device may then be advanced over this
guidewire.

The pigtail catheter (transfemoral or through right brachial/radial) is used to perform an aortogram of the area of interest. After the angiogram is performed, the

proximal neck is evaluated. The length and the diameter of the proximal and distal neck are therefore measured using the pre-operative CT scan, intra-operative IVUS, as well as angiogram. Based on these measurements, the stent graft(s) is(are) chosen and flushed with heparinized solution; the dilator cap (largest hole) is attached to the introducer sheath. The dilator is inserted in sheath until mark is well past (within) the cap introducer sheath and is advanced over the 260 cm length stiff 0.035″ guidewire. The dilator is withdrawn and a clamp applied to the hemostasis pinch valve (Fig. 22.13). The dilator cap is exchanged for a device/balloon cap. The GORE TAG® Device is inserted in the introducer sheath after unclamping the hemostatic pinch valve and advanced into the thoracic aorta and positioned across the aneurysm. Care must be taken to optimize the image intensifier angle. The sheath is stabilized in the patient and the guidewire manipulated to ensure the device is positioned along the outer curve of the flow lumen. A repeat angiogram is commonly performed to reconfirm the positioning of the device within aorta and to serve as a road map. Prior to device deployment, the systolic blood pressure is brought down to 100 mmHg. If the patient is having a landing zone proximal to the left subclavian artery (zone 2 and higher), adenosine (36 mg for the first dose, 18 mg for subsequent doses) is administrated to gain a 4–5 s cardiac arrest. The ventilator is stopped for the deployment in intubated patients. These two measures improve deployment accuracy by reducing aortic pulsatile pressure dp/dt. The device is deployed using

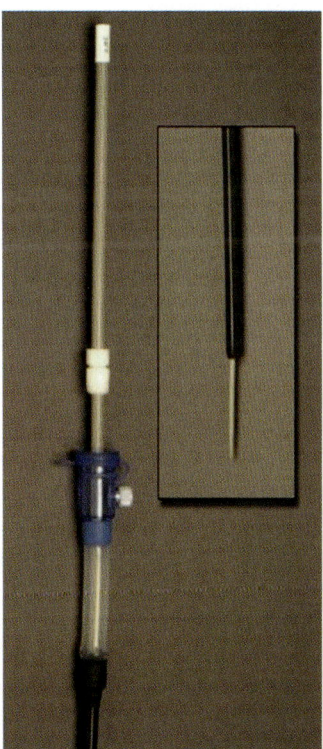

Fig. 22.13 Gore introducer sheath with silicone pinch valve. Catalogue number: 20 Fr – TS2030; 22 Fr – TS2230; 24 Fr – TS2430. All sheaths are 30 cm in length

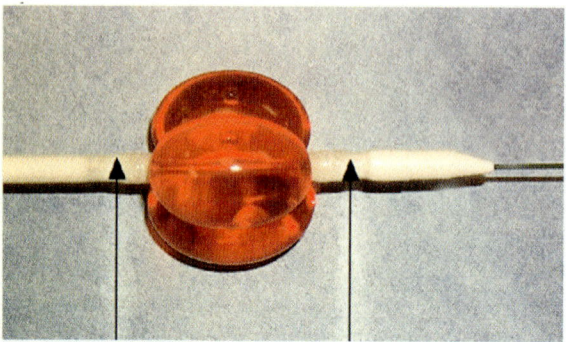

Fig. 22.14   Gore tri-lobed balloon catheter

• Designed for continuous flow BC2640
• Three-lobed silicone balloon
• 108 cm working length
• Stopcock on inflation port
• One size for all GORE TAG® Devices

a two-person deployment technique. A GORE Tri-lobe Balloon (Fig. 22.14) is used to balloon angioplasty the distal neck first, proximal neck second, then overlap areas to mould endoprosthesis to the thoracic aorta.

An IVUS interrogation of the entire stent graft and surrounding aortic branches is performed. This will detect any circumferential stent mal-apposition to the proximal or distal landing zone that may lead to endoleak. A completion angiogram is performed to confirm lack of gross endoleak. However, a single aortogram may miss endoleak due to projection overlap. A biplane aortogram is more reliable in excluding any significant intra-procedural endoleak. When multiple endoprostheses are used to compensate for aortic taper or treatment length, adhere to the sizing guide in conjunction with the recommended guidelines below: When using two endoprostheses of differing diameters, the larger device can be one or two sizes larger than the smaller device. Always deploy the larger diameter endoprosthesis into the smaller diameter endoprosthesis. Use of multiple devices with differing diameters requires a treatment length of ≥13 cm. Overlapping length is measured from gold band to gold band: 5 cm minimum for devices of same diameter and 3 cm minimum for devices of differing diameters.

Once completion of the angiogram is performed, the introducer sheath is removed carefully leaving the wire in the aorta. If there is any concern about iliac artery injury, an iliac artery angiogram is performed. If no angiogram was performed, and the patient remains hemodynamically stable, an intact iliac artery can be assumed. In this case, the wire is removed, and the femoral artery is repaired in standard fashion. If an iliac artery conduit has been performed the conduit can be tunneled through the groin and sewn to the femoral artery as an ilio-femoral bypass or transected and oversewn. The distal pulses are checked and if they correspond to pre-operative baseline, the heparin is reverse and the sterile endovascular wires/catheters may be disposed.

22.8 Patient Follow-Up and Recommendation

Regular follow-up of all patients treated with this device is required. As stated in the IFU, patients with specific clinical findings such as endoleaks and/or enlarging aneurysm should receive enhanced follow-up. Physicians should tailor patient follow-up to the needs and circumstances of each individual patient. CT/CTA film sets should include all sequential images at lowest possible slice thickness ($\leq$3 mm). Ultrasound and MRI/MRA can be used (e.g., patients with contrast sensitivity or intolerance). The GORE TAG® Device is compatible with MR follow-up. Recommended follow-up includes the following: A contrast CT with delayed non-contrast scan is performed at 1 month, 3 months, 6 months, 1 year, and annually thereafter to evaluate for endoleak, migration, device structural deterioration, etc. The close follow-up and the chance of post-operative issues requiring reintervention have to be discussed with the patient as part of the informed consent.

22.9 Preference Card

22.9.1 Sheaths

- 12 Fr sheath (Terumo/Cordis12 Fr × 10 cm Pinnacle Sheath) is used for initial femoral artery access (to accommodate large diameter balloon in case of acute rupture, it will accommodate the IVUS as well).
- 5 Fr sheath (Terumo/Cordis 5 Fr × 10 cm Pinnacle Sheath) used for percutaneous access of contralateral femoral artery.
- 5 Fr sheath (Terumo/Cordis 5 Fr × 10 cm Pinnacle Sheath) used for right brachial/radial artery (for zone 0–2 deployment in the aortic arch).
- Micro-Puncture Introducer Set (Cook, Inc. 4 Fr, MPIS-401).
- 20–24 Fr sheath as per stent graft manufacturer's IFU.

22.9.2 Catheters

- 5 Fr Bern (Boston Scientific 5 Fr × 100 cm Imager II Selective-Berenstein tip) or angled tip catheter used for initial femoral access.
- 5 Fr pigtail catheter (Cook, Inc., 5 Fr × 90 cm Pigtail-Royal Flush Plus) used in the contralateral femoral artery (if brachial is not available).
- 5 Fr Bern (Boston Scientific 4 Fr × 100 cm Imager II Selective) or angled tip catheter (if brachial artery access is used).

- 5 Fr pigtail catheter (Cook, Inc., 4 Fr × 90 cm Pigtail-Royal Flush Plus) when using brachial artery.
- 8.2 Fr IVUS catheter (Volcano, 8.2 Fr × 90 cm Vision PV, 8.2 Fr, 8–12 MHz).

22.9.3 Guidewires

- 0.035 × 180 cm Bentson Starter guidewire (Boston Scientific 0.035 × 180 cm Bentson).
- 0.035 (or 0.025) × 260 cm Stiff type guidewire with soft tip (Boston Scientific 0.025 × 260 cm Platinum Plus ST Guidewire; Boston Scientific 0.035 × 260 cm Amplatz Super Stiff Guidewire, 6 cm tip length; Boston Scientific 0.035 × 260 cm Meier Guidewire, 10 cm tip length; Cook, Inc., 0.035 × 260 cm TFE-coated Lunderquist Guidewire, 15 cm tip; ev3, Inc. 0.035 × 260 cm Nitrex wire).
- 0.035 × 180 cm hydrophilic guidewire (Terumo 0.035 × 180 cm Glide wire).
- 0.035 × 450 cm hydrophilic guidewire (Terumo 0.035 × 450 cm Glide wire).

22.9.4 Balloons

- 8 mm × 8 cm angioplasty balloon (Boston Scientific 8 mm × 8 cm Ultrathin Diamond Balloon).
- Large diameter (~40 mm) compliant occlusion balloons (Medtronic 12 Fr Reliant Stent Graft Balloon, 46 mm max diameter; Cook, Inc., 14 Fr CODA Balloon Catheter, 40 mm max diameter, 20 Fr Gore Tri-lobe Balloon 40 mm max diameter).

22.9.5 Miscellaneous

- Dilator (Endovascular Dilator Set, Cook, Inc., 20–24 Fr).
- Snare (Medical Device Technologies 27–45 mm EN Snare).
- Luer-Lock (Boston Scientific FloSwitch HP).
- Needle for initial arterial access (Boston Scientific Arterial Entry Needle 18 G, $2\frac{3}{4}$ in., Cook 18 G $2\frac{3}{4}$ in.).

References

1. Makaroun MS, Dillavou ED, Kee ST, et al. Endovascular treatment of thoracic aortic aneurysms: results of the phase II multicenter trial of the GORE TAG thoracic endoprosthesis. *J Vasc Surg.* 2005;41:1–9.
2. Diethrich EB, Ramaiah VG, Kpodonu J, Rodriguez-Lopez JA. *Endovascular and Hybrid Management of the Thoracic Aorta. A Case Based Approach.* West Sussex: Wiley-Blackwell; 2008.

3. Casserly IP, Sacher R, Yadav JS, eds. *Manual of Peripheral Vascular Intervention*. Philadelphia, PA: Lippincott Williams and Wilkins; 2005.

4. Zelenock GB, ed. *Mastery of Vascular and Endovascular Surgery*. Philadelphia, PA: Lippincott Williams and Wilkins; 2006.

5. Kpodonu J, Rodriguez-Lopez JA, Ramaiah VG, Diethrich EB. Use of the right brachio-femoral wire approach to manage a thoracic aortic aneurysm in an extremely angulated and tortuous aorta with an endoluminal stent graft. *Interact Cardiovasc Thorac Surg.* 2008;7(2):269.

Chapter 23
Gore TAG Multicenter Phase II Trial

23.1 Gore TAG Thoracic Endoprosthesis

The Gore excluder thoracic endoprosthesis (Gore & Associates, Flagstaff, AZ) was the first thoracic endograft to enter clinical trials in the United States in 1998 with a feasibility trial. This was followed by the pivotal study in 1999. The Gore TAG excluder device gained FDA approval in March 2005 for the commercial use for the treatment of thoracic aortic aneurysms (TAA) (Fig. 23.1).

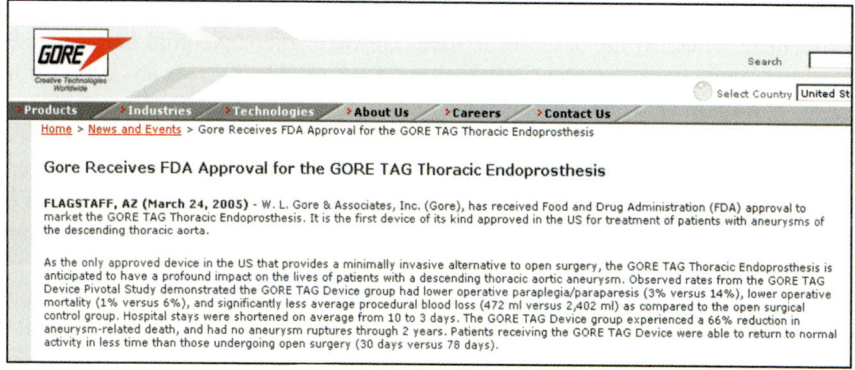

Fig. 23.1 Federal drug administration approves use of thoracic endoluminal graft for treatment of thoracic aneurysms

23.2 Device Design

The TAG endoprosthesis is a symmetrical expanded PTFE (ePTFE) tube reinforced with ePTFE/fluorinated ethylene propylene (FEP) film and an external nickel–titanium (nitinol) self-expanding stent along the entire surface of the graft (Fig. 23.2). The stent is attached to the graft with ePTFE/FEP bonding tape. A circumferential PTFE sealing cuff is located on the external surface of the endograft at the base of each flared, scalloped end. Flares are designed to help with conforming to

J. Kpodonu, *Manual of Thoracic Endoaortic Surgery*,
DOI 10.1007/978-1-84996-296-4_23, © Springer-Verlag London Limited 2010

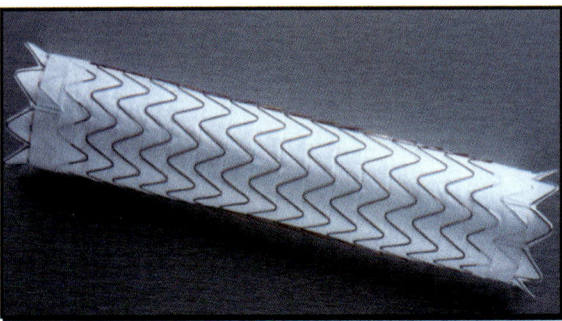

Fig. 23.2 Gore TAG thoracic endoprosthesis

tortuous anatomy. Each cuff is circumferentially attached on one edge with FEP, thus allowing the other end to remain free to enhance sealing of the endoprosthesis to the aortic wall and help eliminate endoleaks.

The original TAG device graft material was constructed from two ePTFE layers with two longitudinal wires for support during deployment. The modified TAG device is constructed from three ePTFE layers. The additional layer, similar to that incorporated into the excluder bifurcated endoprosthesis, is sandwiched between the two original layers and provides support that was formerly provided by the deployment wires. At the base of the flares are two radiopaque gold bands, which serve as a guide during implantation and in follow-up. The devices are available in 26–40 mm diameters that accommodate aortic diameters between 23 and 37 mm and require 20–24 Fr introducer sheaths, depending on the device size. Recently a 45 mm diameter device has been introduced under investigational device protocol.

Deployment of the TAG device is unique. A sleeve made of ePTFE/FEP film is used to constrain the endograft. A deployment knob is located at the control end of the delivery catheter and has a deployment line that runs the entire length of the catheter connecting it to the sleeve. Turning and pulling the deployment knob removes the deployment line from the endograft, thereby deploying it. The device is deployed rapidly from the middle of the endograft toward both ends of the prosthesis. The device is then secured in position with a specially designed tri-lobed balloon, which allows continuous blood flow during inflation.

23.3 Feasibility Study

The first trial to be conducted in the United States was the feasibility study to establish preliminary device safety data. This study was performed at two sites in the United States and enrolled a total of 28 patients between 1998 and 1999. The 30-day mortality rate was 3.6% ($n = 1$). At 1 year, the mortality rate was 21% without any paraplegia or stroke. Renal failure and myocardial infarction were noted in one patient each (3.6%). Through a 5-year follow-up period, two additional adverse events were reported between 2 and 5 years. All-cause mortality at 5 years was 25%. Endoleaks were noted at any time in 21% of the patients, and aneurysm sac growth was noted in 18%. Stent fractures were noted in 32%. There was one conversion and there were two reinterventions over time to place additional devices. No aneurysm ruptures, device migration, extrusion, erosion, lumen obstruction, or branch vessel occlusions were reported.

Once device safety was demonstrated with the feasibility study the pivotal phase II trial was undertaken.

23.4 Pivotal (Phase II) Trial

23.4.1 Objectives and Hypotheses

The objectives were to determine the safety and efficacy of the TAG endoprosthesis for the treatment of DTA as compared with open surgical repair controls. The primary safety hypothesis was that the percentage of subjects with one or more major adverse events (MAEs) through 1 year after treatment would be lower in the TAG group as compared with the surgical control group. The primary efficacy hypothesis was that freedom from any major device-related events through 1 year of follow-up for the TAG device group would be better than 80%. A predefined point estimate of 80% for the endovascular group was considered to be a reasonable efficacy outcome, because the device was expected to show a considerable improvement in safety profile. The efficacy for the surgical procedure was assumed to be 100%. The secondary hypotheses were that the procedural blood loss, intensive care unit (ICU) and hospital stay, and convalescence to normal activities would be lower in the TAG device group as compared with the surgical control group. The primary efficacy end point of this pivotal study was the percentage of subjects who were free from major device-related events through 1 year of follow-up for the TAG device group.

23.4.2 Study Design

This study was a prospective, nonrandomized, controlled multicenter trial. The study enrolled 140 study patients and 94 control subjects between September 1999 and May 2001 through 17 clinical sites in the United States. The control group consisted of 44 patients acquired prospectively during the study and 50 historical patients acquired by selecting the most recent surgical patients in reverse chronological order. Inclusion and exclusion criteria are detailed in Tables 23.1 and 23.2.

23.4.3 Follow-Up

All patients are to be followed for 5 years. Computed tomography (CT) scans, plain radiographs, and physical examinations were obtained at 1-month, 6-month, and 12-month intervals and yearly thereafter. A 3-month visit with a CT scan was

Table 23.1   Inclusion criteria

Criterion	Gore TAG
Age (years)	>21
Women	Must be infertile
Open surgical candidate	Yes
Neck length	Minimal 2 cm proximal and distal
Aneurysm	Fusiform descending thoracic aorta at least twice the size of normal thoracic aorta; saccular
Penetrating ulcer	No
Proximal landing zone location	20 mm distal to left common carotid artery
Distal landing zone location	20 mm proximal to celiac axis
Landing zone diameter (mm)	23–37

Table 23.2   Exclusion criteria

Criterion	Gore TAG
Creatinine (mg/dl)	>2.0
Unstable rupture	Yes
Mycotic aneurysm	Yes
Connective tissue disease	Yes
Significant landing zone thrombus	Yes
Previous descending aortic surgery or endovascular repair of descending thoracic aneurysm or abdominal aortic aneurysm	N/A
Aortic dissection	Yes
Coagulopathy	Yes
Miocardial infarction/cerebrovascular accident	<6 weeks
Major operation within 30 days	Yes
Participation in another investigational study	<1 year

N/A, not applicable

conducted for patients with early endoleaks. A core laboratory reviewed all imaging studies. Clinical data were reported by individual centers and monitored by sponsor representatives. Major adverse effects were adjudicated by the Clinical Events Committee and defined as clinical events that required therapy or that resulted in an unintended increase in the level of care, prolonged hospitalization, permanent adversity, or death.[1] Minor adverse events were those that did not require any therapy or those with no consequences.

23.4.4 Results of the Pivotal Study

23.4.4.1 Clinical Material

The TAG group and the surgical group were very similar in all major demographic and clinical variables (Table 23.3). The average age of the patients was 71 years in

Table 23.3 Patient demographics

Variable	TAG group	Surgical control
Male (%)	57	51
Age (years)	71	68
Ethnicity (%)		
White	87	86
Black	8	10
Other	5	4
Height (cm)	170	170
Weight (kg)	76	78

the TAG group and 68 years in the control group. Men accounted for 58% of the patients in the TAG group and 51% in the control group.

Baseline aortic morphology was also well matched between the groups, except for the smaller diameter of the proximal and distal necks in the TAG device group, which was expected because of the requirements for sealing. Baseline co-morbidities were also quite similar between the TAG device group and the control group (Table 23.4). Although coronary artery disease seemed to be more prevalent among the TAG group, this difference was not significant. Symptomatic aneurysms, however, were significantly more prevalent in the control group than in the TAG group. The risk classifications performed on the basis of the standard American Society of Anesthesiologists classification and the society of vascular surgery risk score showed no significant difference in either classification.

Table 23.4 Comparison of early complications between TAG and open surgical controls in the Gore pivotal study

Variable	TAG device (%)	Surgical control (%)	*P* value
Coronary artery disease	49	36	0.06
Cardiac arrhythmia	24	31	0.23
Stroke	10	10	>0.95
PVOD	16	11	0.33
Prior vascular intervention	45	55	0.14
Symptomatic aneurysm	21	38	<0.01
Other concomitant aneurysms	28	28	>0.95
COPD	40	38	0.89
Smoking	84	82	0.86
Renal dialysis	1	0	0.52
Hepatic dysfunction	2	1	0.65
Paraplegia	1	0	>0.95
Cancer	19	13	0.21

PVOD, peripheral vascular occlusive disease; COPD, chronic obstructive pulmonary disease

23.4.5 Operative Data

Of 142 patients recruited (140 in the pivotal trial and 2 extended access), 139 (98%) underwent successful implantation of the TAG device. The three failures were all due to poor iliac access. A conduit was placed to facilitate access in 21 patients (15%). More than one device were used in 77 patients (55%); 61 patients (44%) received two devices, 11 patients (8%) received three devices, and 5 patients (4%) received four devices.

Prophylactic left carotid/subclavian bypass grafting was performed in 28 patients in preparation for planned left subclavian artery coverage with the device. Unplanned subclavian artery and visceral artery coverage occurred in one patient each. The latter underwent an open abdominal explantation of the device and redeployment of a new device without sequelae.

23.4.6 Early Adverse Events

23.4.6.1 Mortality

Operative mortality, defined as death within 30 days of the procedure or on the same day of hospital admission, occurred in three patients (2.1%) after TAG implantation (Table 23.5). One death was due to a post-operative stroke and another to a cardiac event that occurred on post-operative day 11. The third death occurred after 7 months of a protracted hospital course as a result of anoxic brain injury after a respiratory arrest. The patient died of septic complications from an aorto-esophageal fistula. Six deaths (6.4%) occurred in the surgical control group.

Table 23.5 Operative complications

Variable	TAG	Open surgical
Death	2.1%	11.7%
Paraplegia/paraparesis	3	14
Stroke	4	4

23.4.7 Spinal Cord Ischemia

Spinal drainage was not routinely used in either group. In the TAG group, spinal cord ischemia (SCI) was noted in four patients. One was noted immediately after the procedure, and the deficit persisted despite all supportive measures. Three were delayed in onset, and all these regained motor function (one complete and two partial) and were ambulatory at last follow-up. It should be noted that multiple pieces of TAG endografts were used in three of four patients and that two of four patients had had previous infra-renal aortic aneurysm repair. The incidence of SCI did not differ between those with and without prior abdominal aortic aneurysm repair (4.7 versus 2%, respectively). The incidence of SCI in the control group was significantly higher (13.8%). Of 13 patients, 8 had paraplegia, of whom 6 died. One case of paraplegia resolved completely.

23.4.8 Cerebrovascular Accidents

Perioperative stroke was noted in five patients (3.5%). One was fatal. Three were right-sided. Four of the five strokes occurred in patients who had proximal aneurysms requiring extension of the TAG to the left carotid and coverage of the subclavian artery; all four underwent carotid/subclavian bypass. Of the 28 patients with proximal aneurysms who had planned subclavian artery coverage, 4 (14%) had a stroke, compared with 1 (1%) of 114 with disease distal to the subclavian artery ($P < 0.001$). The overall incidence of cerebrovascular accident (4.3%) was similar in the two groups.

23.4.9 Endoleaks

Early endoleaks were seen in five patients. One patient had a proximal type I endoleak and was treated with endovascular revision and additional grafts. The remaining endoleaks were thought to be type II.

23.4.10 Other MAEs

The other most common MAEs were bleeding, cardiopulmonary events, and intra-operative vascular injury. Both bleeding and pulmonary events were significantly reduced in the TAG group compared with the surgical control group, due to a high percentage of procedural bleeding and respiratory failure in the latter.

The incidence of vascular injuries was 14% in the TAG group, which was significantly higher than in the control group (4%). This was related to the introduction of large introducer sheaths through the iliac system.

23.4.11 Hospital Length of Stay

The average ICU stay was significantly shorter in the TAG group compared with the control group (2.6 ± 14.6 days versus 5.2 ± 7.2 days; $P < 0.001$), as was total length of stay (7.4 ± 17.7 days versus 14.4 ± 12.8 days; $P < 0.001$).

23.4.12 Late Outcome

23.4.12.1 Late Survival

All-cause mortality through 3 years did not differ in the two groups (Fig. 23.3). The causes of death were commensurate with associated co-morbidities in this elderly population. No ruptures have been reported.

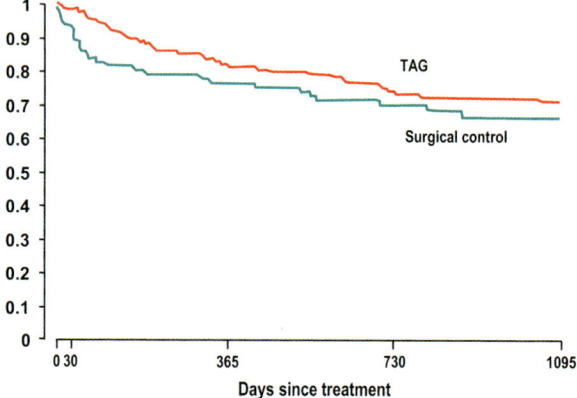

Fig. 23.3 Comparison of Kaplan-Meier estimates for all-cause mortality through the 3-year follow-up between the Gore TAG and surgical control groups

With respect to aneurysm-related mortality, defined as death before hospital discharge, death within 30 days of the primary procedure or within 30 days of any secondary procedure to treat the original aneurysm, or death due to aneurysm rupture, there was one late death in the TAG group. This patient had an aneurysm growth in the setting of graft infection at 2 months. The patient underwent an open conversion and was found to have an aorto-esophageal fistula, which was treated by graft excision and an extra-anatomic bypass, only to experience a respiratory arrest on post-operative day 13 with resultant anoxic brain injury. The patient died 3 days later. In the open surgical group, three additional deaths occurred during the first 6 months of follow-up. Freedom from aneurysm-related mortality through 3 years was 97% for the TAG device group and 90% for the open surgical controls ($P = 0.024$). No mortalities were noted in either group after the first year (Fig. 23.4).[2]

23.4.12.2 Major Adverse Events

The Kaplan-Meier estimates of the probability of freedom from MAEs were significantly higher with TAG treatment (58%) than with open surgical controls: 48 versus 20% at 3 years, respectively (Fig. 23.5). In fact, 70% of all MAEs occurred within 30 days of the original procedure. A similar observation was made in the feasibility study, in which 63% of all events over 5 years were noticed in the first 30 days.

23.4.13 Device-Related Events

During a 3-year follow-up, five patients underwent endovascular revisions, and one patient underwent surgical conversion. Three of the revisions occurred after 24 months of follow-up. Device migrations, three proximal and four components,

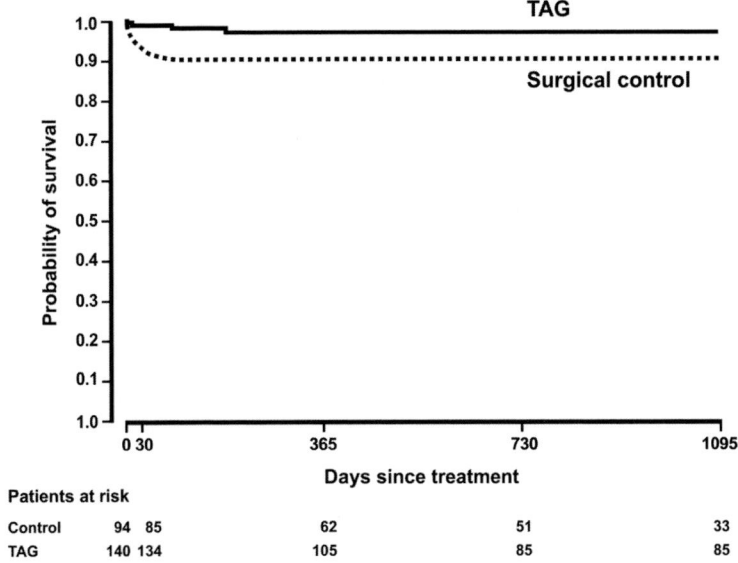

Fig. 23.4 Comparison of Kaplan-Meier estimates for aneurysm-related mortality through 3-year follow-up between the Gore TAG and surgical control groups

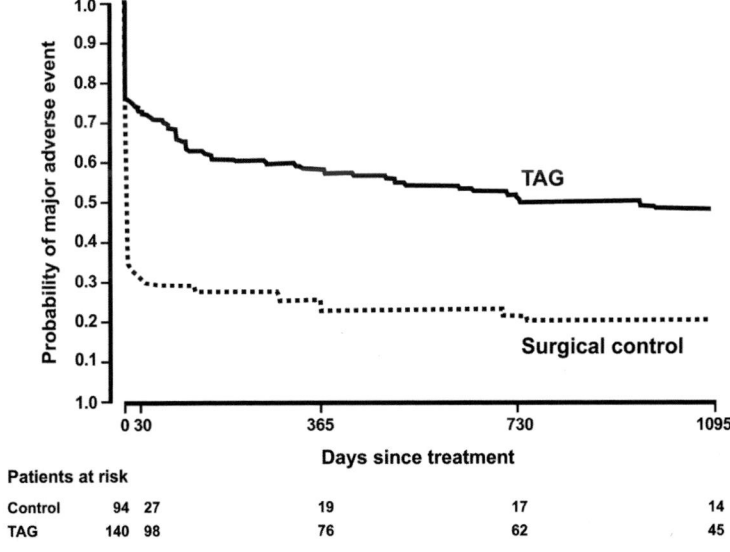

Fig. 23.5 Comparison of Kaplan-Meier estimates for freedom from major adverse events through the 3-year follow-up between the Gore TAG and surgical control groups

were noted without clinical compromise at the 2-year follow-up. Sac shrinkage of greater than 5 mm was observed in 38% (24/64) and sac expansion in 17% (11/64) of patients. Three of the 11 patients with sac enlargement had endoleaks at some point during follow-up. Twenty fractures were noted in 19 patients: 18 in the longitudinal spine and 2 in the apical nitinol support rings. Clinical sequelae developed in only one patient, who developed a type III endoleak that was treated with an endograft. No ruptures were noted at a follow-up extending to 2 years. No device-related deaths were noted through 3 years.

23.4.14 Confirmatory Study

23.4.14.1 Objectives and Hypotheses

The confirmatory study was launched to demonstrate that deployment and early results with the modified device are comparable to those with the original device. The safety and efficacy hypotheses were the same as in the pivotal trial except for using a 30-day end point. This earlier safety end point was chosen as an appropriate measure on the basis of the results of the pivotal study, in which most MAEs occurred within the 30-day period. Almost all major device-related events were also identified in the first 30 days during the pivotal trial. Although 30-day study end points were used, all patients are to be followed up to 5 years. Inclusion and exclusion criteria were identical to those used in the pivotal study.

23.4.14.2 Design

The confirmatory study was a prospective, nonrandomized trial, with all test subjects treated with the modified TAG device. The study was performed at 11 sites, all but one of which had participated in the pivotal trial. Fifty-one patients were enrolled in this study, and their results were compared with the same 94 control subjects used in the pivotal study.

23.4.14.3 Results of the Confirmatory Study

Clinical Materials

Baseline demographics and aortic morphology were quite similar in the TAG device group and the surgical control group. Co-morbidities were also well matched. In this comparison, the symptomatic aneurysm difference did not reach statistical significance. However, there was a higher prevalence of cancer or a history of cancer in the TAG device group compared with the surgical control group. Risk classification according to the American Society of Anesthesiologists was very well matched between the TAG and the surgical control groups. The Society of Vascular Surgery Risk Score was slightly higher in the TAG device group, and this was significant.

Early MAEs

At 30 days, the incidence of MAEs was 12% in the TAG group and 70% in the controls, a highly significant difference corresponding to an 83% risk reduction for those treated with the TAG device. No early deaths were noted in the TAG group. The rate of vascular complications was not significantly different in this cohort compared with the surgical controls.

Kaplan-Meier estimates of the probability of freedom from MAEs through 30 days showed a significant advantage for the TAG device group compared with the surgical control group ($P < 0.001$).

Device-Related Events

No major device-related events were reported through the 30-day follow-up in the test subjects compared with six (4%) reported for the pivotal study test subjects.

Hospital length of stay was shorter with the TAG device compared with the control group (3 versus 10 days, respectively). The time to return to normal activities was shortened in the TAG group to 15 days versus 78 days for the control group.

Results from the Gore TAG trials [3,4] have shown the safety of endovascular repair of thoracic aortic aneurysm is superior to open surgical repair at short-term and mid-term results with operative mortality and morbidity and spinal chord ischemia lower than those observed for open surgical repair. Patients treated with the endovascular approach had a lower length of hospital stay, lower length of ICU stay, lower blood transfusions, rapid recovery rates, lower aneurysm-related deaths and fewer device-related complications.

The incidence of spinal chord ischemic though lower than with open surgical repair is still a major source of morbidity and mortality. Potential risk factors include extensive coverage of the descending thoracic aorta, open abdominal aneurysm repair with extensive coverage of descending thoracic aorta,[1,2,5] and possibly coverage of the left subclavian artery with extensive coverage of the descending thoracic aorta.

Vascular complications were more frequent in the endovascular group compared to the open surgical group. Small access vessels especially in females who comprised 50% of the thoracic aneurysm group are at risk of potential rupture when large sheaths are inserted. Conduits should be readily used as prophylactic procedure when small, tortuous, and calcified vessels are anticipated.

The risk of endoleak requires lifelong surveillance of patients with regular CXR to detect device-related complications like migration or stent fracture and CT scan to follow endoleaks, aneurysm sac regression, or expansion.

In conclusion The Gore TAG US trial has shown the efficacy of the Gore TAG excluder device for the treatment of thoracic aortic aneurysm. The application of this technology to other aortic pathologies is still under investigative trial protocols. Long-term data is required to establish better outcomes in the management of patients with thoracic aortic aneurysms. The evolution of more flexible end grafts, smaller delivery sheaths, and branched endografts would expand the application of this technology to patients with varied thoracic aortic pathologies.

References

1. Gravereaux EC, Faries PL, Burks JA, et al. Risk of spinal chord ischemia after endograft repair of thoracic aortic aneurysms. *J Vasc Surg*. 2001;31:997–1003.
2. Moon MR, Mitchell RS, Dake MD, Zarins CK, Fann JL, Miller DG. Simultaneous abdominal aortic replacement and thoracic stent graft placement for multilevel aortic disease's. *J Vasc Surg*. 1997;25:332–340.
3. Makaroun MS, Dillavou ED, Kes ST, et al. Endovascular treatment of thoracic aortic aneurysms: results of the phase II multicenter trial of the Gore TAG thoracic endoprosthesis. *J Vasc Surg*. 2005;41:1–9.
4. Gore TAG Thoracic Endoprosthesis Annual Clinical Update (April 2010).
5. Greenberg R, Resch T, Nyman U, et al. Endovascular repair of descending thoracic aortic aneurysm: an early experience with intermediate-term follow-up. *J Vasc Surg*. 2000;31: 147–156.

Chapter 24
Five-Year Results of Endovascular Treatment with the Gore TAG Device Compared with Open Repair of Thoracic Aortic Aneurysms

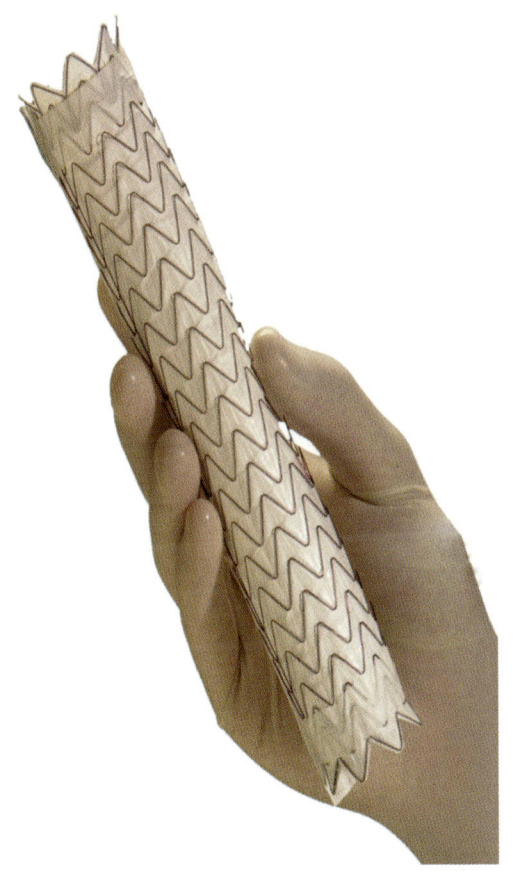

The Gore TAG pivotal trial was a multicenter, prospective, nonrandomized phase II study that recruited surgical candidates with DTA from September 1999 through May 2001. One hundred and forty endovascular patients were enrolled. Ninety-four patients with DTA treated by open surgery were used as a control group. Of the 94 open surgical control patients, 44 were concurrent subjects and 50 were historic

J. Kpodonu, *Manual of Thoracic Endoaortic Surgery*,
DOI 10.1007/978-1-84996-296-4_24, © Springer-Verlag London Limited 2010

controls from the enrolling institutions. Details on the two populations have been previously described in the Gore TAG multicenter phase II Trial.[1,2] The groups were not significantly different on pre-operative co-morbidities or presentation other than there were more symptomatic aneurysm patients in the open surgical group (38 vs. 21%, $P = 0.007$), and there were marginally more patients with cardiac histories in the TAG group (49 vs. 36%, $P = 0.06$). In May 2001, fractures of the longitudinal spine of the TAG graft were noted. The device was modified by eliminating the longitudinal wire and introducing a new stronger and less porous polytetrafluoroethylene (PTFE) material. From January 2004 to June 2004, an additional 51 TEVAR patients were enrolled in a confirmatory TAG arm using the modified device, which is the currently marketed device.

Patients with DTA of at least twice the diameter of the normal thoracic aorta and with 2 cm of non-aneurysmal neck for sealing distal to the left carotid artery and proximal to the celiac artery were eligible for endovascular treatment. TAG devices ranged from 26 to 40 mm in diameter. Open repair was performed according to local protocols at the participating institutions. The extent of the open repair could not extend more proximally than the left carotid artery and more distally than the celiac axis. There were no mandates regarding use of spinal cord protection strategies or use of left heart bypass. High-risk patients, including those with dissection, ruptures, mycotic aneurysms, and trauma, were excluded, as were medically high-risk patients. Follow-up exams, four-view chest x-rays, and spiral computed tomography (CT) scans were performed at 1, 6, and 12 months and yearly thereafter. These assessments were performed at 3 months if an endoleak was present. Five-year follow-up was concluded for all available patients in August 2006.

The primary aims of this nationwide multicenter device trial were to evaluate the safety and efficacy of the TAG endoprosthesis in comparison with open surgical repair as treatment for descending thoracic aortic aneurysms at 1 year, with follow-up scheduled to reach 5 years.[3] Safety was determined by comparing the occurrence of major adverse events between the two treatment groups. Efficacy was measured by the incidence of major device-related events that required intervention. Secondary endpoints of the study were comparisons of the early clinical parameters of blood loss, ICU, and hospital stays and time to return to normal activities.

24.1 Follow-Up

TAG group follow-up was from 3 days to 66 months with a mean of 37 months. Surgical controls were compared with this group with a follow-up of 1 day to 73 months, mean 33 months. Twenty-six percent of TAG patients and 33% of the open controls were lost to follow-up and did not complete 5-year follow-up. These patients were followed for an average of 29 months (TAG) and 30 months (open).

Death occurred in 32% of TAG and 33% of open controls during follow-up. Thirty-six percent of TAG and 24.5% of open patients completed the 5-year follow-up as outlined in the trial protocol.

24.2 Mortality

In up to 66 months after DTA repair, there have been four aneurysm-related deaths (2.8%) in the TAG group, and 11 aneurysm-related deaths (11.7%) in the open surgical group ($P = 0.008$). In the TAG cohort, three of these deaths were within the original hospitalization, resulting from stroke, cardiac causes, and sepsis. One later death occurred 2 months after TAG placement when the patient was found to have an aorto-esophageal fistula. In the open surgical group, deaths were due to respiratory failure ($n = 6$), stroke ($n = 3$), cardiac causes ($n = 1$), and aorto-esophageal fistula ($n = 1$). All deaths occurred within the first year after treatment. The probability of freedom from aneurysm-related death was significantly higher ($P < 0.01$) in the TAG endograft arm versus surgical controls 5 years after treatment (Fig. 24.1).

Death from all causes was similar between the TAG and open surgical groups (Fig. 24.2). Over 60 months, there were 45 deaths in the TAG group and 31 deaths in the surgical cohort, resulting in respective survival rates of 68 and 67% (log-rank test P value $= 0.433$). Cardiac events, respiratory failure, stroke, and malignancy were the leading causes of death in both groups (Table 24.1). There were no known cases of aneurysm rupture in either group although autopsy studies were rarely performed.

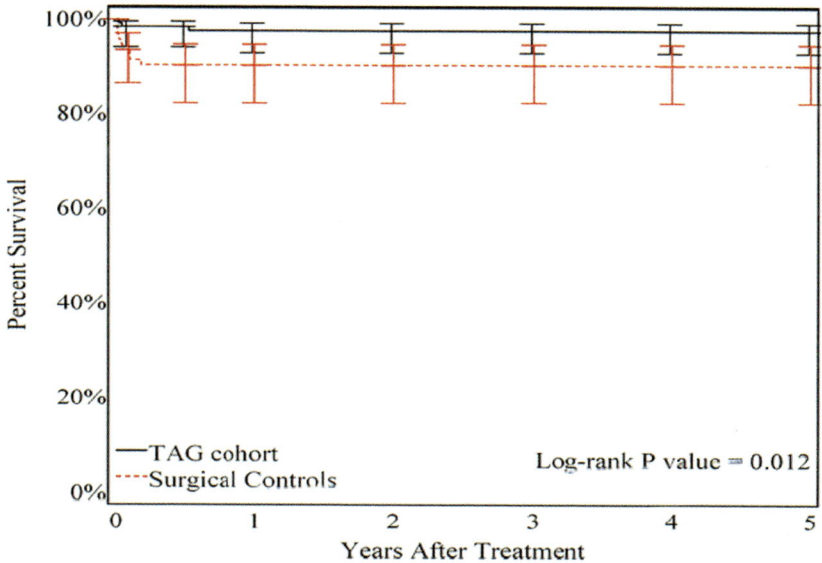

Fig. 24.1 Freedom from aneurysm-related death to 5 years

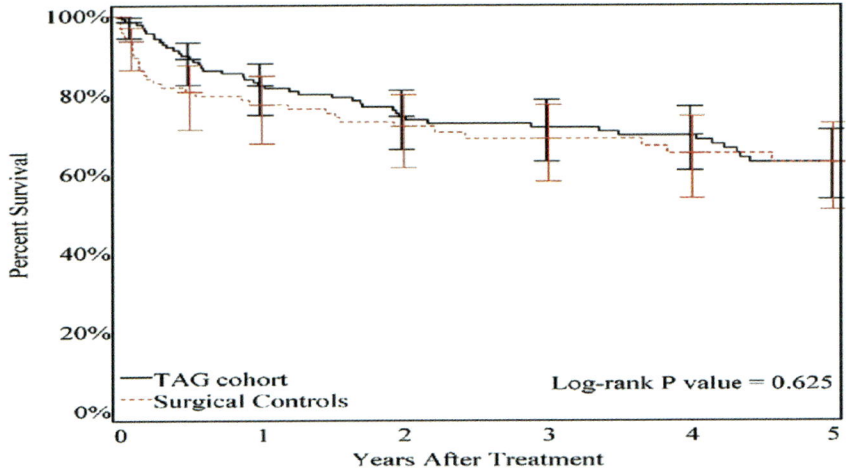

	1 year	2 years	3 years	4 years	5 years
95% C.I. TAG	.749, .879	.662, .811	.632, .787	.609, .770	.534, .712
95% C.I. Control	.677, .848	.617, .800	.582, .776	.538, .746	.509, .728

Fig. 24.2 Freedom from all-cause mortality 5 years after DTA

Table 24.1 Causes of death after descending thoracic aneurysm repair out to 5 years

Aneurysm-related deaths

Cause of death	TAG cohort (number of patients)	Surgical controls (number of patients)
Respiratory failure		6
Stroke	1	3
Cardiac arrest	1	1
Aorto-esophageal fistula	1	1
Respiratory failure after conversion	1	
All-cause mortality		
Cardiac arrest/MI	17	6
Cancer	4	2
Respiratory failure	5	8
Pneumonia	3	1
CHF	4	
Stroke	3	4
Paraplegia		1
Sepsis	4	3
Pulmonary embolism	1	
Ruptured AAA	1	
Mesenteric ischemia	1	
Trauma		1
Unknown	2	5
Total	45	31

MI, myocardial infarction; *CHF*, congenital heart failure; *AAA*, abdominal aortic aneurysm

24.3 Adverse Events

Major adverse events (MAE) after DTA repair primarily occurred in the immediate post-operative period, where 28% of TAG patients and 70% of surgical controls had at least one MAE ($P < 0.001$). The early advantage of fewer TAG MAEs continued throughout follow-up, with 12-month MAE rates of 42% in the TAG group and 77% in the surgical cohort ($P < 0.001$). Kaplan-Meier analysis demonstrated a log-rank value of $P = 0.001$ for differences in the occurrence of MAEs between the TAG and surgical control patients out to 5 years, with 57.9% of TAG and 78.7% of open patients having at least one MAE (Fig. 24.3).

At 5 years, TAG patients were significantly less likely to have had any bleeding, pulmonary, renal, wound, or neurologic complications. TAG patients were more likely to have had vascular complications ($P = 0.004$). Cumulative MAE rates, which plot each MAE rather than the number of patients who had any MAE, showed that the average number of MAEs per patient at 5 years was 2.1 for TAG patients and 3.1 for surgical controls (Fig. 24.4).

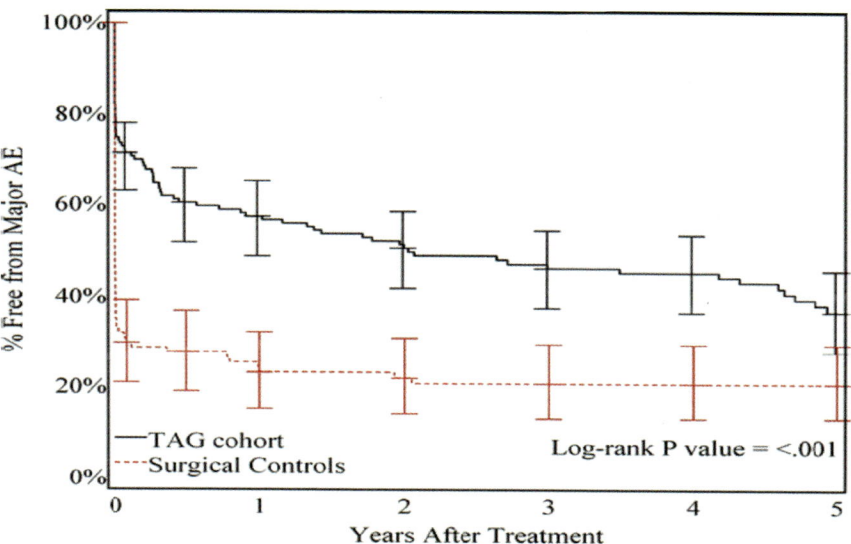

Fig. 24.3 Freedom from major adverse events over time

24.3.1 Endoleaks, Reinterventions, and Secondary Procedures

Endoleaks occurred in 10.6% of pivotal TAG patients at some point during 5 years of follow-up (Table 24.2). Remarkably, very few were suspected to be type II from intercostal arteries, and none of these were treated directly. Most endoleaks were thought to be type I at the attachment sites.

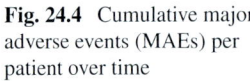
Fig. 24.4 Cumulative major
adverse events (MAEs) per
patient over time

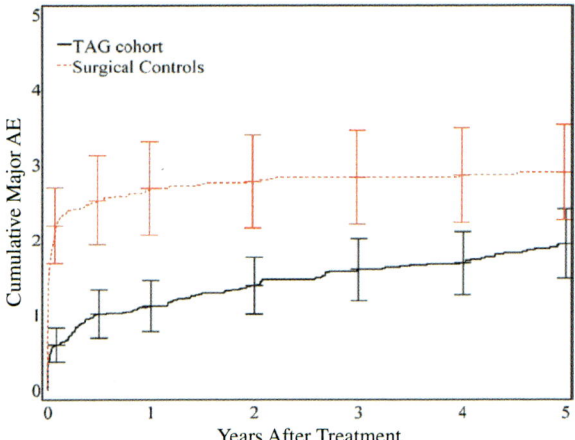

There have been 20 spine fractures seen in 19 TAG patients, with only one patient
(described above) requiring treatment.

Five TAG patients have had additional thoracic reinterventions directly related to
the DTA treated (Table 24.3). Three patients have required a total of five endovascular reinterventions for endoleaks. These additional procedures took place from 45
to 1525 days after the original repairs. One of the patients who had an endovascular
reintervention had a spine fracture in the original endoprosthesis used. This patient
also had a carotid-subclavian bypass to allow for TAG extension and developed
hematoma complications from this at the neck and groin. One patient underwent
conversion to open repair after discovery of an aorto-esophageal fistula 73 days
after TAG placement. He died of respiratory and multisystem failure after the
open procedure. The fifth patient had an open arch aneurysm repair for type 1
endoleak and migration at 5 months. This case of migration was the only one

Table 24.2 Endoleak over time

	Periop	1 month	6 months	12 months	24 months	36 months	48 months	60 months
Patients available for follow-up	81	123	108	103	80	64	57	47
Patients with endoleaks	7 (8.6%)	10 (8.1%)	7 (6.5%)	4 (3.9%)	5 (6.3%)	2 (3.1%)	3 (5.3%)	2 (4.3%)
Type Ia	3	5	4	1	1	–	1	1
Type Ib	1	1	1	1	1	2	2	–
Type II	1	1	1	1	1	–	–	1
Type III	1	1	–	–	1	–	–	–
Indeterminate	1	2	1	1	1	–	–	–

Type Ia, proximal attachment site; *type Ib*, distal attachment site

Table 24.3 All secondary procedures and direct aneurysm reinterventions, reported as number of patients affected. Patients may have had more than one procedure

	TAG	Controls
All secondary procedures		
Additional thoracic aortic procedures	3	2
Empyema/chest wall reconstruction	0	5
Procedures for minor wound complications	8	8
Lumbar drain placement	2	2
Tracheostomy	3	10
Endoscopy or laparotomy for GI issues related to surgery	1	9
Evacuation retroperitoneal bleed	1	0
Cardiac conversion for atrial fibrillation	0	3
Surgery for vocal card paralysis	0	2
Placement dialysis catheter	1	1
Resection of ischemic bowel	0	1
Vascular reconstructions	6	0
Miscellaneous	0	4
Direct aneurysm reinterventions		
Conversion/treatment of graft infection	1	1
Drainage of peri-anastomotic collection		1
Extension for endoleaks	3	0
Evacuation of hematoma after carotid-subclavian bypass, repair of femoral pseudoaneurysm after TAG extension (all same patient as counted above)	1	
Conversion for migration		

seen in 5 years and was probably related to poor proximal neck anatomy (migration incidence 0.7%). The rate of major, direct aneurysm-related reinterventions in the TAG group at 5 years follow-up was 5/140 (3.6%). Reinterventions directly related to open aneurysm repair occurred in two patients, with one having a proximal anastomotic collection drained and one having debridement and drain placement for an aorto-esophageal fistula. The aneurysm reintervention rate was 2.1% for open controls.

There were six patients in the TAG group who needed secondary vascular procedures. Four of these took place on post-operative day 1. Three were related to acute leg ischemia and one was an evacuation of a brachial artery hematoma. Another patient had hematoma complications after carotid subclavian bypass and extension of the TAG device. The final patient had thrombosis of an ilio-femoral conduit on post-operative day 127 and underwent femoral to femoral bypass.

The total number of TAG patients with at least one secondary procedure following but not directly related to the aneurysm repair was 21/140 (15.0%). There have been 30 patients with additional secondary procedures in the surgical control

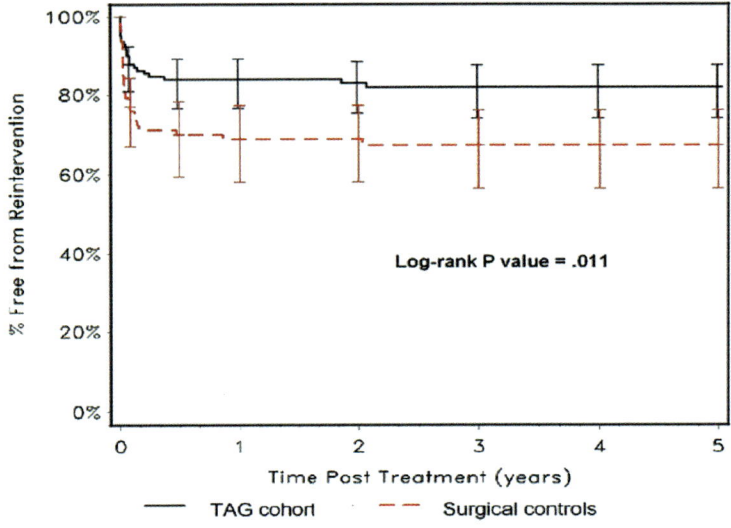

	1 year	2 years	3 years	4 years	5 years
95% C.I. TAG	.766, .891	.754, .883	.741, .875	.741, .875	.741, .875
95% C.I. Control	.581, .773	.581, .773	.564, .761	.564, .761	.564, .761

Fig. 24.5 Freedom from reintervention in TAG and surgical controls at 5 years

group (31.91%). Most of these procedures were related to perioperative complications (Table 24.3). There was one TAG patient who had a secondary procedure
not directly related to aneurysm treatment more than 30 days after the DTA repair.
This was a thrombosis of an ilio-femoral conduit and is described above. In the surgical control group, there were six secondary procedures which took place more
than 30 days after DTA repair, five related to wound issues and one patient with
axillary aneurysm repairs. At 5 years, there were significantly fewer aneurysm-
related secondary procedures in the TAG group ($P = 0.011$). Figure 24.5 shows
all secondary procedures and reinterventions at 5 years.

24.4 Sac Diameter

Change in the aneurysm sac diameter was assessed at each follow-up timepoint,
and most aneurysms were found to increase or decrease over time, with a small
percentage remaining stable at 5 years (Table 24.4). In the pivotal trial, 19% of
patients at 5 years had 5 mm or more of sac enlargement compared with a 1-
month baseline, and 50% had ≥ 5 mm of sac shrinkage. Between 9.1 and 12.5%
of all patients with sac enlargement were noted to have endoleaks between 1 and 60
months post-operatively.

Table 24.4 Aneurysm sac size change over time in TAG group

Change in aneurysm size	1–6 months (N = 85)	1–12 months (N = 87)	1–24 months (N = 71)	1–36 months (N = 57)	1–48 months (N = 50)	1–60 months (N = 26)
Decrease	31(35%)	37(43%)	32(46%)	29(53%)	23(45%)	21(50%)
No change	49(56%)	41(48%)	29(41%)	17(31%)	17(33%)	13(31%)
Increase	8(8%)	8(9%)	9(13%)	9(16%)	11(22%)	8(19%)

The confirmatory patient cohort, treated with the revised low-porosity TAG endograft, exhibited no sac enlargement at 1 year ($P = 0.0548$ versus earlier TAG patients at 1 year), and 2.9% exhibited d5 mm sac enlargement at 2 years ($P = 0.11$ versus earlier TAG patients at 2 years) (Fig. 24.6). Further follow-up data are not yet available for the confirmatory arm. The currently available commercial device is the low-porosity endograft

Fig. 24.6 Original and modified low-porosity TAG endograft sac shrinkage at 2 years

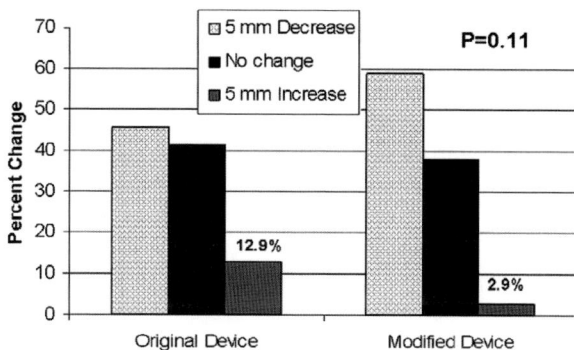

References

1. Makaroun MS, Dillavou ED, Kes ST, et al. Endovascular treatment of thoracic aortic aneurysms: results of the phase II multicenter trial of the Gore TAG thoracic endoprosthesis. *J Vasc Surg*. 2005;41(1):1–9.
2. Gore TAG Thoracic Endoprosthesis Annual Clinical Update (April 2010).
3. Makaroun MS, Dillavou ED, Wheatley GH, Cambria RP; the Gore TAG Investigators. Five-year results of endovascular treatment with the Gore TAG device compared with open repair of thoracic aortic aneurysms. *J Vasc Surg*. 2008;47(5):912–918.

Chapter 25
Technique of Thoracic Endografting for Thoracic Aneurysm Using the Approved Gore TAG Device

The technique of thoracic endografting for the treatment of thoracic aortic aneurysm using a Gore TAG device (W.L. Gore & Associates, Flagstaff, AZ) (Fig. 25.1) is preferably performed in a hybrid operating room (Fig. 25.2) or an endovascular suite provided the patient is an adequate candidate for endovascular repair. The procedure is performed under general anesthesia with spinal drainage selected to patients that have had a previous open surgical repair of an abdominal aortic aneurysm or patients considered high risks for paraplegia. Percutaneous retrograde access of the common femoral artery is obtained in one groin and open retrograde cannulation of

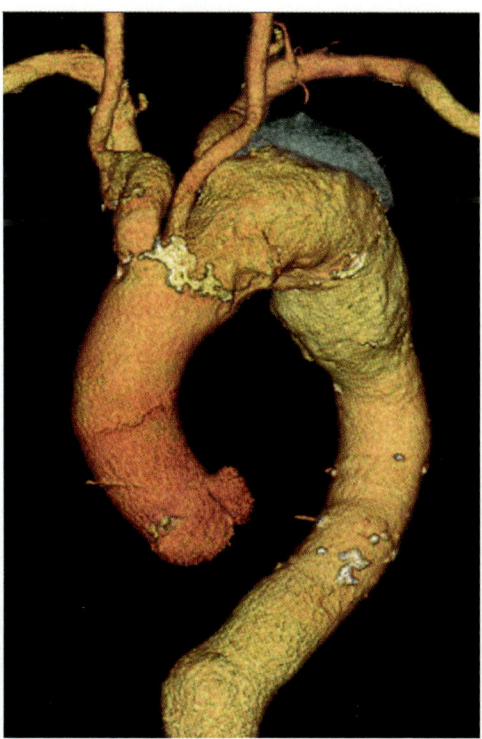

Fig. 25.1 Three-dimensional reconstructed CT scan of the chest demonstrates a thoracic aortic aneurysm

J. Kpodonu, *Manual of Thoracic Endoaortic Surgery*,
DOI 10.1007/978-1-84996-296-4_25, © Springer-Verlag London Limited 2010

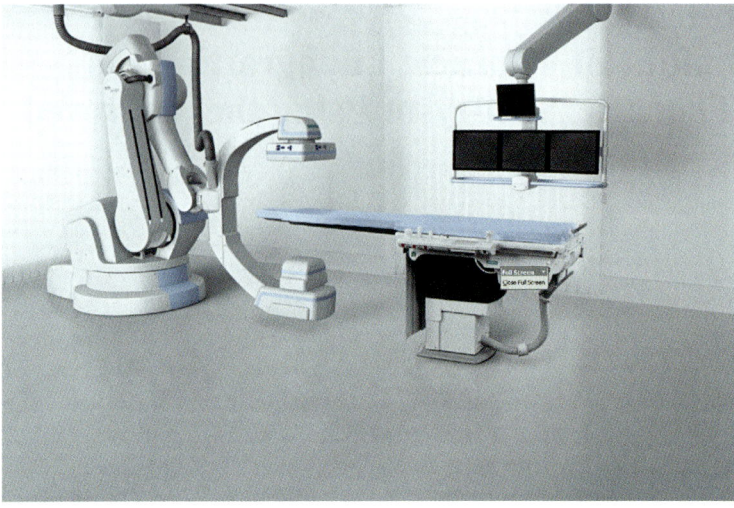

Fig. 25.2 A hybrid room with a fixed imaging system used for the endovascular management of thoracic aortic aneurysms

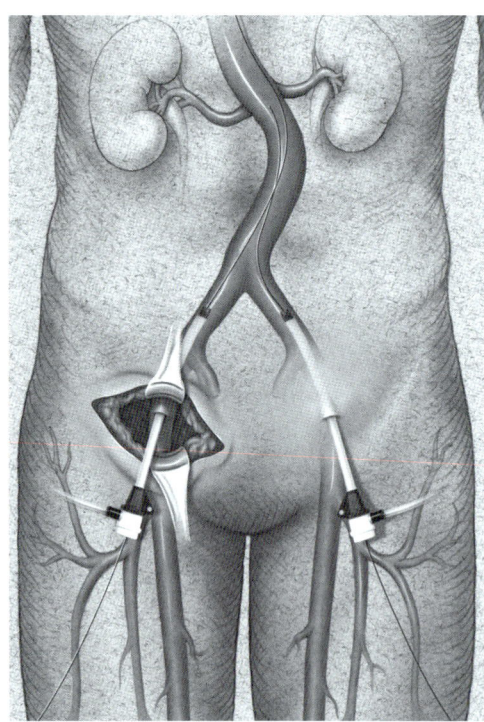

Fig. 25.3 Illustration demonstrates open retrograde cannulation of right groin with an introducer sheath and a retrograde percutaneous access of the left common femoral artery using an 18 G needle

the contralateral common femoral artery performed with an 18 G needle (Fig. 25.3) as previously described.[1] An 0.035 in. soft tip angled glide wire (Medi-tech/Boston Scientific, Natick, MA) is advanced into the distal thoracic aorta (Fig. 25.4). A 9 Fr sheath is usually placed in the open common femoral artery and similarly 5 Fr placed in the percutaneously accessed common femoral artery under fluoroscopic visualization. Five thousand units of heparin is given to keep the activated clotted time greater than 200 s. A 5 Fr pigtail catheter is advanced through the percutaneous sheath into the ascending thoracic aorta for an ascending and arch angiogram and saved as a road map picture (Fig. 25.5). The fluoroscopic C-arm is positioned in a left anterior oblique angle and an oblique thoracic arch aortogram is performed to visualize the arch vessels and the descending thoracic aortic aneurysm (Fig. 25.6). Intravascular ultrasound (IVUS) (Fig. 25.7a, b) can be performed to provide more information on the proximal and distal neck diameter, length of thoracic aorta involved with the aneurysm, presence or absence of thrombus in the neck, and any other pathology that may have been missed on the angiogram or pre-operative CT angiogram of the thoracic aorta (Fig. 25.1). The 5 Fr pigtail catheter is exchanged for an extra stiff 260 cm double-curve Lunderquist wire (Cook, Bloomington, IN). The 9 Fr groin sheath in the open cannulated femoral artery is exchanged for an

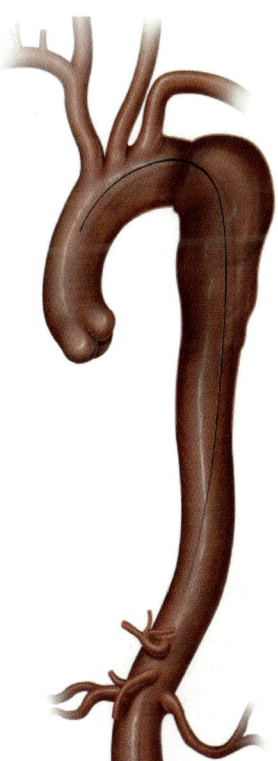

Fig. 25.4 Illustration demonstrates advancement of a glide wire up the aortic arch

Fig. 25.5 Illustration demonstrates advancement of a pigtail angiographic catheter up the aortic arch for a thoracic aortogram

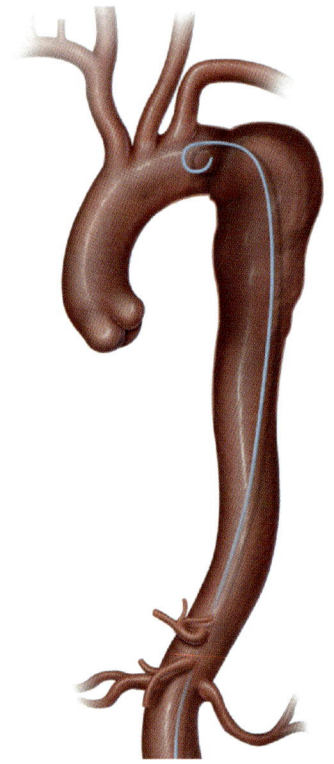

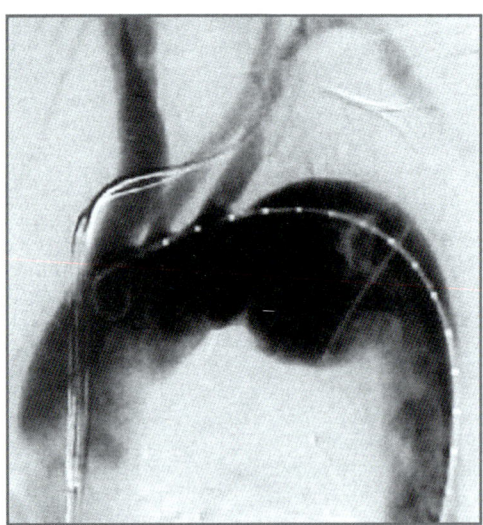

Fig. 25.6 A thoracic aortogram performed with an angiographic pigtail catheter

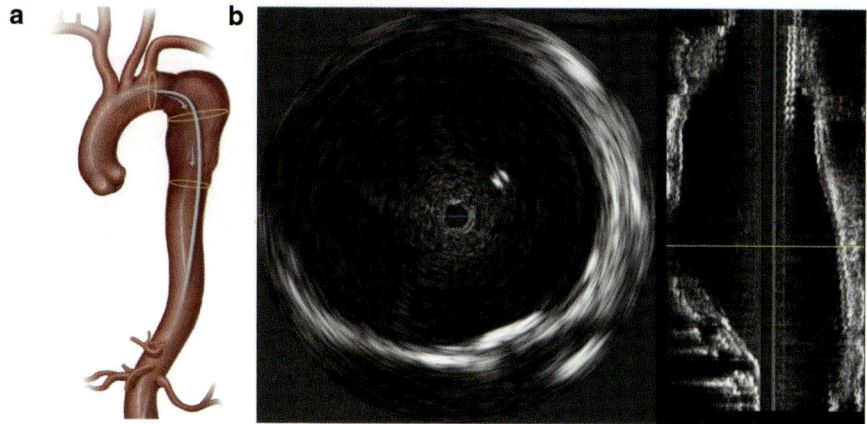

Fig. 25.7 (**a**) Illustration demonstrates intravascular ultrasound catheter advanced into the proximal thoracic aorta to determine proximal and distal landing zone diameters, diameter and length of aneurysm. (**b**) Intravascular ultrasound image of a thoracic aneurysm

appropriate-sized device sheath which is advanced into the distal thoracic aorta (Fig. 25.8). The endograft is subsequently advanced through the device sheath and positioned into the thoracic aorta to exclude the thoracic aneurysm (Fig. 25.9). Prior to deployment, the proximal and distal landing zones identified are marked

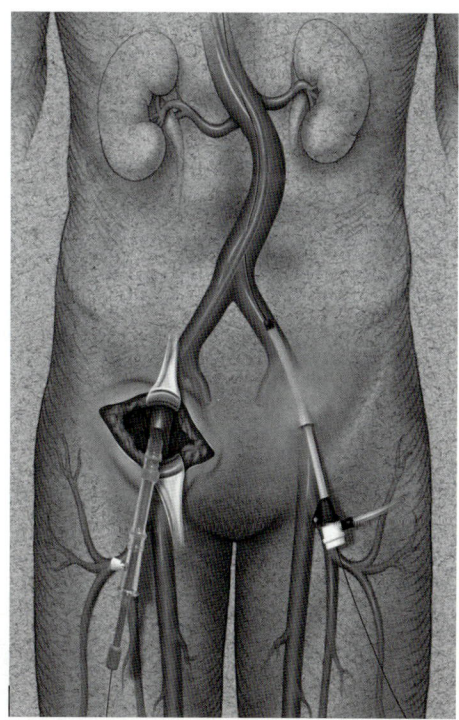

Fig. 25.8 Illustration demonstrates device sheath for endograft advanced into the thoracic aorta

Fig. 25.9 Illustration demonstrates advancement of endoluminal graft and positioning for exclusion of thoracic aneurysm

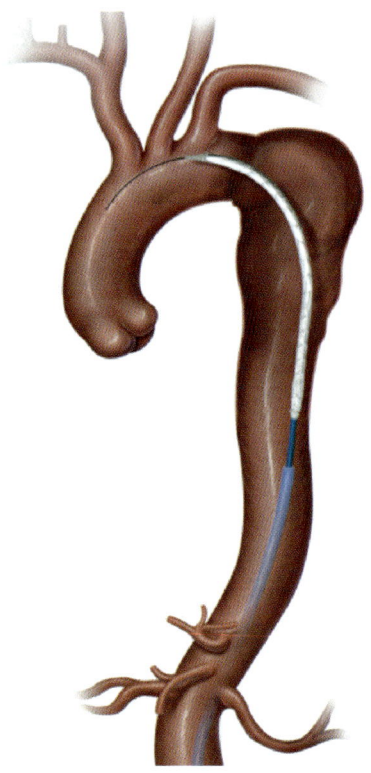

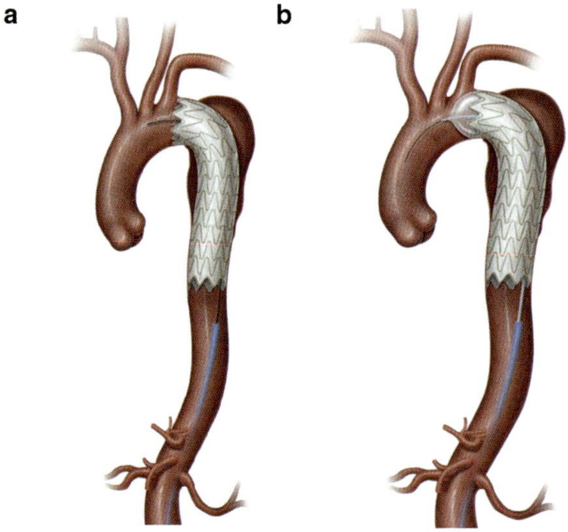

a   b

Fig. 25.10 (**a**) Illustration demonstrates deployment of endoluminal graft to exclude thoracic aneurysm. (**b**) Illustration demonstrates balloon angioplasty of proximal end for adequate fixation to aortic wall to prevent a type 1 endoleak

Fig. 25.11 (**a**, **b**) Completion angiogram and illustration demonstrate adequate position of endograft with exclusion of aneurysm

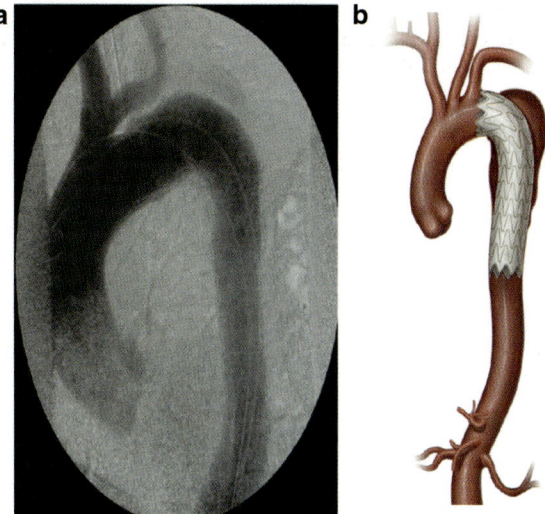

on angiographic road map. At the time of deployment of the endoluminal graft, a systolic blood pressure of 90 mmHg is achieved to decrease the "windsock" effect in the thoracic aorta. We have not felt the need for adenosine-induced asystole. The device is deployed (Fig. 25.10a) and a Gore tri-lobe balloon (Fig. 25.10b) is used to perform post-deployment balloon angioplasty to both the proximal and distal segments of the graft for good fixation and any areas of overlap if more than one graft is deployed. A completion angiogram is then performed to confirm exclusion of the aneurysm and to determine if any endoleak is present (Fig. 25.11a, b). All wires and sheaths were removed from the right common femoral artery with the incision closed in a transverse fashion (Fig. 25.12). A 6 Fr Angioseal vascular closure device (St. Judes Medical, Inc.) is deployed to the common femoral artery that was percutaneously accessed (Fig. 25.13). At the end of the procedure confirmation of the presence of bilateral peripheral pulses is performed, the patient is extubated prior to leaving the operating room and transferred to the recovery room. The blood pressure is kept elevated using a pressor agent if needed to keep the mean arterial pressure greater than 90 mmHg. A post-operative CT scan of the chest (Fig. 25.14) is performed prior to discharge to confirm exclusion of the thoracic aortic aneurysm and to identify any endoleaks that may have been missed on operative angiograms.

25.1 Preference Card

25.1.1 Equipment

– 18 G access needle
– Indeflator for therapeutic ballooning of iliac arteries
– 60 cc syringe for profile ballooning of aorta and graft junctions

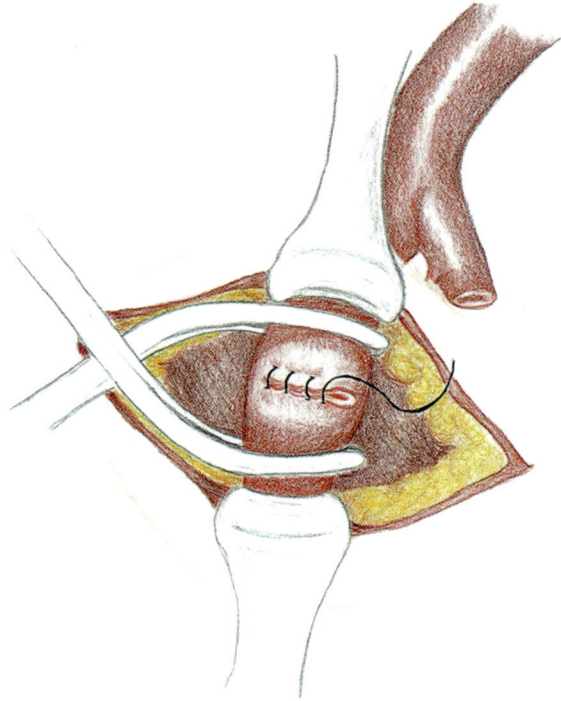

Fig. 25.12 Illustration demonstrates repair of femoral arteriotomy used for device sheath introduction

- Guidewire 0.035 180 cm angled glidewire/260 cm angled for (thoracic)
- Guidewire 0.035 260 cm Cook Lunderquist ({x2} abdominal)/Lunderquist (LES3) for (thoracic {x1})
- Sheath 5, 6, or 9 Fr 11 cm Cordis Brite-tip for percutaneous contra
- Sheath 12 or 14 Fr for post-endoluminal graft ballooning
- Flush catheter 5 or 6 Fr 100 cm TR flush/pigtail/or marker pigtail
- Balloon Cordis OPTA-PRO 80 cm or Abbott FOX PTA 75 cm (for lesions of the iliac vessels/to allow delivery of the ELG) (size to be determined by physician)

Fig. 25.13 Angioseal (St. Judes Medical, Inc.) vascular device closure used to achieve hemostasis of percutaneous retrograde puncture

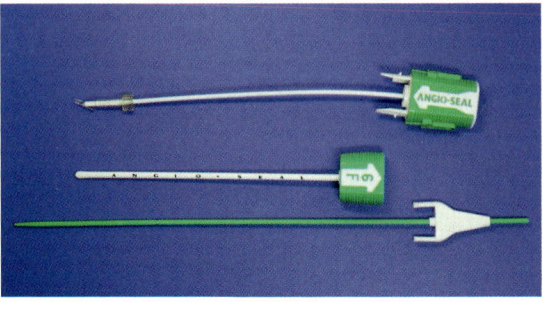

Fig. 25.14 A reconstructed 3D CT scan demonstrates satisfactory exclusion of thoracic aortic aneurysm with no endoleak

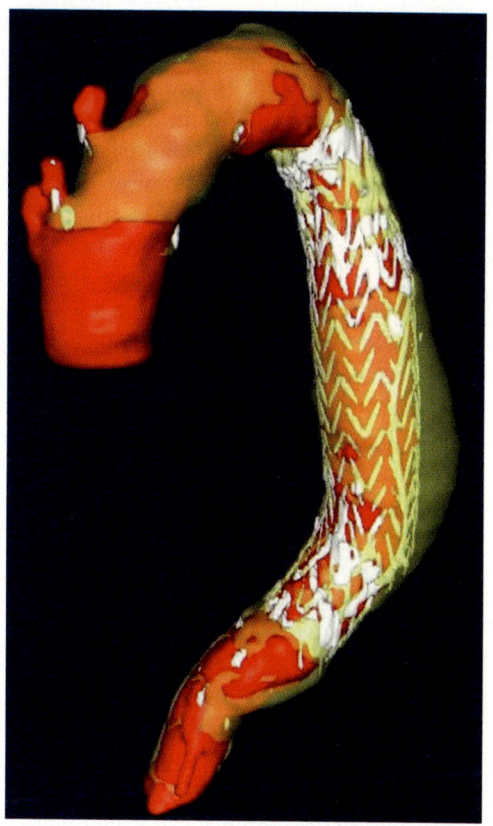

– Balloon Cordis MAXI-LD 14,15,16,18,20,22,25 × 4 cm for graft junction (size to be determined by physician)
– Balloon Cook CODA 32 or 40 mm (size to be determined by physician)
– Endoluminal graft (size to be determined by physician)

25.1.2 Procedure Pearls

– Patient placed supine
– EKG leads and EKG wires are positioned so they do not appear on the fluoroscopic images
– Possibly prep the patient's arm out for brachial–femoral wire (used for difficult access anatomy such as extremely tortuous iliacs)

  1) Oblique incision to expose CFA (thoracic/endologix {x1 side cut down}) (aneurx/excluder/Zenith {x2 side cut down}) Puncture both CFA with 18 G needle
  2) Place 0.035 angled glide wire through needle lumen; under fluoroscopic guidance advance into distal aorta; (*percutaneous*) make a small incision at the

puncture site with a scalpel; leave guidewire in place and remove the needle; while leaving the guidewire in place, dilate the tract with a mosquito hemostat

3) Place the 5, 6, or 9 Fr (IVUS) 11 cm brite-tip sheath over the guidewire and advance well into the vessel; remove the obturator of the sheath leaving the sheath and guidewire in place; flush sheath with heparinized saline; have anesthiologist/CRNA administer 3000–5000 units of heparin i.v.

 If sheath is not able to be advanced, place a Cordis 4 Fr dilator over the wire and exchange the wire for a stiffer 0.035 guidewire (EG. 0.035 75 cm Amplatz); remove the dilator keeping the wire in place; then place sheath over the stiff guidewire and advance well into the vessel; replace the stiff guidewire with the original glide wire

4) Under fluoroscopic guidance advance the glide wire into thoracic aorta

6) Place 5 or 6 Fr flush catheter over the guidewire and advance into the proximal abdominal aorta at the level of (L1–L2 vertebral space for renal artery visualization (ABD): advance into ascending thoracic aorta to visualize the great vessels (thoracic)

7) Position image intensifier for imaging (ABD) AP with a 10–15° cranial angulation (thoracic) 40–60° LAO angulation

8) Shoot an aortagram to determine if you have adequate length landing zone (*road map for IVUS measurements*)

9) Place the Lunderquist guidewire into flush catheter and remove flush catheter leaving the Lunderquist in place

10) Place 8.2 Fr PV IVUS probe over the wire and perform IVUS examination (take diameter measurements/evaluate plaque and thrombus burdens/perform longitudinal pull-through/take length measurement)

11) Remove IVUS probe leaving the Lunderquist wire in place

12) Shoot a retrograde angiogram through the sheath to evaluate the access vessels (if needed perform angioplasty)

13) Through contralateral sheath place flush catheter in position to perform aortagram prior to ELG deployment

14) Choose the appropriate-sized ELG

15) Introduce ELG delivery sheath or ELG delivery device into the CFA over the Lunderquist wire (follow the sheath/delivery system as it passes through the aorta and iliac vessels)

16) Rotate the C-arm to appropriate angle for aortagram (see #7)

17) Shoot aortagram (road map) to deploy the ELG

18) Place a needle at the proximal landing zone

19) Deploy the ELG (small puffs of contrast through the flush catheter aid in accurate deployment)

20) Follow the IFU for each specific device deployment step

21) After ELG is deployed removed the flush catheter from behind the ELG by placing the angled glide wire through the catheter

22) If the ELG is a bifurcated abdominal ELG, cannulate the contralateral gate; select the appropriate limb and deploy according to the device-specific IFU

23) Profile balloon the landing zones and overlapping areas with MAXI-LD balloon(s) or Coda balloon

24) Reintroduce the flush catheter and check for endoleaks

25) Perform retrograde angiogram through the sheaths to check for distal seal of the ELG

26) Deployment of closure device in access vessels with sheaths less than 12 Fr. Repair of access vessels with sheath size larger than 12 Fr.

Reference

1. Diethrich EB, Ramaiah VG, Kpodonu J, Rodriguez JA. *Endovascular and Hybrid Management of the Thoracic Aorta. A Case Based Approach.* 1st ed. West Sussex: Wiley-Blackwell; 2008.

Part VII
Medtronic Talent/Valiant Thoracic Endovascular Stent Graft

Chapter 26
Talent Thoracic Stent Graft

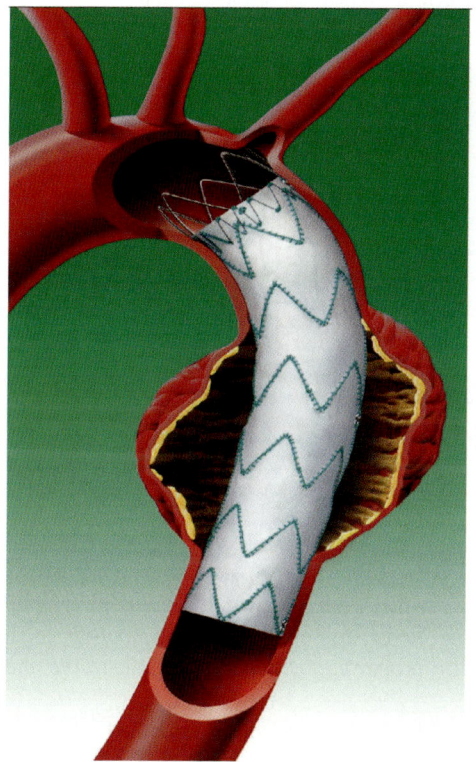

26.1 The Talent Device

The Talent device is a preloaded stent graft incorporated into a Coil-Trac delivery system.[1] It is composed of a polyester graft (Dacron; C.R. Bard, Haverhill, PA) sewn to a self-expanding nitinol wire frame skeleton. Radiopaque "figure-of-8" markers are sewn to the graft material to aid in visualization during fluoroscopy. The

J. Kpodonu, *Manual of Thoracic Endoaortic Surgery*,
DOI 10.1007/978-1-84996-296-4_26, © Springer-Verlag London Limited 2010

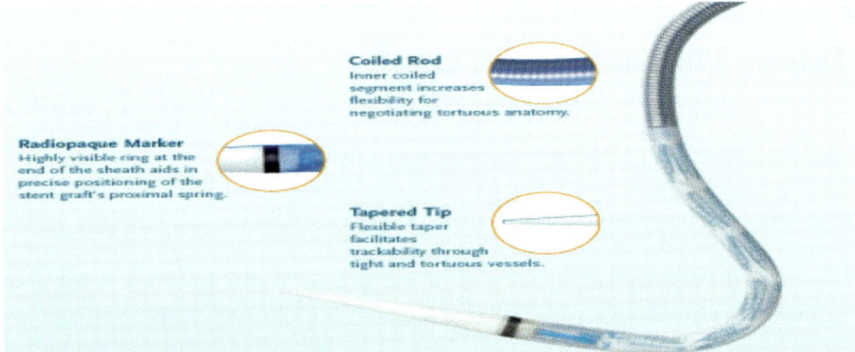

Fig. 26.1 The CoilTrac delivery system for Talent stent graft

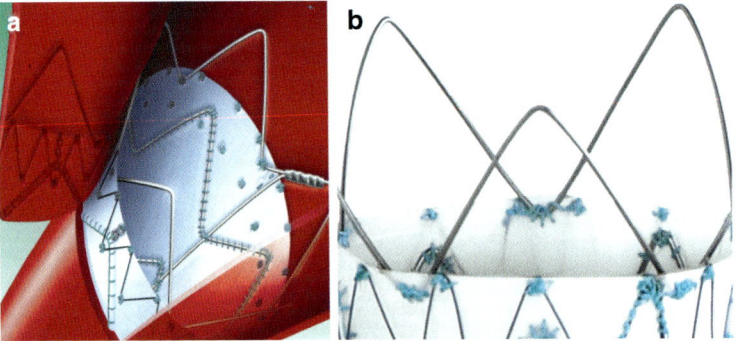

Fig. 26.2 (**a, b**) Illustration of a Talent device which consists of self-expanding, nitinol wire scaffolding incorporated into a low-profile polyester monofilament weave graft. The Talent graft has five flared crown geometry to provide a high radial force to maintain fixation to the aorta over time

CoilTrac delivery system (Fig. 26.1) is sheathless and push rod based. Preloaded onto an inner catheter, the Talent device is deployed by pulling back an outer catheter, allowing the device to self-expand and contour to the aorta. A balloon may be used to ensure proper apposition of the graft to the aneurysmal aorta after deployment.

The Talent device (Fig. 26.2) is a modular system; 47 different configurations are available, ranging from a diameter of 22 to 46 mm and covering lengths from 112 to 116 mm. To accommodate the size differences often found between the proximal and distal portions of the aorta in thoracic aneurysms, tapered grafts are available for better aneurysmal conformability and prevention of junctional endoleaks. Four configuration categories are available: proximal main, proximal extension, distal main, and distal extension. The proximal configurations and the distal extension are offered with a bare spring design (FreeFlo), which allows placement of the device across the origins of the arch vessels proximally and the celiac artery distally for supra-subclavian and infra-celiac fixation, respectively.

26.2 Talent Graft Dimensions

Talent graft dimensions consist of two main sections: a proximal main straight tube with a proximal FreeFlo system with an open web system and a distal section which is a taped tube with 4 mm difference from top to bottom; the proximal portion being open web and the distal portion close web (Fig. 26.3).

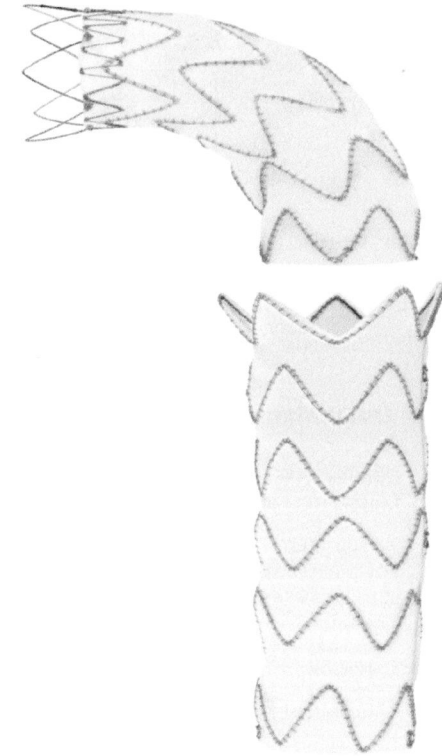

Fig. 26.3 Image of an open web Talent (Medtronic) stent graft system demonstrating a proximal and distal component

The Talent stent graft system comes in a variety of diameter range. The proximal component has diameters of 22–46 mm and length 112–116 mm (Fig. 26.4). The distal component has diameter range 22–46 mm and length 110–114 mm (Fig. 26.5).

26.3 Stent Graft Sizing Guidelines

The recommended choice of thoracic stent graft should be oversized up to 20% when treating thoracic aortic aneurysms. Recommended vessel diameters and thoracic stent graft diameters are illustrated in Fig. 26.6.

Proximal Main Sections Diameter 22-46mm, Length 112-116mm

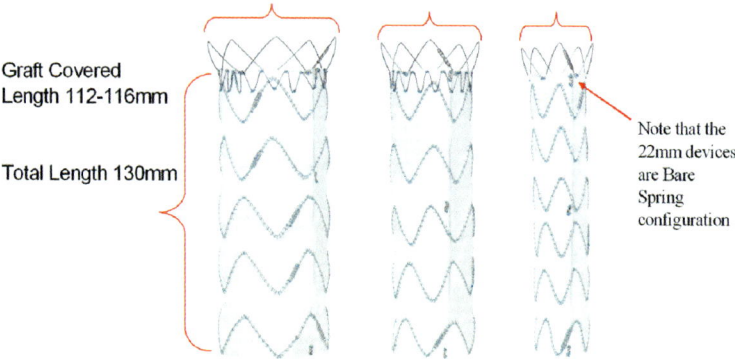

Graft Covered
Length 112-116mm

Total Length 130mm

Note that the
22mm devices
are Bare
Spring
configuration

Fig. 26.4   Proximal components of the Talent stent graft system

Distal Main Sections Diameter 26-46mm, Length 110-114mm

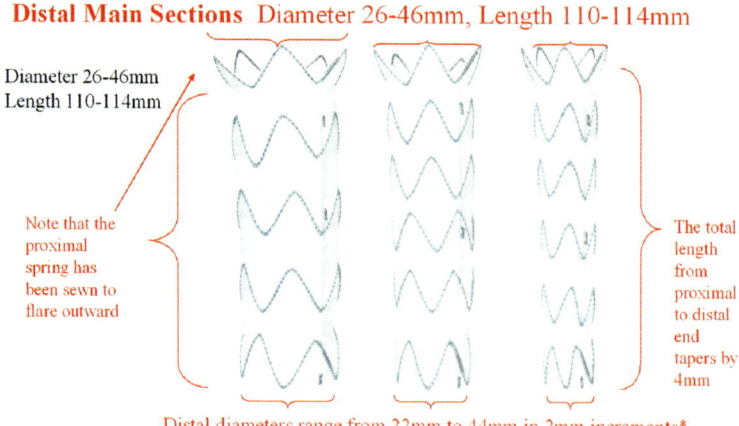

Diameter 26-46mm
Length 110-114mm

Note that the
proximal
spring has
been sewn to
flare outward

The total
length
from
proximal
to distal
end
tapers by
4mm

Distal diameters range from 22mm to 44mm in 2mm increments*

Fig. 26.5   Distal components of the Talent stent graft system

26.4 Delivery System Insertion of the Talent Stent Graft System

The introducer system of the Talent stent graft system is advanced over a 0.035″
stiff guidewire to the target landing zone (Fig. 26.7).

Fig. 26.6 Chart for recommended Talent graft oversizing to aortic neck diameter

VESSEL DIAMETER	TALENT OVERSIZING	VESSEL DIAMETER	TALENT OVERSIZING
18mm	22mm	31mm	34mm
19mm	22mm	32mm	36mm
20mm	24mm	33mm	38m
21mm	24mm	34mm	38mm
22mm	26mm	35mm	40mm
23mm	26mm	36mm	40mm
24mm	28mm	37mm	42mm
25mm	28mm	38mm	42mm
26mm	30mm	39mm	44mm
27mm	30mm	40mm	44mm
28mm	32mm	41mm	46mm
29mm	32mm	42mm	46mm
30mm	34mm		

Fig. 26.7 Talent stent graft system advanced over a 0.035″ extra stiff guidewire

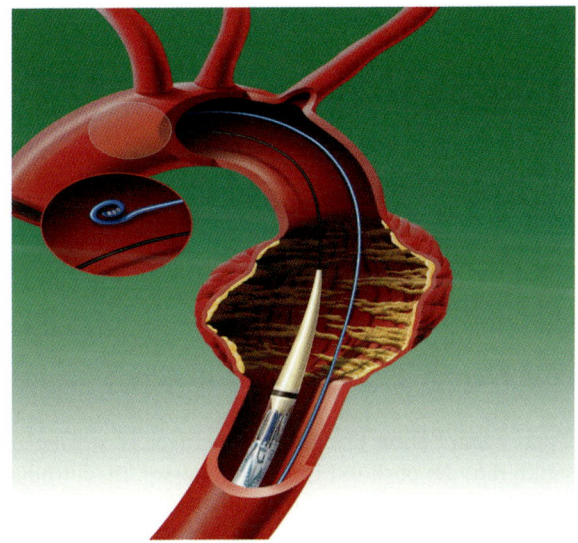

26.5 Stent Graft Positioning

The position of proximal markers is verified with confirmation that the connecting bar is aligned on the outside of the most severe angle. The cup plunger is checked to ensure that it is still encapsulating the distal stent graft spring and that the Touhy Borst is tightened (Fig. 26.8).

Fig. 26.8 Positioning of stent graft system with verification of proximal markers

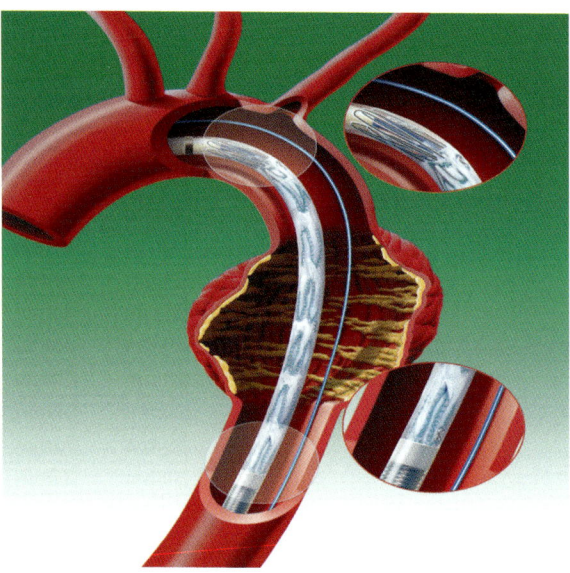

26.6 Deploy Proximal End

The push rod is held stationary with one hand, and the introducer sheath slowly withdrawn with the other hand. The initial force will be high, but greatly reduced once the sheath begins moving. Stop deployment once the bare spring and first covered spring are deployed to reconfirm stent graft position using angiography (Fig. 26.9).

26.7 Deploy Remaining Stent Graft

Upon confirmation that the cup plunger is still encapsulating the bottom of the stent graft, the push rod is held stationary; the introducer sheath is then withdrawn until the distal spring is completely deployed. The marker band position is verified (Fig. 26.10).

26.8 Remove Delivery System

The Touhy Borst valve is loosened and the inner catheter is withdrawn into the introducer sheath establishing a smooth transition between the tapered tip and the sheath.

The Touhy Borst is the tightened and the entire system gently removed (Fig. 26.11).

Fig. 26.9 Introducer sheath
slowly withdrawn to uncover
proximal bare springs

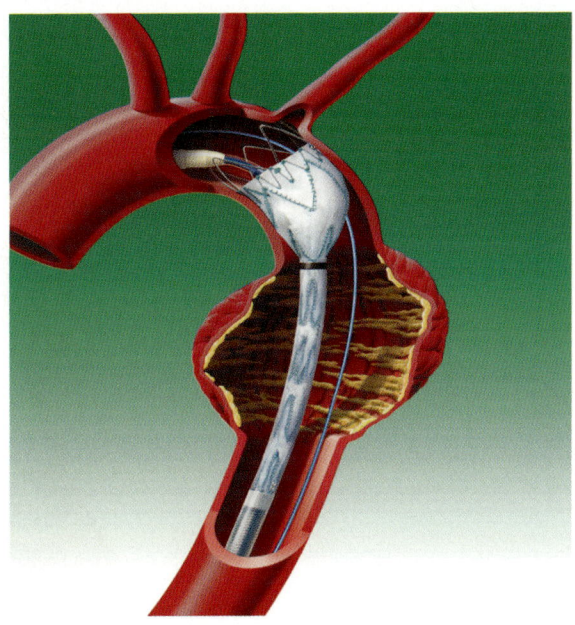

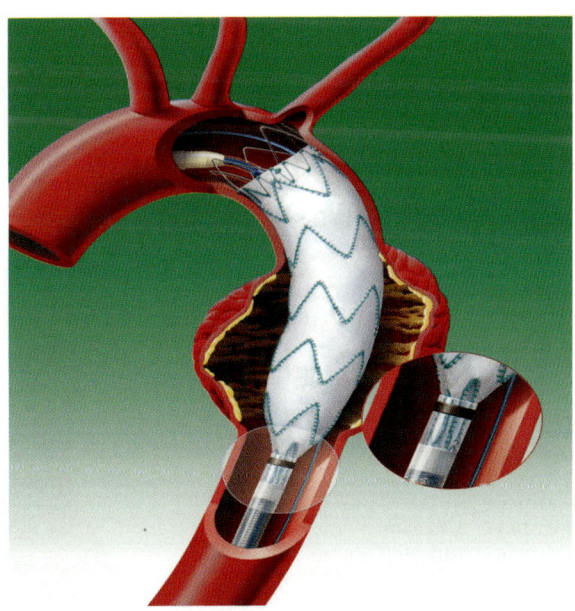

Fig. 26.10 Continue to
withdraw introducer sheath
till distal component is
deployed

Fig. 26.11 Introducer sheath is removed over the 0.0035″ extra stiff guidewire

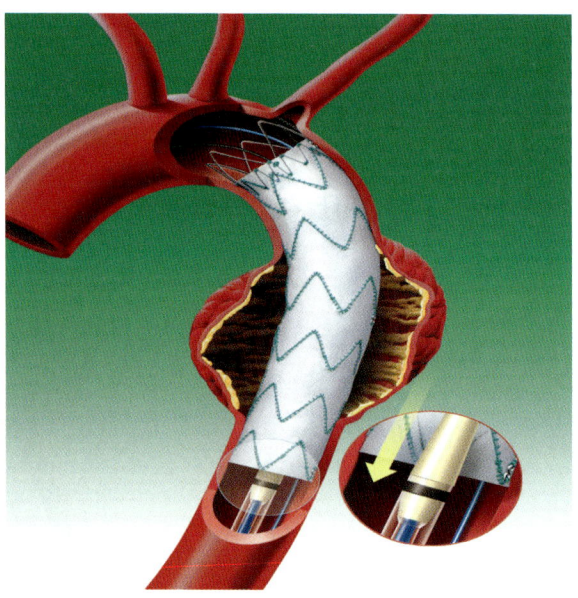

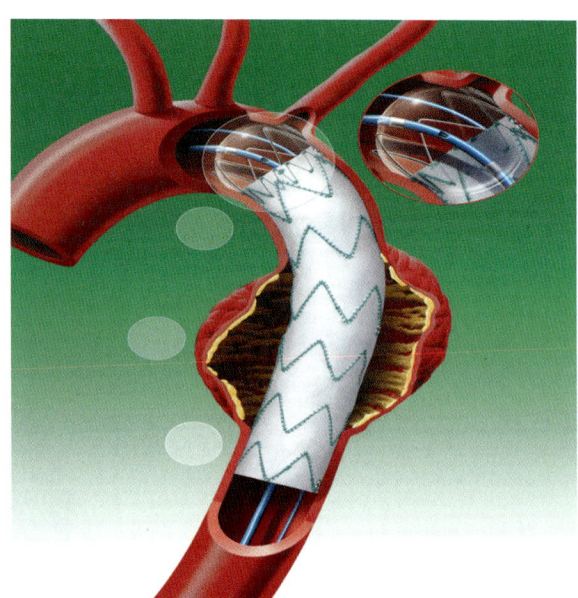

Fig. 26.12 A Reliant (Medtronic) balloon is used to mold the proximal and distal ends of the Talent stent graft

26.9 Model Graft to Vessel

A compliant balloon (Reliant, Medtronic) is then inflated and deflated from the proximal covered spring to the distal covered spring, to smooth wrinkles in the graft material. Care is taken not to inflate the balloon more than 1 atm (Fig. 26.12).

26.10 Final Angiogram

A completion angiogram is performed and leaks that remain after ballooning may require extension cuff placement. *Caution: It is not recommended to make high-pressure injections of contrast media at the edges of the stent graft immediately after implantation.* Introducer and guidewire from patient are removed and seal entry sites are closed using standard surgical closure techniques.

Reference

1. *Medtronic Talent Thoracic Physician Reference Manual.*

Chapter 27
Valiant Thoracic Stent Graft

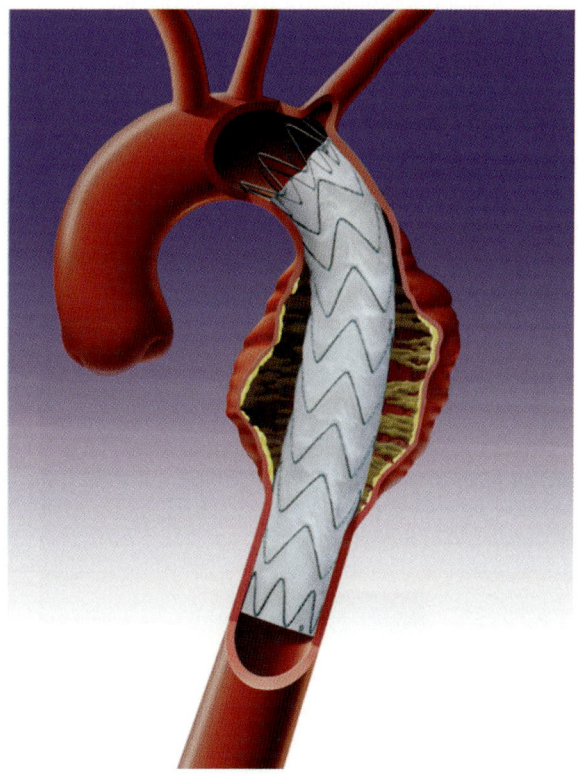

The valiant thoracic stent graft is a self-expanding stent graft with nitinol wire scaffolding attached to a low-profile polyester monofilament weave (Fig. 27.1). There is no connecting bar which therefore eliminates the need to rotationally orient device. There are 8-peak springs which distribute radial force across more points of contact

J. Kpodonu, *Manual of Thoracic Endoaortic Surgery*,
DOI 10.1007/978-1-84996-296-4_27, © Springer-Verlag London Limited 2010

Fig. 27.1 Illustration of a valiant stent graft system

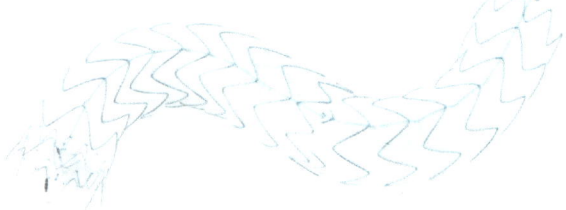

with less force and stress per point. Springs sewn to outside of graft material raised surface may provide better opportunity for tissue incorporation.

Graft lengths range from 100 to 227 mm and proximal neck diameters range from 24 to 46 mm. Closed web devices in both a straight and a tapered configuration are available as a distal extender. The advantage of the distal bare spring device is significant when apposition near the celiac axis is required. The graft is fully MRI (magnetic resonance imaging) safe. There is no additional risk to a patient with the valiant thoracic stent graft with respect to movement, dislodgment, or migration using an MR system with a static magnetic field of 3 T or less. The delivery system in the valiant device is 2 Fr size smaller compared with the Talent device and allows for controlled ratcheted precise deployment using the refined Xcelerant delivery system (Fig. 27.2). Currently the valiant stent graft system is in a clinical trial in the United States.

Stent graft length, diameter, and proximal and distal configurations are outlined in Table 27.1.

If using more than one piece, at the overlapping area, the graft going inside of the other graft must have a closed web configuration. At the joint, the distal graft

Fig. 27.2 The Xcelerent delivery system of the Talent thoracic stent graft device allows stable and accurate deployment

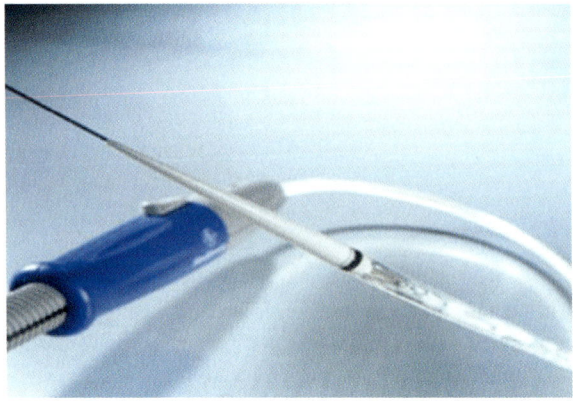

Table 27.1 Stent graft size guidelines and product codes

Vessel diameter (mm)	Valiant stent graft oversizing (mm)	Vessel diameter (mm)	Valiant stent graft oversizing (mm)
20	24	32	36
21	24	33	38
22	26	34	38
23	26	35	40
24	28	36	40
25	28–30	37	42
26	30	38	42
27	30–32	39	44
28	32	40	44
29	32–34	41	46
30	34	42	46
31	34–36		

piece should have a diameter of 4 mm greater than the diameter of the proximal graft end. Tapered grafts can be used so that the overall diameter does not expand over the length of the covered aorta. The second piece graft is used when the stent graft junction is supported by tissue (e.g., dissections) in such scenarios less than 4 mm oversizing may be appropriate.

Recommended overlap distance:

Proximal diameter of stent graft (mm)	Overlap distance (mm)
24	50
26	50
28	55
30	55
32	55
34	55
36	60
38	60
40	60
42	60
44	65
46	65

Product code: Proximal Free Flo straight:

Product Code	Proximal Aortic Diameter (mm)		Distal Aortic Diameter (mm)	Graft Covered Length (mm)	Stent Graft Total Length (mm)	Catheter Diameter (F)
TF 24	24	C	100 X	115	127	22
TF 26	26	C	100 X	115	127	22
TF 28	28	C	100 X	120	132	22
TF 30	30	C	100 X	120	132	22
TF 32	32	C	100 X	120	132	22
TF 34	34	C	100 X	110	122	24
TF 36	36	C	100 X	110	122	24
TF 38	38	C	100 X	110	122	24
TF 40	40	C	100 X	110	122	24
TF 42	42	C	100 X	115	127	25
TF 44	44	C	100 X	115	127	25
TF 46	46	C	100 X	115	127	25
TF 24	24	C	150 X	155	167	22
TF 26	26	C	150 X	155	167	22
TF 28	28	C	150 X	160	172	22
TF 30	30	C	150 X	160	172	22
TF 32	32	C	150 X	160	172	22

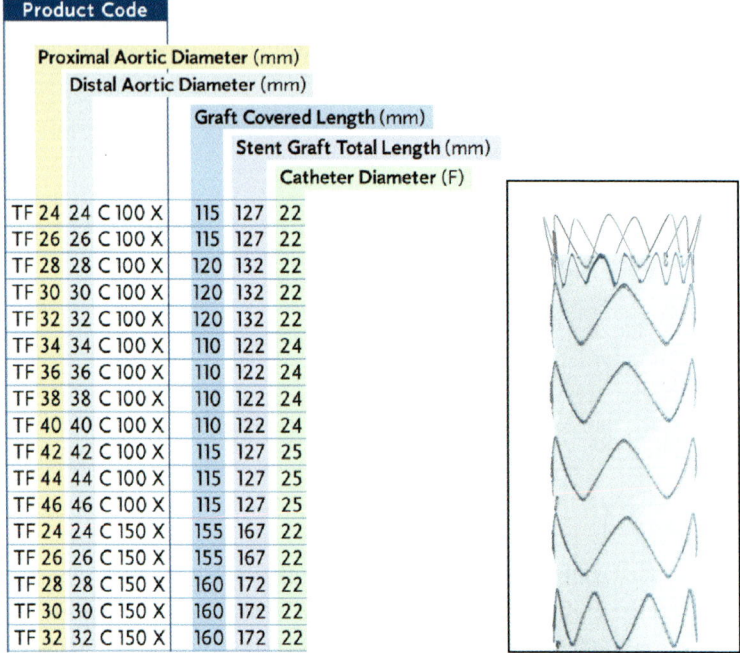

Products code: Distal bare spring straight:

Product Code	Proximal Aortic Diameter (mm)		Distal Aortic Diameter (mm)	Graft Covered Length (mm)	Stent Graft Total Length (mm)	Catheter Diameter (F)
TF 24	24	C	100 X	115	127	22
TF 26	26	C	100 X	115	127	22
TF 28	28	C	100 X	120	132	22
TF 30	30	C	100 X	120	132	22
TF 32	32	C	100 X	120	132	22
TF 34	34	C	100 X	110	122	24
TF 36	36	C	100 X	110	122	24
TF 38	38	C	100 X	110	122	24
TF 40	40	C	100 X	110	122	24
TF 42	42	C	100 X	115	127	25
TF 44	44	C	100 X	115	127	25
TF 46	46	C	100 X	115	127	25
TF 24	24	C	150 X	155	167	22
TF 26	26	C	150 X	155	167	22
TF 28	28	C	150 X	160	172	22
TF 30	30	C	150 X	160	172	22
TF 32	32	C	150 X	160	172	22

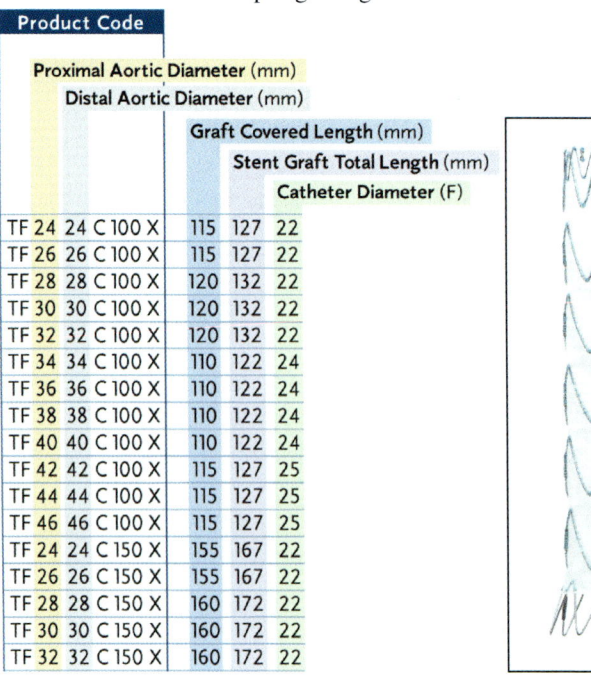

Product guide: Close web straight distal:

Product Code	Proximal Aortic Diameter (mm)	Distal Aortic Diameter (mm)	Graft Covered Length (mm)	Stent Graft Total Length (mm)	Catheter Diameter (F)
TC 24 24 C 100 X	105	105	22		
TC 26 26 C 100 X	105	105	22		
TC 28 28 C 100 X	110	110	22		
TC 30 30 C 100 X	110	110	22		
TC 32 32 C 100 X	110	110	22		
TC 34 34 C 100 X	100	100	24		
TC 36 36 C 100 X	100	100	24		
TC 38 38 C 100 X	100	100	24		
TC 40 40 C 100 X	100	100	24		
TC 42 42 C 100 X	105	105	25		
TC 44 44 C 100 X	105	105	25		
TC 46 46 C 100 X	105	105	25		
TC 24 24 C 150 X	145	145	22		
TC 26 26 C 150 X	145	145	22		
TC 28 28 C 150 X	150	150	22		
TC 30 30 C 150 X	150	150	22		
TC 32 32 C 150 X	150	150	22		

Product guide: Close web tapered distal:

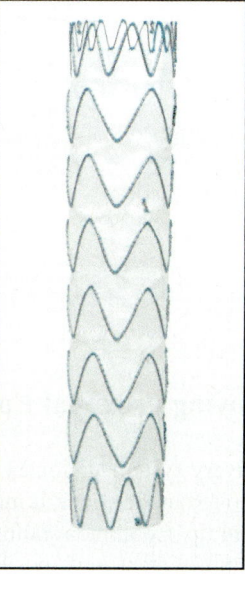

Product Code	Proximal Aortic Diameter (mm)	Distal Aortic Diameter (mm)	Graft Covered Length (mm)	Stent Graft Total Length (mm)	Catheter Diameter (F)
TC 28 24 C 150 X			150	150	22
TC 30 26 C 150 X			150	150	22
TC 32 28 C 150 X			150	150	22
TC 34 30 C 150 X			160	160	24
TC 36 32 C 150 X			160	160	24
TC 38 34 C 150 X			160	160	24
TC 40 36 C 150 X			160	160	24
TC 42 38 C 150 X			150	150	25
TC 44 40 C 150 X			150	150	25
TC 46 42 C 150 X			155	155	25

27.1 Device Implantation

Slowly insert the system over an 0.035″ stiff guidewire. Advance the system to the target landing zone; if patient does not have calcification or excessive thrombus, it is recommended to begin deployment several millimeters proximal to intended landing zone (Fig. 27.3).

Verify position of proximal and distal markers is where intended deployment should occur. At physician's discretion, it may be appropriate to temporarily decrease mean arterial blood pressure to approximately 80 mmHg to avoid inadvertent displacement of the stent graft upon withdrawal of graft cover. *Caution*: Do not place the proximal edge of the graft material beyond the top of the aortic arch or the distal edge of the left common carotid artery (Fig. 27.4).

Fig. 27.3 Advancement of stent graft system in thoracic aorta

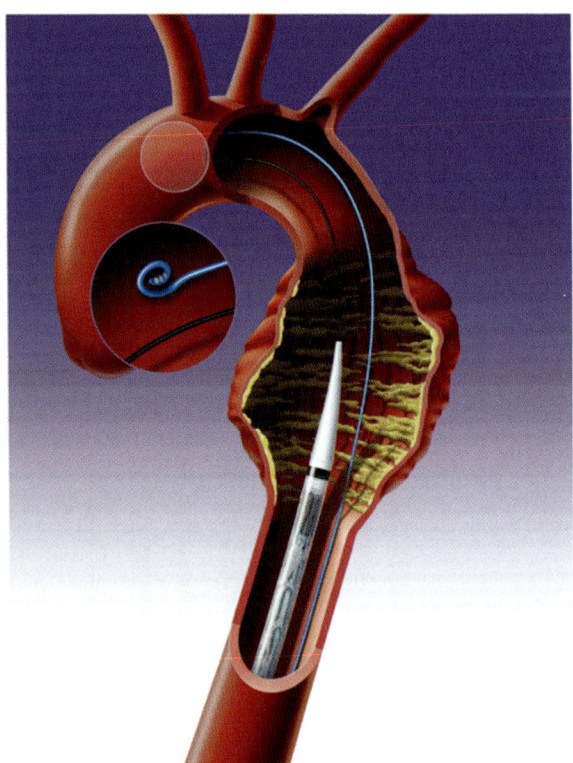

27.2 Deploying Proximal End

Hold the delivery system stationary with one hand on the front grip with the other hand, begin to rotate the slider; it may take multiple rotations before the graft cover separates from tip. Continue rotating until the first *two stents* (bare or covered) are deployed. Confirm stent graft position using angiography. System may be pulled distally to reposition if necessary (Fig. 27.5).

Fig. 27.4 Positioning of
stent graft

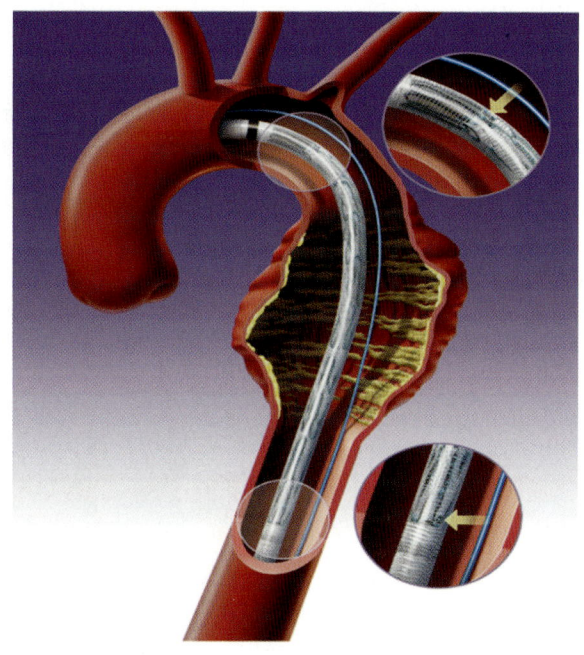

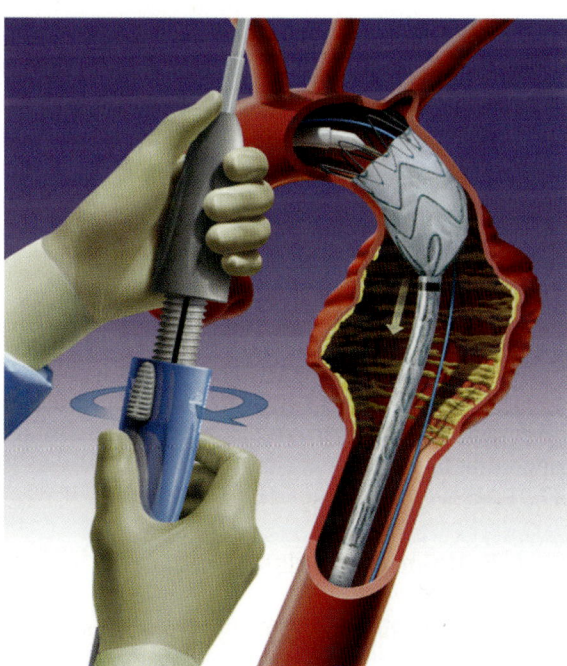

Fig. 27.5 Slow deployment
of thoracic stent graft

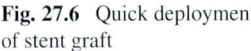**Fig. 27.6** Quick deployment
of stent graft

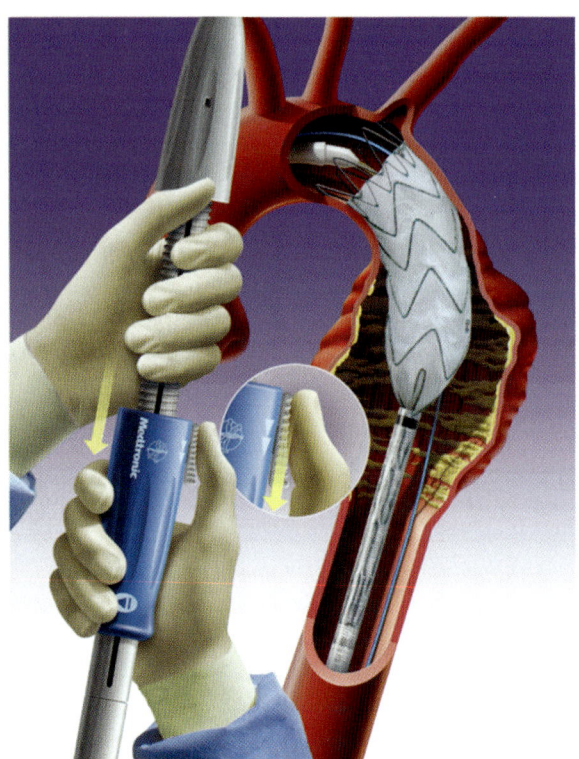

Physician may deploy the remaining graft more quickly: Front hand is placed in front of blue handle to brace system against potential recoil. Using rear hand, pull back on trigger and retract blue handle to deploy graft. When necessary, trigger can be reengaged and rotation used to continue deployment of stent graft (Fig. 27.6).

27.3 Removal of Delivery System

Depress Quick Disconnect button and pull section of handle back to retract tapered tip into graft cover. After reestablishing a smooth transition between tip and graft cover, pull entire delivery system back and remove it from patient. Do not remove guidewire (Fig. 27.7).

27.4 Balloon Angioplasty

Flush guidewire lumen. Aspirate air from balloon. Advance over guidewire to target location. Inflate balloon with contrast solution (*75% sodium chloride/25% contrast*).

Fig. 27.7 Recapture of tapered tip prior to retrieval of delivery system

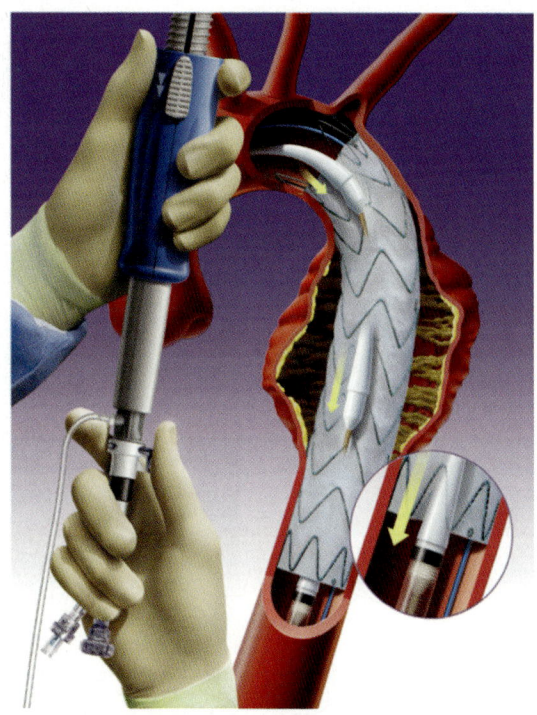

Fig. 27.8 Balloon angioplasty of proximal and distal ends of graft

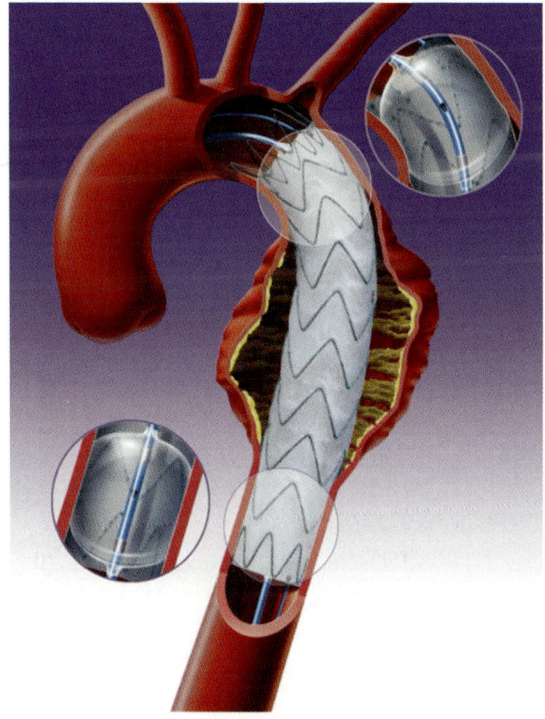

Fig. 27.9 Completion
angiogram demonstrates
satisfactory exclusion or
thoracic aneurysm

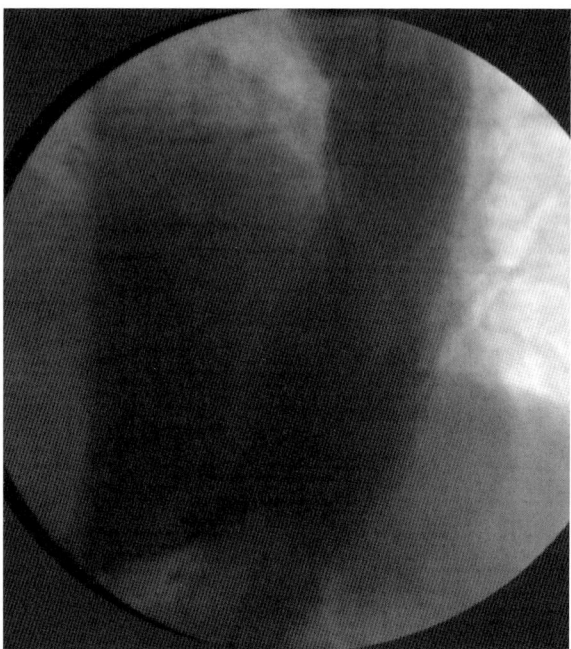

Rapidly deflate balloon. Repeat inflations and deflations as required. Remove catheter from patient (Fig. 27.8).

Completion angiogram is performed and if satisfactory device and guidewires are removed and seal entry sites repaired using standard surgical techniques (Fig. 27.9).

Chapter 28
Pivotal Results of the Medtronic Vascular Talent Thoracic Stent Graft System: The VALOR Trial

Abbreviations

CABG	coronary artery bypass grafting
DBP	diastolic blood pressure
Dip-Thal	dipyridamole thallium scan
ECG	electrocardiogram
EF	ejection fraction
FEV1	forced expiratory volume in 1 s
MI	myocardial infarction
PFT	pulmonary function tests

The VALOR trial was a prospective, nonrandomized, multicenter clinical study conducted in the United States to evaluate the safety and efficacy of the Medtronic Vascular Talent Thoracic Stent Graft in the treatment of thoracic aortic diseases. Enrollment occurred from December 2003 to June 2005 at 38 institutions across ed States This report focuses on the pivotal test group population, which included patients diagnosed with TAAs. These patients were considered candidates for open surgical repair and were low to moderate risk (0, 1, and 2) per the modified Society for Vascular Surgery and the American Association for Vascular Surgery criteria. (The anatomic and medical inclusion and exclusion criteria are presented in Table 28.1.)

Surgical candidates with a fusiform thoracic aortic aneurysm ≥ 5 cm or ≥ 2 times the diameter of the non-aneurysmal aorta, as well as focal saccular thoracic aneurysms (penetrating atherosclerotic ulcers), were considered for inclusion. The aneurysm had to be at least 20 mm distal to the left common carotid and 20 mm proximal to the celiac artery, have a proximal and distal non-aneurysmal aortic neck diameter of between 18 and 42 mm, and proximal and distal non-aneurysmal aortic neck lengths of at least 20 mm. A notable exclusion criterion was previous surgical or endovascular treatment of an infra-renal aortic aneurysm.

Standard follow-up evaluations were performed at 1, 6, and 12 months and annually thereafter. Follow-up visits included a CT scan, chest radiograph, and

J. Kpodonu, *Manual of Thoracic Endoaortic Surgery*,
DOI 10.1007/978-1-84996-296-4_28, © Springer-Verlag London Limited 2010

Table 28.1 Anatomic and medical inclusion and exclusion criteria

Inclusion criteria
- Age between 18 and 85 years
- SVS/AAVS criteria 0, 1, or 2
- Women with negative pregnancy test 7 days before implant
- Fusiform focal TAA ≥5 cm or ≥2 times non-aneurysmal aorta and/or focal saccular TAA or penetrating atherosclerotic ulcer
- TAA 20 mm distal to origin of left common carotid artery and 20 mm proximal to the origin of the celiac artery
- Proximal and distal neck diameter 18–42 mm
- Proximal and distal aneurysm neck length >20 mm
- TAA confirmed by CTA/MRA with optional 3D reconstruction 3 months before screening
- Subject must be able and willing to undergo follow-up imaging and examinations at 1, 6, and 12 months and annually thereafter

Exclusion criteria
- Planned placement of the covered portion of the stent graft in zones 0 or 1
- Access vessel precludes safe insertion of the delivery system
- Planned aortic conduit
- TAA with contained rupture
- Connective tissue disease (e.g., Marfan syndrome, medial degeneration)
- Mycotic aneurysm or is suspected of having systemic infection
- Previous stent and/or stent graft or previous surgical repair in the DTA
- Treatment of an infra-renal aneurysm at the time of implant
- Previous surgical or endovascular treatment of an infra-renal aortic aneurysm
- History of bleeding diathesis, coagulopathy, or refuses blood transfusions
- Vascular interventional procedure or major surgery 30 days before enrollment
- Planned vascular interventional procedure or major surgery ≤30 days of the implant procedure
- Cerebrovascular accident ≤3 months
- Currently participating in an investigational drug or device clinical trial
- Known allergy or intolerance to the device components
- Known hypersensitivity or contraindication to anticoagulants or contrast media, which is not amenable to pretreatment
- Significant and/or circumferential aortic mural thrombus at proximal or distal attachment sites
- Medical condition that may cause noncompliance with the protocol, confound the data interpretation, or a limited life expectancy of <1 year

CTA, computed tomography angiography; *DTA*, descending thoracic aorta; *MRA*, magnetic resonance angiography; *SVS/AAVS*, Society for Vascular Surgery/American Association for Vascular Surgery; *TAA*, thoracic aortic aneurysm

physical examination. All clinical data were reported by the investigative center on case report forms and monitored by the sponsor. A Clinical Events Committee adjudicated major adverse events (MAEs) for device and procedure relatedness. Medical Metrx Solutions (M2S; West Lebanon, NH) served as the imaging core laboratory and provided critical and comprehensive data evaluation of all imaging studies, ensuring third-party assessment of graft effectiveness. Endoleaks were defined according to the well-established type I to IV nomenclature.[1] In the event the core laboratory could not identify the source, the endoleak was classified as unknown. Migration was defined as >10 mm proximal or distal movement of the stent graft relative to fixed anatomic landmarks, and aneurysm expansion was defined as >5 mm increase in diameter from the 1-month to 12-month follow-up visit. An MAE was defined as death due to the procedure, any death ≤30 days of the procedure, respiratory complications, renal insufficiency or failure, cardiac events, neurologic events, aneurysm rupture, bowel ischemia, major bleeding, or vascular complications. An MAE that was identified as a serious adverse event by the clinical investigator was defined as serious MAE. Aneurysm-related death was defined as any death ≤30 days from initial implantation or occurring as a consequence of an aneurysm rupture, a conversion to open repair, or any other secondary endovascular procedure relative to the aneurysm that was treated by the Talent Thoracic Stent Graft System as evidenced by CT scan, angiography, or direct observation at surgery or autopsy. Excluded were aneurysms in anatomic areas other than the targeted segment treated by the Talent Thoracic Stent Graft System. Aneurysm-related death after open repair included any death ≤30 days from the surgical procedure or any death caused by reintervention of the targeted aortic segment or by complications related to the graft or the procedure. Summary statistics presented for categorical variables are the number in each category and the percentage of known values that this number represents. For continuous variables, the mean and standard deviation are provided; P values were calculated using standard t-tests. In some cases the median is provided as well. Kaplan-Meier curves were used to plot freedom from event over time.

28.1 Results

28.1.1 Demographics

The VALOR trial enrolled 195 patients. Figure 28.2 details patient accountability of the 195 test group patients at 12 months of follow-up. A total of 189 patients were identified as retrospective open surgical subjects. Subject demographics, baseline history, and aneurysm dimensional characteristics for VALOR test group and the open surgery group are presented in Tables 28.2, 28.3, and 28.4. Compared with the open surgery group, the subjects in the VALOR test group had similar age and gender distributions but had lower TAA size and were less likely to have a previous abdominal aortic aneurysm (AAA) or AAA repair. At the time of enrollment, 51 of 195 patients (26%) in the VALOR test group had aneurysm-related symptoms. The mean aneurysm length was 121.4 ± 72.7 mm as measured by the core laboratory. These data were not available for the open surgery group.

28.2 Procedure and Hospital Course

Vessel access and deployment of the study device at the intended site was successful in 194 (99.5%) of the 195 patients enrolled in the VALOR trial. One patient did not receive a study device because of access failure. Iliac conduits were required

Table 28.2 Subject demographics: VALOR test group versus open surgery

Variable	VALOR test group	Open surgery
Age		
Total population		
N	195	189
Mean ± SD (years)	70.2 ± 11.1	69.6 ± 9.1
Median	73.0	71.0
Min–max	27–86	27–85
Male		
N	115	99
Mean ± SD (years)	69.3 ± 11.7	69.9 ± 8.5
Median	72.0	71.0
Min–max	27–85	40–84
Female		
N	80	90
Mean ± SD (years)	71.6 ± 10.1	69.3 ± 9.8
Median	74.0	71.0
Min–max	38–86	27–85
Sex, % (no.)		
Males	59.0 (115)	52.4 (99)
Females	41.0 (80)	47.6 (90)
Ethnicity, % (no.)		
White, non-Hispanic	83.1 (162)	93.7 (177)
Black, non-Hispanic	12.8 (25)	5.8 (11)
Hispanic (white or black)	2.6 (5)	0.5 (1)
Asian/Pacific Islander	1.0 (2)	0 (0)
Native American	0 (0)	0 (0)
Other[a]	0.5 (1)	0 (0)

SD, standard deviation; *VALOR*, Evaluation of the Medtronic Vascular Talent Thoracic Stent Graft System for the Treatment of Thoracic Aortic Aneurysms
[a]One subject had ethnicity specified as "none given"

for arterial access in 21.1% of the patients. A mean number of 2.7 ± 1.3 stent graft devices (range 1–7) were implanted per patient. Approximately 25% of the patients had proximal main Talent Thoracic Stent Graft components implanted with diameters <26 mm (3 patients, 1.9%) or >40 mm (49 patients, 23.2%). The highest implantation zone (Fig. 28.1) of the bare spring segment of the most proximally implanted device was zone 1 in 6.7% of patients, zone 2 in 26.8%, zone 3 in 35.6%, and zone 4 in 30.9%.

The decision to revascularize the LSA was left to the implanting physician and was performed before the initial stent graft procedure in 10 of 194 patients (5.2%). At the conclusion of the procedure, the 194 patients with a device implanted had patent stent grafts, with integrity maintained and freedom from twisting or kinking. Clinical utility measures for the VALOR test group and the open surgery group are compared in Table 28.5. The VALOR test group showed superiority in regard to subjects requiring blood transfusion, procedural blood loss, and length of procedure, as well as intensive care unit and overall hospital stay ($P < 0.001$).

Table 28.3 Baseline medical history: VALOR test group versus open surgery

Medical history	VALOR test group % (m/n)	Open surgery % (m/n)
Cardiovascular		
Angina	14.4 (28/195)	22.8 (26/114)
Arrhythmias	26.7 (52/195)	20.3 (37/182)
Congestive heart failure	8.7 (17/195)	11.2 (21/187)
CABG	10.3 (20/195)	13.3 (25/188)
Coronary artery disease	40.5 (79/195)	49.2 (91/185)
Hypertension	87.2 (170/195)	88.8 (166/187)
Myocardial infarction	13.8 (27/195)	20.9 (39/187)
Peripheral vascular disease	16.4 (32/195)	37.4 (70/187)
AAA	19.0 (37/195)	37.0 (70/189)
AAA repair	2.1 (4/195)	27.5 (52/189)
Gastrointestinal conditions	53.8 (105/195)	NA
Renal insufficiency	17.4 (34/195)	16.0 (30/187)
Musculoskeletal conditions	53.8 (105/195)	NA
Neurologic		
Cerebral vascular accident	9.7 (19/195)	13.4 (25/186)
Paraplegia	1.0 (2/195)	0.5 (1/186)
Paraparesis	0.5 (1/195)	NA
Transient ischemic attack	7.7 (15/195)	NA
Pulmonary		
COPD	36.9 (72/195)	42.6 (80/188)
Tobacco use	76.9 (150/195)	75.9 (142/187)
Other abnormal body systems		
Hyperlipidemia	43.6 (85/195)	NA
Diabetes	15.9 (31/195)	8.6 (16/187)
Bleeding disorders	2.6 (5/195)	NA

AAA, abdominal aortic aneurysm repair; *CABG*, coronary artery bypass grafting; *COPD*, chronic obstructive pulmonary disease; *NA*, not available; *VALOR*, Evaluation of the Medtronic Vascular Talent Thoracic Stent Graft System for the Treatment of Thoracic Aortic Aneurysms

Mortality: Four of 195 VALOR patients (2.1%) died ≤30 days after implantation. Causes of death of these patients included atheroembolic multisystem failure, stroke, peri-procedural cardiac arrest, and complications from a myocardial infarction and perforated ulcer. Table 28.6 describes the 30-day mortality rates for the VALOR test group compared with the open surgery group. The VALOR test group experienced a significantly lower rate of early mortality (2% versus 8%, $P < 0.01$). All-cause mortality at 12 months is presented in Table 28.7 (16.1% versus 20.6%, $P = $ NS). Freedom from all-cause mortality is presented for both groups in Fig. 28.2. Predictors of all-cause mortality at 12 months in the VALOR patients included prior stroke, with an odds ratio of 4.45 ($P = 0.019$), chronic obstructive lung disease, with an odds ratio of 3.72 ($P = 0.008$), and aneurysm length, with an odds ratio of 1.008 ($P = 0.017$) for each additional millimeter.

Aneurysm-related mortality: Six of 192 patients (3.1%) in the VALOR test group died of an aneurysm-related cause through 12 months of follow-up. Four patients died ≤30 days of the procedure. Two additional late deaths were adjudicated as aneurysm-related. In the open surgery group, 22 of 189 patients (11.6%)

Table 28.4 Baseline maximum aneurysm diameters: VALOR test group versus open surgery

Aneurysm diameter (mm)	Site reported, % (m/n)[a]	Core lab reported, % (m/n)[b]	Open surgery, % (m/n)
10–17	0 (0/188)	0 (0/187)	0 (0/189)
18–29	0 (0/188)	0.5 (1/187)	0 (0/189)
30–39	4.3 (8/188)	7.5 (14/187)	0 (0/189)
40–49	10.6 (20/188)	20.3 (38/187)	0.5 (1/189)
50–59	34.6 (65/188)	34.8 (65/187)	13.8 (26/189)
60–69	33.5 (63/188)	24.6 (46/187)	40.7 (77/189)
70–79	12.2 (23/188)	10.2 (19/187)	24.3 (46/189)
80–89	3.2 (6/188)	2.1 (4/187)	16.9 (32/189)
90–99	1.1 (2/188)	0 (0/187)	0.5 (1/189)
100–109	0.5 (1/188)	0 (0/187)	1.6 (3/189)
110–119	0 (0/188)	0 (0/187)	0.5 (1/189)
120+	0 (0/188)	0 (0/187)	1.1 (2/189)

VALOR, Evaluation of the Medtronic Vascular Talent Thoracic Stent Graft System for the Treatment of Thoracic Aortic Aneurysms
[a]Denominator is 188 subjects with site reported data
[b]Denominator is 187 subjects with evaluable scans

Fig. 28.1 Zones of stent graft implantation for thoracic aortic aneurysms

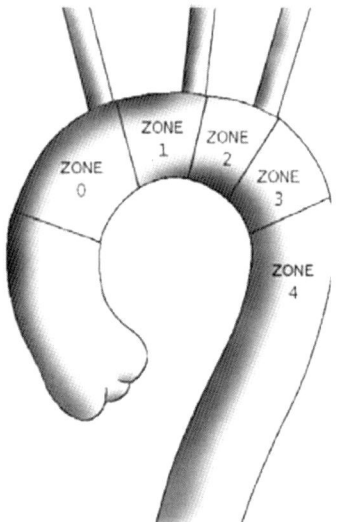

died of aneurysm-related causes, and this difference was statistically significant at $P < 0.002$. Freedom from aneurysm-related death for both groups is presented in Fig. 28.3.

Conversion to surgery: One patient (0.5%) was converted to open surgical repair approximately 9 months after implantation for complications related to an apparent infection in the stented segment of the aorta. This patient was alive and fully evaluable at the 12-month post-implantation follow-up.

Table 28.5   Acute procedural data: VALOR test group versus open surgery

Variable	VALOR test group	Open surgery	P^a
Subjects requiring blood transfusion, % (m/n)	22.7 (44/194)	93.7 (164/175)	<0.001
Blood loss during procedure, mean ± SD (ml)[b]	371.2±514.4	3054.9±1702.4	<0.001
Duration of implant procedure, mean ± SD (min)	154.2±76.0	303.3±97.6	<0.001
Length of stay, mean ± SD			
ICU (accessible subjects) (h)	46.8±114.3	185.3±204.7	<0.001
Overall hospital (days)	6.4±11.5	16.7±15.0	<0.001

SD, standard deviation; VALOR, Evaluation of the Medtronic Vascular Talent Thoracic Stent Graft System for the Treatment of Thoracic Aortic Aneurysms
[a]For difference between groups. Percentage of subjects requiring blood transfusion was compared using the Fisher exact test. Other variables were compared using the Wilcoxon test
[b]Only one open surgical site could provide blood loss during procedure data

Table 28.6   All-cause mortality at 30 days

Group	30-day mortality, % (m/n)*
VALOR test group	2.1 (4/195)
Open surgery	7.9 (15/189)

*$P < 0.01$
VALOR, Evaluation of the Medtronic Vascular Talent Thoracic Stent Graft System for the Treatment of Thoracic Aortic Aneurysms

Table 28.7   All-cause mortality at 12 months

Group	12 month mortality, % (m/n)*
VALOR test group	16.1 (31/192)
Open surgery	20.6 (39/189)

*$P = 0.29$
VALOR, Evaluation of the Medtronic Vascular Talent Thoracic Stent Graft System for the Treatment of Thoracic Aortic Aneurysms

Major adverse events: One or more MAEs occurred in 41% (80 of 195) of the VALOR patients ≤30 days after implantation compared with 84.4% (151 of 179) in the open surgery group ($P < 0.001$; Table 28.8). Most of the individual MAE categories in the endovascular group were lower, but vascular complications were higher in the VALOR patients, at 21% (41 of 195), compared with the open surgery patients, at 12.3% (22 of 179). Freedom from MAEs is presented in Fig. 28.4.

Cerebrovascular accidents: Seven VALOR patients (3.6%) had a peri-procedural stroke. Three patients had resolution of stroke-related disability at 12 months, death, or last follow-up. Logistic regression analysis was performed on the occurrence of stroke ≤30 days after the implantation procedure. Patients who had a history

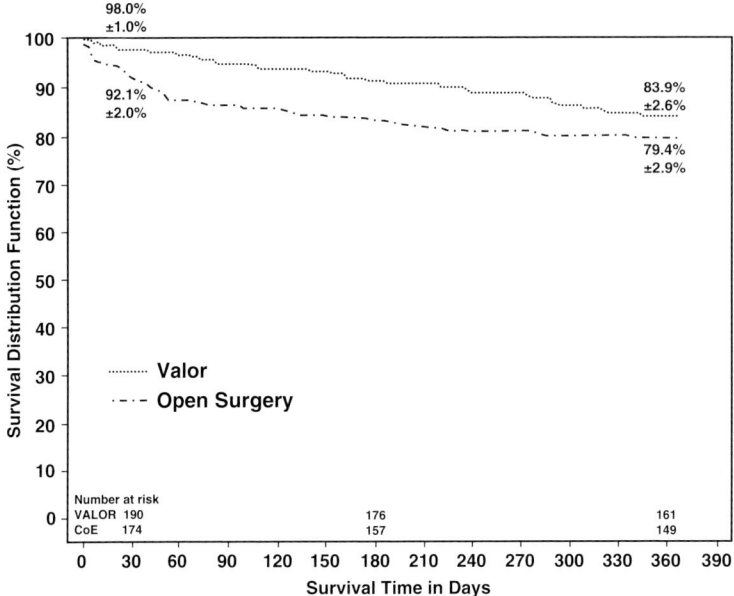

Fig. 28.2 Kaplan-Meier plot of freedom from all-cause mortality for Evaluation of the Medtronic Vascular Talent Thoracic Stent Graft System for the Treatment of Thoracic Aortic Aneurysms (*VALOR*) trial participants (*solid line*) and the open surgery cohort (*dashed line*)

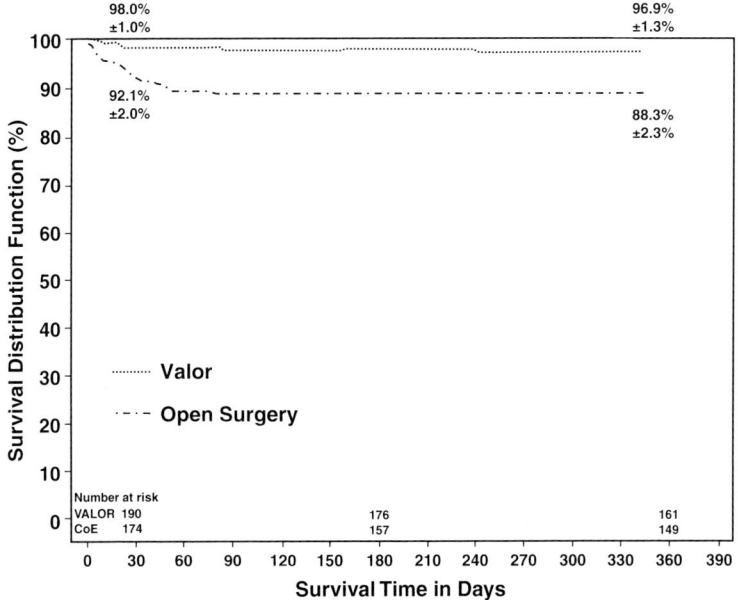

Fig. 28.3 Kaplan-Meier plot of freedom from aneurysm-related mortality for Evaluation of the Medtronic Vascular Talent Thoracic Stent Graft System for the Treatment of Thoracic Aortic Aneurysms (VALOR) trial participants (*solid line*) and the open surgery cohort (*dashed line*)

Table 28.8 Major adverse events for VALOR test group versus open surgery group at 30 days

Category	VALOR test group, % (m/n)	Open surgery % (m/n)
Respiratory complications	13.3 (26/195)	46.9 (84/179)
Pneumonia	9.2 (18/195)	22.3 (40/179)
Pulmonary embolism	0.5 (1/195)	0.6 (1/179)
Pulmonary edema	2.1 (4/195)	24.6 (44/179)
Respiratory failure	6.2 (12/195)	26.8 (48/179)
Renal complications	6.2 (12/195)	29.1 (52/179)
Renal insufficiency	1.5 (3/195)	16.2 (29/179)
Renal failure	4.6 (9/195)	19.6 (35/179)
Cardiac complications	12.3 (24/195)	44.7 (80/179)
Myocardial infarction	1.5 (3/195)	5.6 (10/179)
Unstable angina	0.5 (1/195)	0.6 (1/179)
New arrhythmia	8.7 (17/195)	41.3 (74/179)
Exacerbation of CHF	3.1 (6/195)	5.6 (10/179)
Neurologic complications	11.8 (23/195)	20.1 (36/179)
New CVA/embolic events	3.6 (7/195)	7.3 (13/179)
Paraplegia	1.5 (3/195)	3.4 (6/179)
Paraparesis	7.2 (14/195)	12.8 (23/179)
Gastrointestinal complications	1.0 (2/195)	0.6 (1/179)
Bowel ischemia	1.0 (2/195)	0.6 (1/179)
Bleeding complications	15.4 (30/195)	48.0 (86/179)
Coagulopathy	5.6 (11/195)	20.1 (36/179)
Procedural/Post-procedural	14.4 (28/195)	37.4 (67/179)
Vascular complications	21.0 (41/195)	12.3 (22/179)
Expanding hematoma at access site	1.5 (3/195)	2.2 (4/179)
Pseudo/false aneurysm at access site	2.1 (4/195)	1.1 (2/179)
AV fistula	0.5 (1/195)	0 (0/179)
Retroperitoneal bleed	2.6 (5/195)	1.1 (2/179)
Thrombosis	0 (0/195)	6.1 (11/179)
Arterial occlusion	2.1 (4/195)	2.2 (4/179)
Vessel rupture/dissection	6.2 (12/195)	1.7 (3/179)
Vessel disruption	7.7 (15/195)	0.6 (1/179)
Embolism	5.1 (10/195)	1.1 (2/179)
Re-op for limb ischemia	1.0 (2/195)	0.6 (1/179)
Vascular surgical repair or ultrasound compression required	14.4 (28/195)	3.4 (6/179)
Target lesion aneurysm rupture	0 (0/195)	0.6 (1/179)
Total major adverse events	41.0 (80/195)	84.4 (151/179)

CHF, congestive heart failure; *CVA*, cerebrovascular accident; *VALOR*, Evaluation of the Medtronic Vascular Talent Thoracic Stent Graft System for the Treatment of Thoracic Aortic Aneurysms

of AAA had an odds ratio of 7.1 for the occurrence of stroke ($P = 0.031$), and implantation in zone 1 or zone 2 had an odds ratio of 15.2 for the occurrence of stroke ($P = 0.018$).

Spinal ischemia: Post-operative paraplegia occurred ≤30 days in three of 195 VALOR patients (1.5%) and in a fourth patient at 32 days after implantation. All

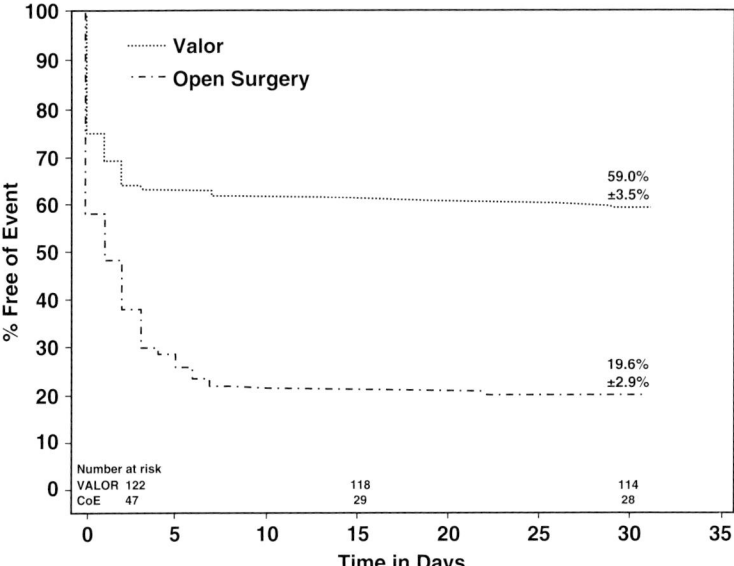

Fig. 28.4 Kaplan-Meier plot of freedom from major adverse events at 30 days for Evaluation of the Medtronic Vascular Talent Thoracic Stent Graft System for the Treatment of Thoracic Aortic Aneurysms (VALOR) trial participants (*solid line*) and the open surgery cohort (*dashed line*)

patients had placement of a lumbar drain at the time neurologic deficits were identified. None of these patients experienced recovery at the 1-year follow-up or by the time of death, and none of the patients with paraplegia had a previously treated AAA. Onset of paraparesis occurred ≤30 days in 14 VALOR patients (7.2%). The proportion of patients with unresolved paraparesis within 12 months or last known follow-up fell to 3.1% (6 of 192). Logistic regression analysis was performed on the incidence of paraplegia or paraparesis within ≤30 days after the implantation procedure. The only covariate that was found to be a significant predictor was the use of a conduit for access, with an odds ratio of 4.13 ($P = 0.020$).

Stent graft effectiveness: The core laboratory identified seven patients with a type I endoleak by the 30-day follow-up visit, as noted in Table 28.9. Most endoleaks were type II. Sixteen patients had 17 additional endovascular procedures, of which

Table 28.9 Endoleaks at 1 and 12 months (core laboratory)

Device-related event	At 1-month visit, % (m/n)	At 12-month visit, % (m/n)
Endoleak of any size	25.9 (45/174)	12.2 (15/123)
Type I	4.0 (7/174)	4.9 (6/123)
Type II	15.5 (27/174)	4.9 (6/123)
Type III	1.7 (3/174)	0 (0/123)
Type IV	0 (0/174)	0 (0/123)
Indeterminate	4.6 (8/174)	2.4 (3/123)

two procedures (1.0%) occurred in the 30-day period before discharge and 15 procedures (8.1%) occurred at 31–365 days. Fourteen procedures were performed to resolve an endoleak. One patient had a procedure to resolve migration and to cover a pseudoaneurysm. One patient was treated for an aneurysmal expansion, and one patient was treated for a second aneurysm.

The core laboratory noted four stent graft migrations ≤12 months. Two migrations involved the proximal end of the graft moving distally, and two involved the distal end of the graft moving proximally. Only one patient required an additional intervention related to the migration. Aneurysm sac diameter was stable or shrinking in 91.4% of patients. In 11 patients (8.5%), the increase in maximal aneurysm diameter was >5 mm during this interval, and seven of these patients had endoleaks during follow-up. No study patient had loss of stent graft patency or instances of compression or collapse of the endograft ≤12 months. In two patients the core laboratory confirmed stent fractures ≤12 months. Neither patient had adverse events related to these fractures.

Appendix A   Catalog stent graft specifications and configurations

Variables	Main sections	Additional distal main sections	Proximal extensions	Distal extensions
Diameters (2-mm increments)				
Proximal	22–46	26–46	26–46	26–46
Distal	22–46	22–44	26–46	26–46
Total covered length of device, mm[a]	112–116	110–114	46–54	46–54
Proximal configurations	FreeFlo[b] (Bare Spring)	Open Web	FreeFlo[b]	Open Web
Distal configurations	Closed Web	Closed Web	Open Web	Bare Spring[b]

[a]The maximum total length cannot exceed 130 mm
[b]"Bare Spring" and "FreeFlo" refer to the configuration in which the terminating spring has no fabric coverage. Bare Spring is the term used for devices having a proximal diameter <24 mm, while FreeFlo is the term used for devices having a proximal diameter ≥24 mm. FreeFlo devices feature a support spring to prevent fabric infolding

Reference

1. Fairman RM, Criado F, Farber M, et al.; VALOR Investigators. Pivotal results of the Medtronic vascular talent thoracic stent graft system: The VALOR Trial. *J Vasc Surg*. 2008:48(3);546–554.

Part VIII
Endografting for Thoracic Aortic Aneurysms

Chapter 29
Endovascular Management of Thoracic Aortic Aneurysm Using a Cook Zenith TX2 Endograft

Cook Zenith TX2 Thoracic Endovascular Graft

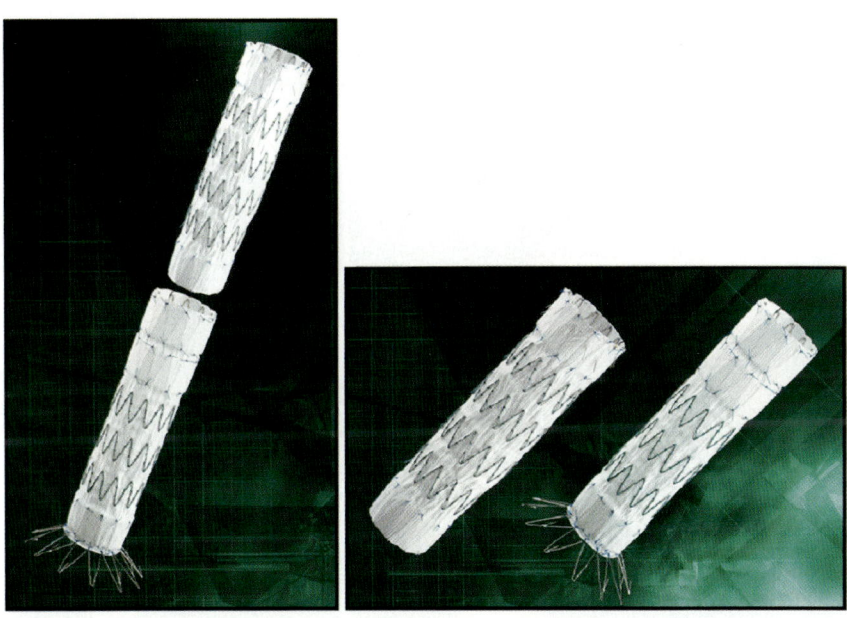

29.1 Introduction

With the introduction of the first commercially available endograft, two additional endoprosthesis are in the process of being evaluated for FDA approval. The Cook TX2 stent graft is designed as a two-piece system that incorporates hooks and barbs, distal fixation, and a proximal controlled deployment. Thoracic stent graft treatment of thoracic aortic pathologies, including thoracic aortic aneurysms, has been associated with migration of both proximal and distal fixation points,[1] erosion of

J. Kpodonu, *Manual of Thoracic Endoaortic Surgery*,
DOI 10.1007/978-1-84996-296-4_29, © Springer-Verlag London Limited 2010

uncovered proximal portion through the aortic arch,[2] and component separation with modular devices.[2,3] These problems have been described with most of the thoracic endoprosthesis implanted for thoracic aortic pathologies.[3-5] The ideal thoracic stent graft currently does not exist but would need to be flexible enough to accommodate the tortuosity of the arch, incorporate a fixation system that is secure both proximally and distally, seal within both straight and tortuous segments, be readily deliverable, and have favorable effects on the excluded region of the aorta. Additionally, delivery of the device would optimally not require the induction of hypotension or bradycardia even in the setting of extreme tortuosity. The Cook TX1 and TX2 device has been designed to attempt to solve some of these issues but currently at this time is not approved as a commercial device in the United States.

29.2 Case Scenario

An 60-year-old man with a 40 pack year smoking history was found to have a thoracic aortic aneurysm of the mid and descending thoracic aorta on a chest X-ray

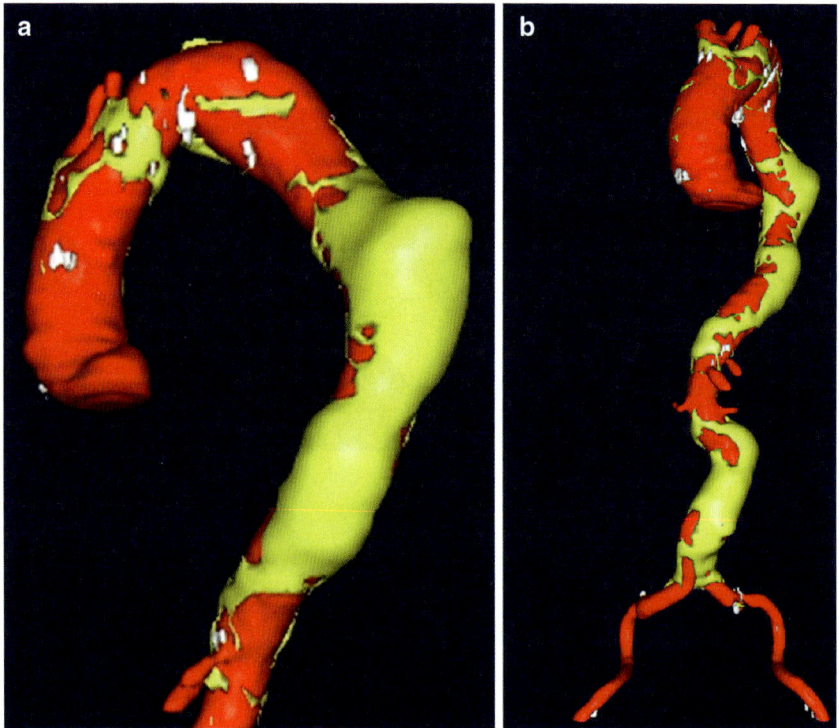

Fig. 29.1 (**a**, **b**) Reconstructed CT scan of the chest demonstrating a thoracic aortic aneurysm measuring 6.0 cm in diameter with adequate-sized iliac vessels with minimal tortuosity and calcium

performed for evaluation of a lung nodule. A CT scan of the chest performed demonstrated a 6.0 cm thoracic aortic aneurysm with mural thrombus (Fig. 29.1). Due to the extensive co-morbidities he was felt to be a high-risk candidate for open surgical repair and enrolled in the multicenter TX2 trial.

29.3 Endovascular Procedure

The right common femoral artery was exposed through a small oblique incision and cannulated with a 9 Fr sheath. Percutaneous access of the left common femoral artery was performed and a 5 Fr sheath was introduced. Oblique thoracic aortogram was performed through the left groin sheath via a 5 Fr pigtail angiographic catheter to delineate the arch and the descending thoracic aorta aneurysm (Fig. 29.2a). Intravascular ultrasound was performed using a (Volcano Therapeutics, Inc.) 8.2 Fr probe through the right groin sheath to confirm the size of aneurysm, presence or absence of thrombus, proximal neck diameter and length, and distal neck diameter and length. The proximal neck and distal neck diameter were measured at 30 mm. Based on the measurements, a 36 mm Cook Zenith TX2 thoracic endoluminal graft was chosen for exclusion of the thoracic aortic aneurysm. An extra stiff Lunderquist wire (Cook Bloomington, IN, USA) was exchanged through the IVUS catheter. The right 9 Fr sheath was exchanged for a Cook Zenith TX2 device (Bloomington, IN) measuring 36 mm × 152 mm and deployed 2 cm distal to the left subclavian artery with at least a 3 cm proximal neck. A second Cook Zenith device 36 mm × 136 mm was deployed distally with adequate overlap between grafts to a level just above

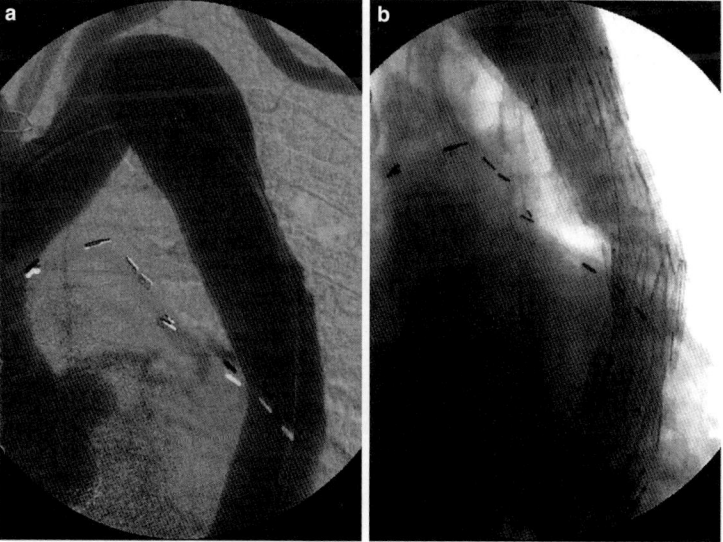

Fig. 29.2 (**a, b**) A pre- and post-thoracic aortogram demonstrating an angulated and tortuous arch and exclusion of the aneurysm

Fig. 29.3 (**a, b**)
Post-operative CT scan of the
chest demonstrating
satisfactory exclusion of
aneurysm

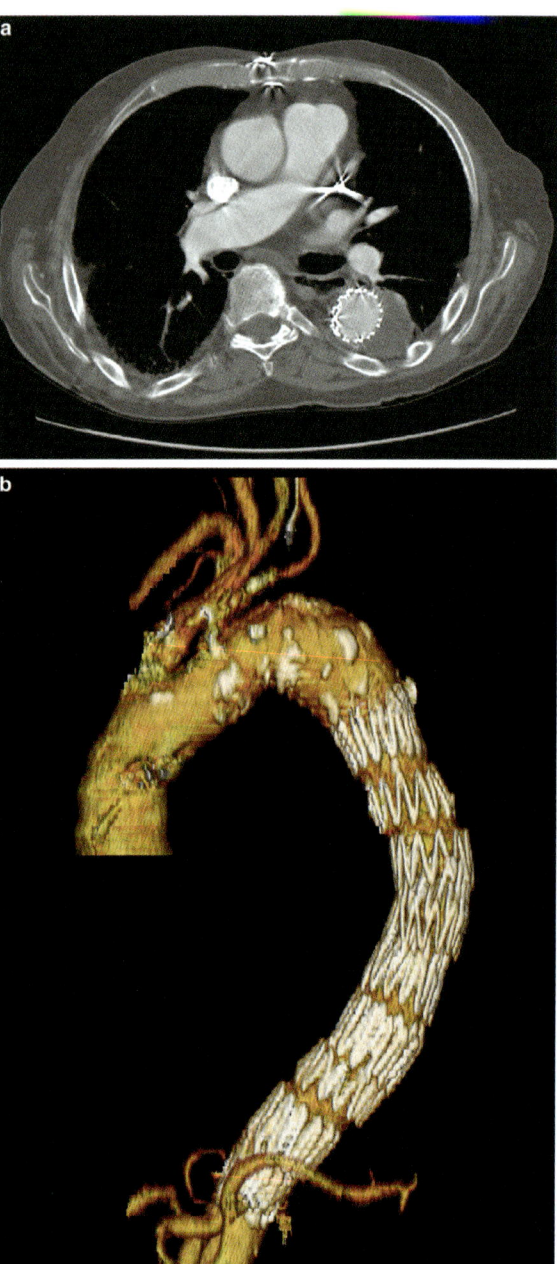

the celiac trunk. A completion angiogram demonstrated satisfactory exclusion of
the thoracic aortic aneurysm with no endoleak (Fig. 29.2b). All wires and sheaths
were removed. The right common femoral artery was closed in a transverse fashion
with restoration of flow. A vascular closure device was deployed to the left common

femoral artery with satisfactory results. The patient had bilateral palpable pulses at the end of the procedure was extubated and transferred to recovery room. A postoperative CT scan demonstrated adequate exclusion of thoracic aortic aneurysm with no endoleak (Fig. 29.3a).

References

1. Greenberg R, Resch T, Nyman U, et al. Endovascular repair of descending thoracic aortic aneurysms (an early experience with intermediate-term follow-up). *J Vasc Surg.* 2000;31(1):147–156.
2. Malina M, Brunkwall J, Ivancev K, et al. Late aortic arch perforation by graft-anchoring stent (complication of endovascular thoracic aneurysm exclusion). *J Endovasc Surg.* 1998;5(3):274–277.
3. Criado FJ, Clarke NS, Barnaton M. Stent-graft repair in the aortic arch and descending thoracic aorta (a 4-year experience). *J Vasc Surg.* 2002;36:1121–1128.
4. White RA, Donayre CE, Walot L, Kopchok G, Woody J. Endovascular exclusion of descending thoracic aortic aneurysms and chronic dissections (initial clinical results with the AneuRx device). *J Vasc Surg.* 2001;33:927–934.
5. Dake MD, Miller DC, Mitchell RS. The first generation of endovascular stent grafts for patients with descending thoracic aortic aneurysms. *J Thorac Cardiovasc Surg.* 1998;116:689–704.

Chapter 30
Management of a Patient with Thoracic Aortic Aneurysm Using Gore TAG Device

Patients with asymptomatic descending aortic aneurysm larger than twice the size of the normal distal aortic arch in an orthogonal projection (at least 5 cm), with no history or evidence of connective tissue disorder require repair. Symptomatic aneurysms mandate endovascular or open repair, regardless of size. The patient should have proximal (distal to left common carotid) and distal neck of at least 2 cm without significant calcification or thrombus; the patient should have access vessels of at least 8 mm luminal diameter and without extreme tortuosity. Depending on device availability, the patient's landing zone diameter has to be within the manufacturer's instruction for use (IFU), e.g., for the Gore TAG device the proximal and distal landing zones should not be smaller than 23 mm or larger than 37 mm.

30.1 Case Scenario

A 71-year-old lady presented with a descending thoracic aneurysm (DTA) of 6.0 cm × 5.3 cm (Fig. 30.1). Due to the expansion of the aneurysm and her

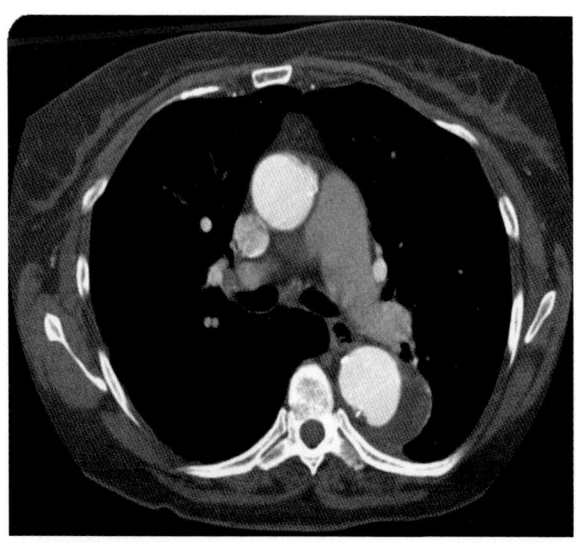

Fig. 30.1 CT scan of the chest with IV contrast demonstrating a descending thoracic aneurysm with mural thrombus measuring 6.0 cm × 5.3 cm in diameter

J. Kpodonu, *Manual of Thoracic Endoaortic Surgery*,
DOI 10.1007/978-1-84996-296-4_30, © Springer-Verlag London Limited 2010

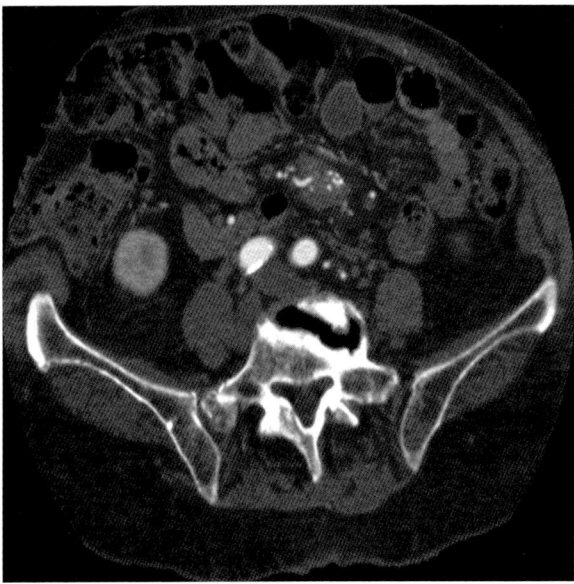

Fig. 30.2 An axial CT image demonstrating adequate-sized iliac arteries with mild calcification in the posterior wall of right iliac artery

prohibitive medical history CT imaging of the iliac vessels (Fig. 30.2) showed appropriate sizing for endovascular repair.[1]

30.2 Recommendation

Measurements obtained from the diagnostic CT scans of the chest, abdomen, and pelvis indicated that the patient met the criteria for endoluminal stent grafting using the preoperative work sheet (Fig. 30.3).

30.3 Procedure

Under general anesthesia, open retrograde cannulation of the right common femoral artery was performed with an 18 G needle and a 0.035 in. soft tip angled glide wire (Medi-tech/Boston Scientific, Natick, MA) was passed into the distal thoracic aorta and exchanged for a 9 Fr sheath under fluoroscopic visualization. Percutaneous access of the left common femoral artery was similarly performed with a 5 Fr sheath. Five thousand units of heparin was given to keep the activated clotted time greater than 200 s. A 5 Fr pigtail catheter was advanced through the left groin sheath into the thoracic aorta. The fluoroscopic C-arm was positioned in a left anterior oblique angle and an oblique thoracic arch aortogram was performed to visualize the arch

Fig. 30.3 A pre-operative worksheet to evaluate the candidacy for stent graft placement. A, proximal implantation site – 30 mm; B, 1 cm proximal to implantation site; C, 2 cm from implantation site – 32 mm; D, aneurysm diameter – 60 mm; E, secondary aneurysm – N/A; F, 2 cm distal to implantation site; G, 1 cm from distal implantation site – 29 mm; H, distal implantation site – 28 mm; M, aneurysm length – 5 cm; N, distal neck, distance from aneurysm to celiac axis – 3 cm; O, total treatment length 9 cm

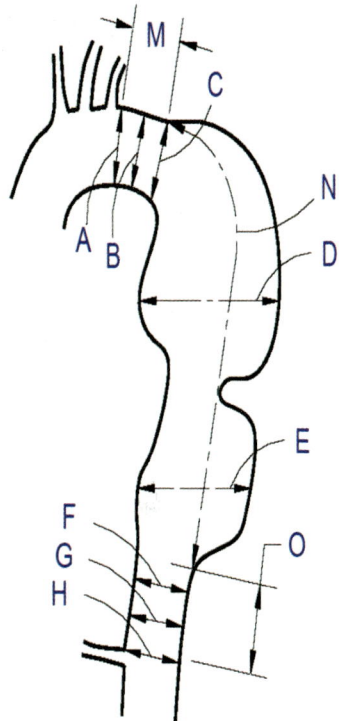

vessels and the descending thoracic aortic aneurysm (Fig. 30.4). Intravascular ultrasound (IVUS) is routinely performed in our institution using an IVUS (Volcano Therapeutics, Inc.) 8.2 Fr probe. The IVUS probe was advanced through the right groin sheath to confirm the size of the aneurysm, presence or absence of thrombus, proximal neck diameter and length, and distal neck diameter and length. The 34 mm × 15 cm TAG stent graft was chosen. The IVUS catheter was exchanged for an extra stiff 260 cm double-curve Lunderquist wire (Cook, Bloomington, IN). The right 9 Fr sheath was exchanged for a 22 Fr Gore sheath and a 34 mm × 15 cm TAG stent graft device was advanced through the Gore sheath (Fig. 30.5). Prior to deployment, the proximal and distal landing zones were identified and marked on angiographic road map. At the time of deployment of the endoluminal graft, a systolic blood pressure of 90 mmHg is achieved to decrease the "windsock" effect in the thoracic aorta. We have not felt the need for adenosine-induced asystole. A Gore trilobe balloon was used to perform post-deployment balloon angioplasty to both the proximal and distal segments of the graft for good fixation. A completion angiogram demonstrated exclusion of the aneurysm with no endoleak (Fig. 30.6). All wires and sheaths were removed from the right common femoral artery with the incision closed in a transverse fashion. A 6 Fr Angioseal vascular closure device (St. Judes Medical, Inc.) was deployed to the left common femoral artery. At the end, the

Fig. 30.4 An aortogram
demonstrating a descending
thoracic aortic aneurysm with
adequate proximal and distal
neck length

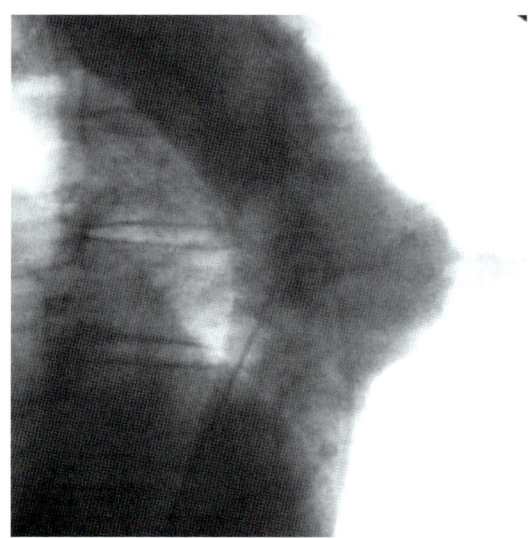

patient had bilateral peripheral pulses, was extubated prior to leaving the OR, and
transferred to the recovery room. She was discharged on post-operative day (POD)
#2 in satisfactory condition. A CT scan of the chest performed on POD #1 showed
exclusion of the 6 cm aneurysm with no evidence of an endoleak (Fig. 30.7a, b).

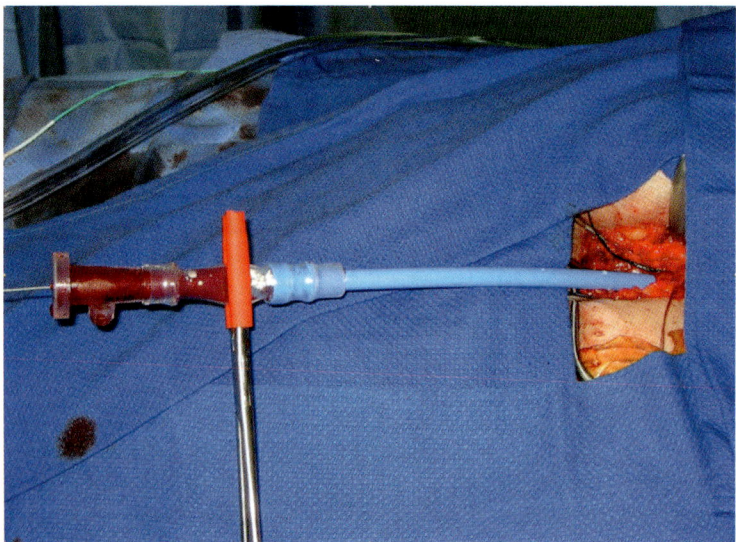

Fig. 30.5 22 Fr Gore delivery sheath introduced through the femoral artery for deployment of
endoluminal graft

Fig. 30.6 A post-deployment angiogram demonstrating exclusion of the thoracic aneurysm

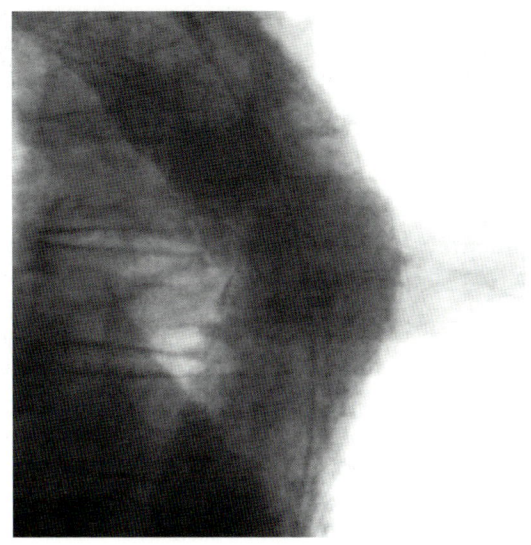

30.4 Discharge CT Scan

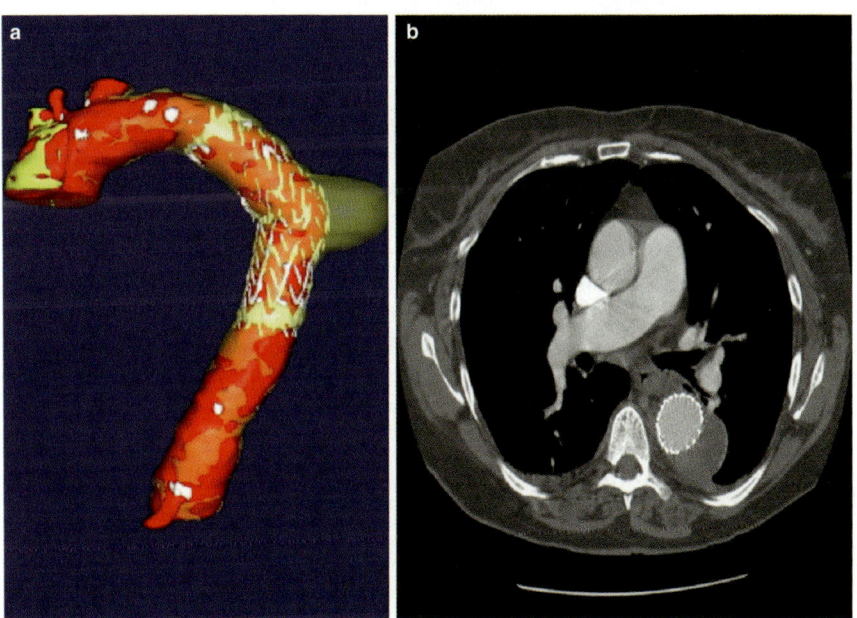

Fig. 30.7 (**a**, **b**) CT scan showing successful exclusion of the descending thoracic aneurysm

30.5 Discussion

Thoracic endoluminal grafting has recently gained wide acceptance as a treatment modality for managing various aortic pathologies including DTA's.[1–5] From September 1999 through May 2001, 140 patients with descending thoracic aneurysms were evaluated and enrolled at 17 sites across the United States. An open surgical control arm consisting of 94 patients was identified by enrolling both historical controls and concurrent subjects. Results of this US multicenter comparative trial (TAG 99-01)[5] showed a perioperative mortality in the endograft arm of 2.1% ($n = 3$) versus 11.7% ($n = 11$, $P < 0.001$) in the open surgery cohort. A 30-day analysis revealed a statistically significant lower incidence of the following complications in the endovascular cohort versus surgical cohort: spinal chord ischemia (3 versus14%), respiratory failure (4 versus 20%), and renal insufficiency (1 versus 13%). The endovascular group had a higher incidence of peripheral vascular complications (14 versus 4%). The mean intensive care and hospital stay were shorter in the endovascular cohort group. Accepted commercial indications for a thoracic ELG include DTA's deemed to warrant surgical repair, fusiform aneurysm >2 times diameter of normal adjacent aorta, and saccular aneurysms. A minimum of a 2 cm non-aneurysmal segment in both the proximal and distal landing areas is needed for successful deployment of a thoracic ELG. Angles less than 60° between the aortic arch and the descending thoracic aorta may require additional length of non-aneurysmal segment, and coverage of the left subclavian artery may be required. Late complications associated with endografting include aortic wall perforation from the proximal bare spring configuration of earlier devices, device collapse from oversizing the endograft >20% of the thoracic aortic neck diameter metal fracture, fabric erosion, and suture breakage associated with circumferential, radial, and tensional stresses from repetitive aortic pulsations.[6] Two-year follow-up data from the Tag 01 US multicenter trial showed a 6% endoleak rate detected at 1 year and 9% endoleak at 2 years post-procedure. During that time, three reinterventions in the endograft cohort were done with none in the open surgical cohort.[7] Five-year follow-up data show freedom from device-related complications to be very low with no aneurysm-related deaths, conversions, or ruptures for the control subjects enrolled in the pivotal and confirmatory studies (TAG 99-01 and TAG 03-03). Recommendations for endograft surveillance include a four-view chest X-ray to assess for device migration or stent fracture and a CT scan of the chest at periodic intervals (1 month, 6 months, 1 year, and annually thereafter).

References

1. Dietrich EB, Ramaiah VG, Kpodonu J, Rodriguez JA. *Figures Courtesy Endovascular and Hybrid Management of the Thoracic Aorta. A Case Based Approach.* 1st ed. West Sussex: Wiley-Blackwell; 2008.
2. Bavaria JE, Appoo JJ, Makaroun MS, Verter J, Zi-Fan Y, Scott Mitchell RS. Endovascular stent grafting versus open surgical repair of descending thoracic aortic aneurysms in low-risk patients: a multicenter comparative trial. *J Thorac Cardiovasc Surg.* 2007;133:369–377.

3. Gore TAG Thoracic Endoprosthesis Annual Clinical Update (April 2010).
4. Makaroun MS, Dillavou ED, Kes ST, et al. Endovascular treatment of thoracic aortic aneurysms: results of the phase II multicenter trial of the Gore TAG thoracic endoprosthesis. *J Vasc Surg*. 2005;41:1–9.
5. Wheatley GH 3rd, Gurbuz AT, Rodriguez-Lopez JA, et al. Midterm outcome in 158 consecutive Gore TAG thoracic endoprostheses: single center experience. *Ann Thorac Surg*. 2006;81(5):1570–1577; discussion 1577.
6. Kasirajan K, Milner R, Chaikof E. Late complications of thoracic endografts. *J Vasc Surg*. 2006;43:94A–99A.
7. Makaroun MS, Dillavou ED, Wheatley GH, Cambria RP; the Gore TAG Investigators. Five-year results of endovascular treatment with the Gore TAG device compared with open repair of thoracic aortic aneurysms. *J Vasc Surg*. 2008;47(5):912–918.

Chapter 31
Management of a Thoracic Aortic Aneurysm Using a Talent Stent Graft

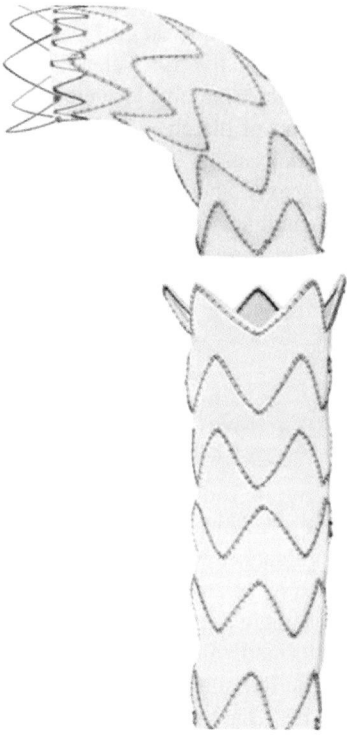

The Talent thoracic stent graft system is composed of a self-expanding serpentine-shaped nitinol endoskeleton inlaid in a woven polyester graft. The Talent has a longitudinal support bar throughout the length of the endograft, which provides column strength while maintaining device flexibility to accommodate tortuous vessels. Individual stents are secured to the graft with suture. Between individual stents is an unsupported graft to allow for flexibility. The proximal end of this stent graft is made in two configurations, which include either a serrated (open web configuration) or

J. Kpodonu, *Manual of Thoracic Endoaortic Surgery*,
DOI 10.1007/978-1-84996-296-4_31, © Springer-Verlag London Limited 2010

an open bare stent segment (FreeFlo configuration). The bare stent FreeFlo configuration allows device implantation across the orifice of the left subclavian or common carotid artery while maintaining antegrade blood flow. A similar bare wire configuration is also available in the distal stent graft, which permits the uncovered device to anchor across the celiac artery. The delivery systems for the Talent have profiles between 22 and 25 Fr. The Talent system consists of two device components. The proximal device is a straight tube stent graft with proximal FreeFlo configuration. The proximal device is available in diameters of 22–46 mm with a 2 mm increment.

31.1 Case Scenario

A 44-year-old woman with past medical history significant of hypertension and diabetes mellitus presented to an outside facility with severe chest and lower back pain. Her cardiac workup was negative for ischemic heart disease.[1] Her physical examination was significant for moderately elevated blood pressure with equal bilateral femoral pulses. A CT scan of the chest and abdomen demonstrated a type B dissecting thoracic aneurysm measuring 9 cm with a dissecting flap distal to the left subclavian artery to the celiac axis. She was felt to be at high risk for an open surgical repair and considered a candidate for endoluminal graft therapy. An angiogram and an intravascular ultrasound were scheduled to determine the pathophysiology of the dissection in relation to the aneurysm and to determine proximal and distal landing zones.

31.2 Intravascular Ultrasound and Angiogram

Patient was taken to the operating room; after local sedation, percutaneous access of the right common femoral artery was performed with the introduction of a 9 Fr sheath under fluoroscopic guidance. A 5 Fr pigtail catheter (Cordis Corporation, a Johnson & Johnson Company, Miami, FL) was advanced into the thoracic arch. The fluoroscopic C-arm was angled in a left anterior oblique view and an oblique thoracic aortogram was performed which demonstrated a large thoracic aortic dissecting aneurysm distal to the left subclavaian artery with adequate proximal and distal landing zones (Fig. 31.1). The ascending aorta was normal and the innominate, left common carotid and the left subclavian arteries appeared within normal limits. Two dissecting thoracic aortic aneurysms were identified distal to the left subclavian artery. The angiographic pigtail catheter was exchanged for an 8.2 Fr (Volcano Therapeutics, Inc.) intravascular ultrasound probe and advanced into the thoracic aorta to determine the length of thoracic aorta to be covered, proximal and distal neck length, and diameter. The thoracic dissecting aneurysm originated about 3.5 cm distal to the left subclavian artery. The bigger aneurysm measured 9 cm with mural thrombus present in the aneurysm sac with the smaller aneurysm measured at 4.5 cm. A proximal neck diameter of 29 mm × 29 mm was measured and a distal

Fig. 31.1 Thoracic
aortogram demonstrating a
descending thoracic aortic
aneurysm measuring 9.0 cm
in its maximum diameter

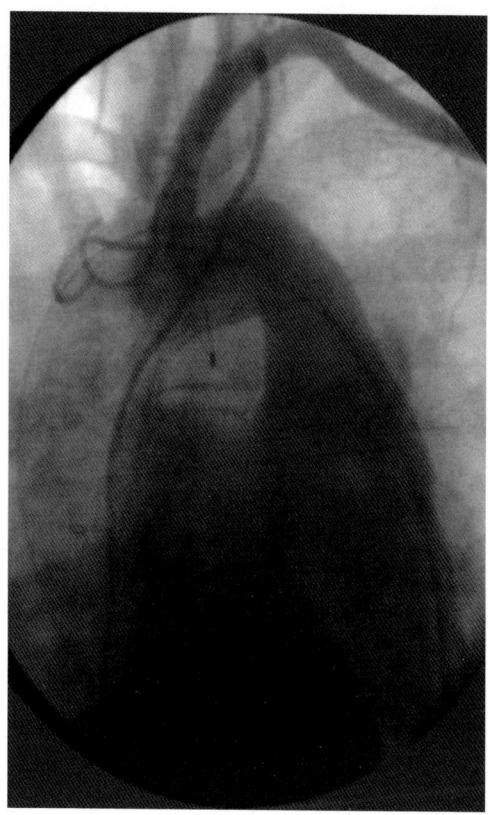

neck diameter of 23 mm × 20 mm about 6 cm proximal to the celiac axis. The total
length of thoracic aorta to be excluded was measured at 30 cm. The right common
iliac artery was measured at 9 mm and was mildly calcified. The measurements
obtained were used for the selection of an appropriate-sized endoluminal graft.

31.3 Surgical Planning

1. *Proximal neck diameter D1*: Based on the proximal neck diameter, a Talent
(Medtronic, Santa Rosa, CA) endoluminal graft 34 mm × 15 cm was chosen. The
presence of 3.5 cm neck length was adequate for a proximal landing zone without
the need to cover the left subclavian artery. The lack of a tortuous thoracic aortic
arch and descending thoracic aorta would allow the device to track smoothly along
the thoracic aortic curve with good apposition of the endograft to the aortic wall
(Fig. 31.2a, b).

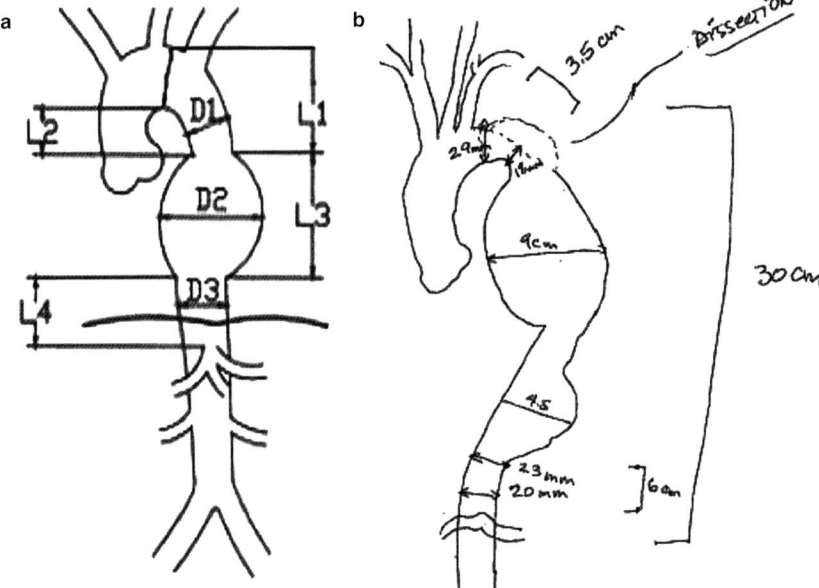

Fig. 31.2 (**a**) Planning sheet for Talent (Medtronic, Santa Rosa, CA) endograft. (**b**) An actual diagram for the patient treated with a Talent endograft

2. *Distal neck diameter D3*: Due to the difference in the proximal and distal neck diameters, two different sized devices need to be used with deployment of the larger 34 mm × 28 mm × 15 cm device proximally and telescoping the second device 32 mm × 28 mm × 15 cm device into the more proximal device.

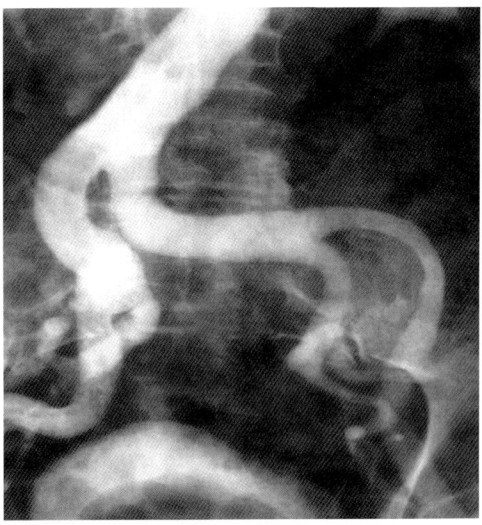

Fig. 31.3 Tortuous iliac vessels

3. *Tortuous, calcified iliac artery*: An iliac artery of 9.0 mm would tolerate the passage of a 25 Fr sheath which is needed to deploy the largest 44 mm diameter Talent thoracic endograft. The presence of tortuous vessels may make tracking of the device sheath more difficult than usual and any difficulty encountered should prompt urgent conversion to a retroperitoneal conduit with a 10 mm limb for delivery of endoluminal graft to the thoracic aorta (Fig. 31.3).

31.4 Endovascular Procedure

Open retrograde cannulation of the right common femoral artery was performed with an 18 G needle and a 0.035 in. soft tip angled glide wire (Medi-tech/Boston Scientific, Natick, MA) was passed into the distal thoracic aorta and exchanged for a 9 Fr sheath under fluoroscopic visualization. Percutaneous access of the left common femoral artery was similarly performed and a 5 Fr sheath introduced. Five thousand units of heparin was given to keep the activated clotted time greater than 200 s. A 5 Fr pigtail catheter was advanced through the left groin sheath into the thoracic aorta. The fluoroscopic C-arm was positioned in a left anterior oblique angle and an oblique thoracic arch aortogram was performed to visualize the orifices of the arch vessels and the descending thoracic aortic dissecting aneurysm.

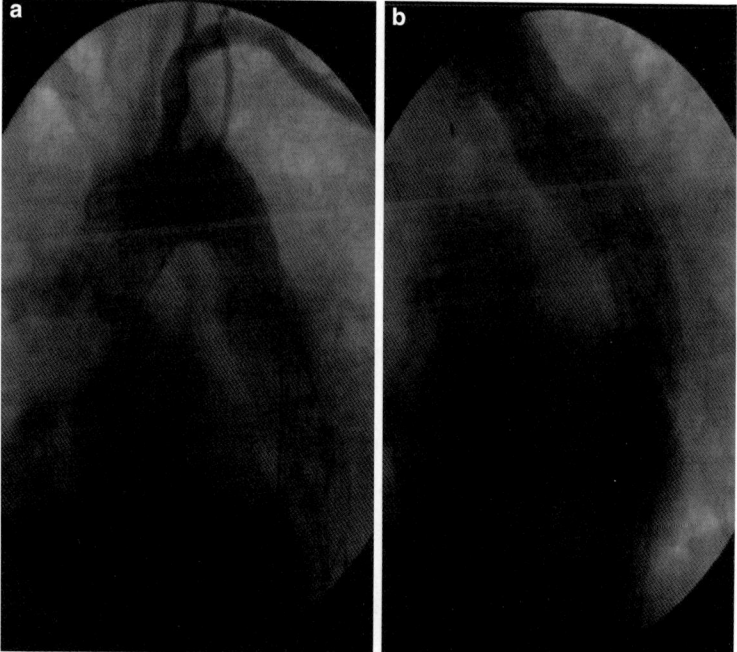

Fig. 31.4 (**a, b**) Completion angiogram demonstrating exclusion of thoracic aortic dissecting aneurysm with a Talent endograft

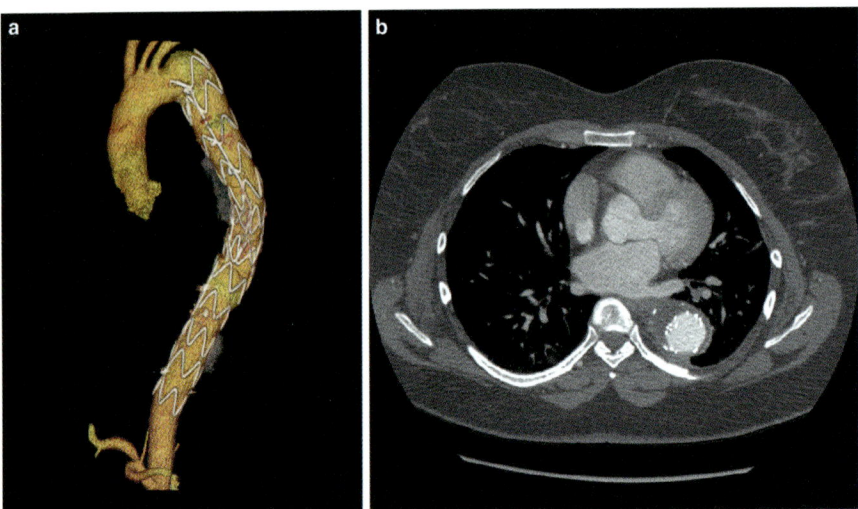

Fig. 31.5 (**a**, **b**) Post-operative CT scan demonstrating exclusion of aneurysm with no visualized endoleak and satisfactory position of endoluminal graft

Intravascular ultrasound (IVUS) performed previously using an IVUS (Volcano Therapeutics, Inc.) 8.2 Fr probe confirmed the location of the type B dissection to be 3.5 cm distal to the left subclavian artery with a 29 mm proximal and a 23 mm distal neck diameter with 30 cm of thoracic aorta to be covered to exclude the two aneurysms measured at 9.0 and 4.5 cm. An extra stiff 260 cm wire Lunderquist (Cook, Bloomington, IN) was advanced into the thoracic aorta with the help of a guiding catheter. The right 9 Fr sheath was exchanged for a 34 mm × 28 mm × 150 cm Talent device which was advanced into the thoracic aorta and deployed distal to the left subclavian artery as demarcated on an earlier road map angiogram. A second device 32 mm × 28 mm × 150 mm Talent stent graft device was deployed 2 cm proximal to the celiac trunk by telescoping the device with 3 cm of overlap between devices. Balloon angioplasty with a 40 mm balloon of the proximal and distal segments and area of overlap of the grafts was performed for aortic wall fixation. A completion angiogram demonstrated exclusion of the aneurysm with no endoleak (Fig. 31.4a, b). All wires and sheaths were removed from the right common femoral artery and closed in a transverse fashion with restoration of flow. Patient was discharged on post-operative day (POD) #2 in satisfactory condition. A CT scan of the chest performed on POD #1 showed exclusion of the 9 cm aneurysm with no identifiable endoleak (Fig. 31.5a, b).

Reference

1. Diethrich EB, Ramaiah VG, Kpodonu J, Rodriguez-Lopez JA. *Case Scenario Courtesy of Endovascular and Hybrid Management of the Thoracic Aorta. A Case Based Approach.* West Sussex: Wiley-Blackwell; 2008.

Chapter 32
Endovascular Management of a Thoracic Aortic Aneurysm Using a Retroperitoneal Conduit

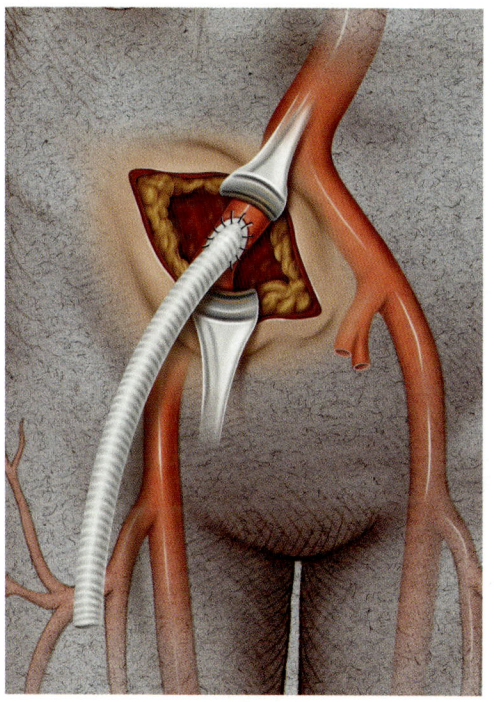

32.1 Introduction

Problems related to vascular access for stent grafts occur in up to 28% of cases and are related to ilio-femoral occlusive disease, small vessel size, and excessive ilio-femoral tortuosity.[1,2] Patients with calcified, tortuous, and small vessel size

Case scenario courtesy of Endovascular and Hybrid management of the Thoracic Aorta. A Case based Approach. Diethrich EB, Ramaiah VG, Kpodonu J, Rodriguez-Lopez JA. Wiley-Blackwell 2008 1st edition.

Table 32.1 Graft and delivery sheath sizes for descending thoracic aortic stent grafts currently available in the United States

Endograft	Graft size available (diameter) (mm)	Sheath size required (diameter)
Gore TAG	26–40	20–24 Fr (7.6–9.2 mm)
Zenith TX1/TX2	28–42	20–22 Fr (7.6–8.3 mm)
Talent	22–46	22–25 Fr

Table 32.2 Recommended iliac diameters for the introduction of Gore sheaths

Size (Fr)	ID (mm)	OD (mm)
20	6.7	7.6
22	7.3	8.3
24	8.1	9.1

may not be candidates for endoluminal graft therapy due to sub-optimal vascular access, aortic arch angulation, and landing zone inadequacies. Retroperitoneal exposure with construction of a 10 mm ilio-femoral conduit is a technique that permits delivery of large sheaths in patients with tortuous, calcified and small iliac vessels or vessels with severe ilio-femoral vascular occlusive disease. Current endoluminal graft devices in the United States require delivery sheaths ranging from 20 to 25 Fr depending on the size of the graft required to treat the aorta (Table 32.1). Current recommendations for the Gore TAG device delivery through a Gore sheath is re-summarized in Table 32.2.

32.2 Case Scenario

An 81-year-old female was admitted to the hospital for chest and abdominal pain. She had a past medical history significant for diverticulitis, chronic bronchitis with steroid dependence, history of a small abdominal aortic aneurysm, and a strong history of smoking.[3] A CT scan of the chest abdomen and pelvis was ordered for evaluation of her pain and a 6.0 cm descending thoracic aortic aneurysm in association with a 3.2 cm infra-renal abdominal aortic aneurysm was identified (Fig. 32.1). She was noted to have small tortuous and calcified iliac arteries on her CT scan (Fig. 32.2). Due to her co-morbidities she was felt to be a high-risk surgical candidate and enrolled in a single site investigational device exemption study for endoluminal graft placement.

32.3 Hybrid Endovascular Technique

Under general anesthesia, open exposure of the right common femoral artery was performed. The right common femoral artery was noted to be small and heavily calcified. Open retrograde puncture of the right common femoral artery was performed

Fig. 32.1 A reconstructed CT image demonstrating a descending thoracic aortic aneurysm of 6.0 cm in diameter

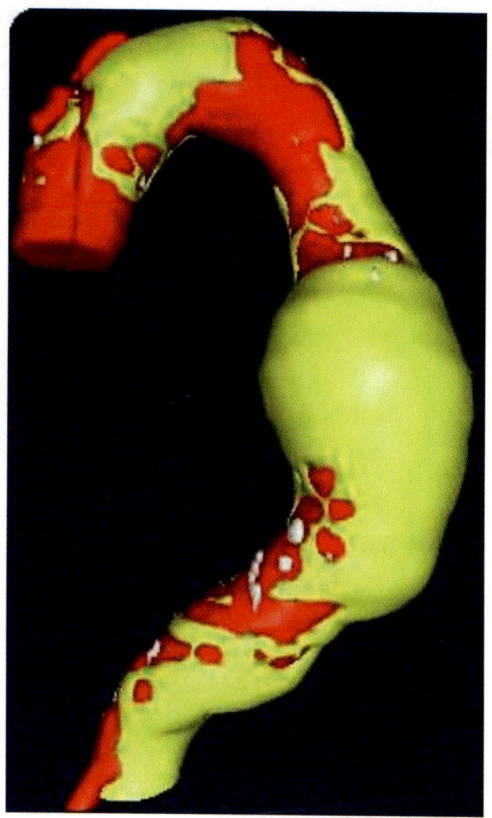

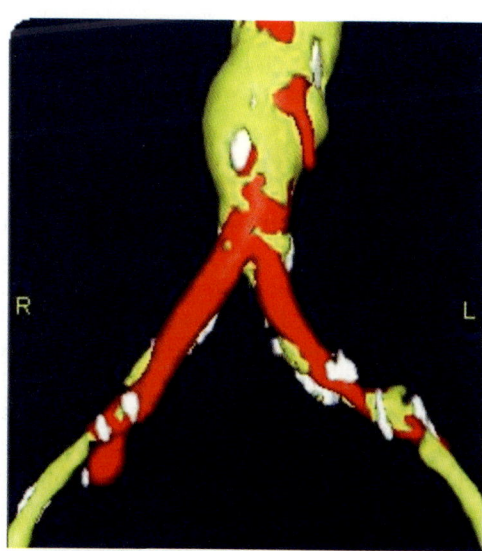

Fig. 32.2 A reconstructed CT scan demonstrating small-sized iliac vessels with diffuse calcification and stenosis of bilateral external iliac arteries

Fig. 32.3 An angiogram demonstrating small, tortuous iliac vessels

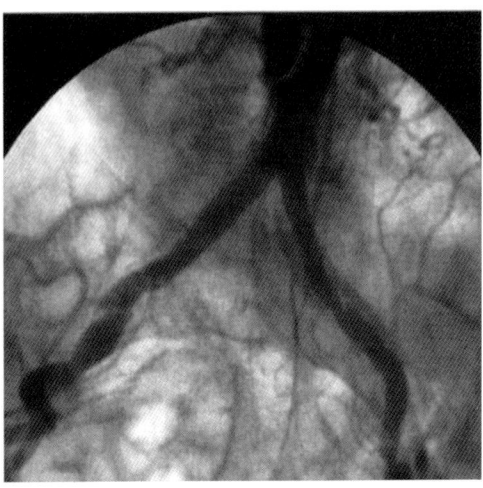

with an 18 G (Cook, Inc., IN) needle and attempts to cannulate the right common iliac artery with a 0.035 in. soft tip glide wire under fluoroscopic guidance beyond the external iliac artery were met with resistance with an area of dissection created from the wire.

Percutaneous access of the left common femoral artery was performed with an 18 G needle and a 0.035 glide wire could not be advanced. A retrograde percutaneous left brachial approach was performed with a 6 Fr sheath. Using a 5 Fr guiding catheter, a 0.035 in. soft tip angled glide wire was advanced into a very tortuous aorta with two curvatures. A 5 Fr pigtail angiographic catheter was exchanged for the guiding catheter and an aortogram demonstrated a very tortuous aorta, a large thoracic aortic aneurysm, and small bilateral common iliac arteries with near total occlusion of both external iliac arteries (Fig. 32.3). The right common iliac artery was measured to be 7.0 mm, with 6.5 mm on the left side. It was evident that both iliac arteries were prohibitive in nature for the delivery of the device sheath. A retroperitoneal conduit was the only way to deliver an endograft into the thoracic aorta in this patient.

32.4 Construction of Retroperitoneal Conduit

A 15 cm semilunar right flank incision was made 4 finger breaths above the right groin crease. Division of the external oblique, internal oblique, and transversus abdominus muscle was performed. The peritoneum was identified and gently retracted medially with the help of a retractor. The right common iliac artery and the hypogastric and the external iliac arteries were identified and mobilized. Care was taken to spare the right urether which crossed the common iliac artery before diving into the pelvis. Rummel tourniquets were applied at the proximal right common iliac artery, right external iliac artery, and origin of the hypogastric artery. Five thousand units of heparin was given to the patient. An arteriotomy was made on the right common iliac artery close to the bifurcation with the hypogastric artery and a 10 mm conduit sewn in an end-to-side fashion using 5-0 prolene suture. The 10 mm graft was subsequently tunneled through the retroperitoneal space beneath the inguinal ligament and brought out through the right groin incision that had been performed to expose the right common femoral artery. The graft was flashed and clamped at the right groin incision and the Rummel tourniquets released from the right common iliac artery, external iliac artery and hypogastric artery. The 10 mm conduit was looped with a Rummel tourniquet and punctured with an 18 G Cook (Bloomington, IN, USA) needle; a 0.035 glide wire was advanced under fluoroscopic guidance into the thoracic arch and the needle exchanged for a 9 Fr sheath. A pigtail catheter was advanced up the thoracic arch and an oblique thoracic aortogram was performed and saved as a road map for deployment of endograft (Fig. 32.4). An 8.2 Fr intravascular ultrasound (IVUS) probe was advanced through the conduit sheath again to confirm the measurements of the neck diameter. A Lunderquist wire (Cook, Bloomington, IN, USA) was exchanged through the IVUS catether. A 22 Fr sheath was exchanged for the 9 Fr sheath through the 10 mm conduit and under fluoroscopic guidance deployment of 34 mm × 20 cm Gore TAG (W.L. Gore & Associates, Flagstaff, AZ, USA) thoracic endoluminal grafts was deployed distal to the left subclavian artery excluding the thoracic aortic aneurysm (Fig. 32.5). Completion angiogram demonstrated complete exclusion of the thoracic aortic aneurysm with no endoleak (Fig. 32.6). Wires and sheaths were removed from the 10 mm conduit. The conduit was clamped. Adequate exposure of the left common femoral artery was performed, proximal and distal control of the right common femoral artery was achieved, and an arteriotomy was made with the right 10 mm iliac limb conduit sewn as an end-to-side anastomosis on the right common femoral artery (Fig. 32.7). Adequate flushing

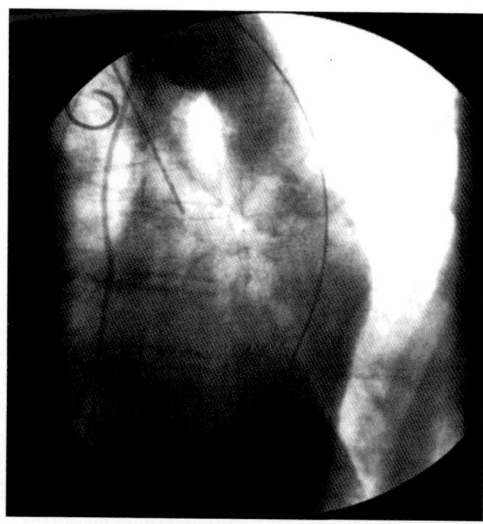

Fig. 32.4 An angiogram demonstrating a thoracic aortic aneurysm measuring 6.0 cm in diameter

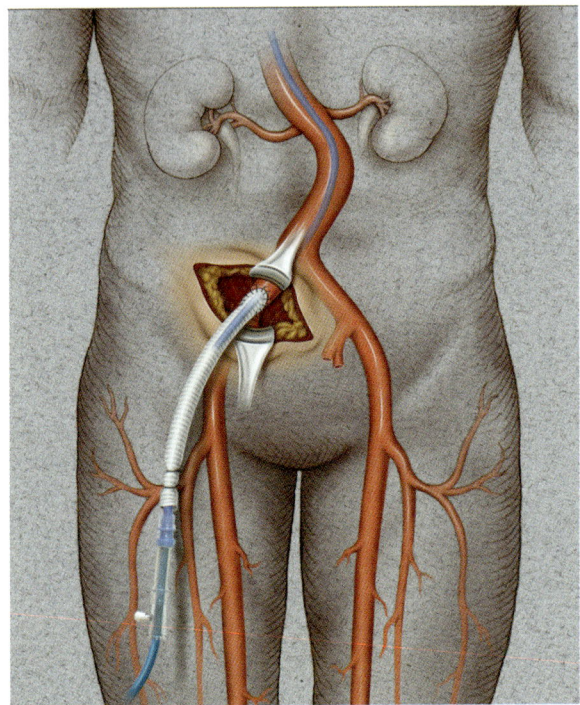

Fig. 32.5 A right retroperitoneal incision with a 10 mm conduit sewn to the right common iliac artery and connected to a device delivery sheath for deployment of endoluminal graft to the thoracic aorta

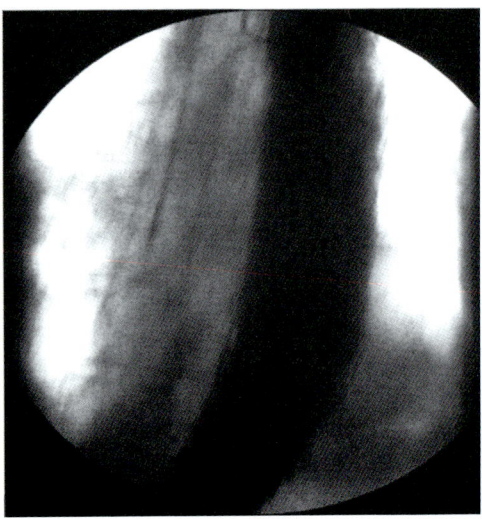

Fig. 32.6 Completion angiogram demonstrating satisfactory exclusion of thoracic aortic aneurysm with no endoleak

Fig. 32.7 A retroperitoneal iliac conduit sewn as an end-to-side bypass graft to the right common femoral artery as an ilio-femoral bypass graft

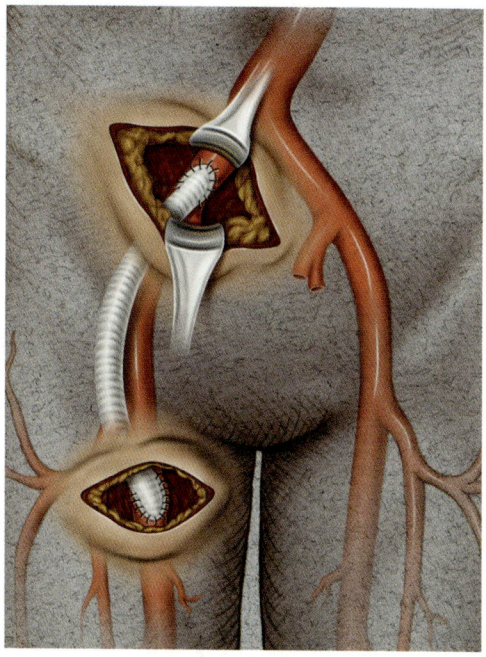

maneuvers were performed prior to completion of the anastomosis. The right groin incision was approximated. The right sheath was removed and a closure device used to achieve hemostasis. The right flank incision was irrigated, a 10 Fr Jackson-Pratt drain was placed, and the incision closed in layers. The patient was returned to the

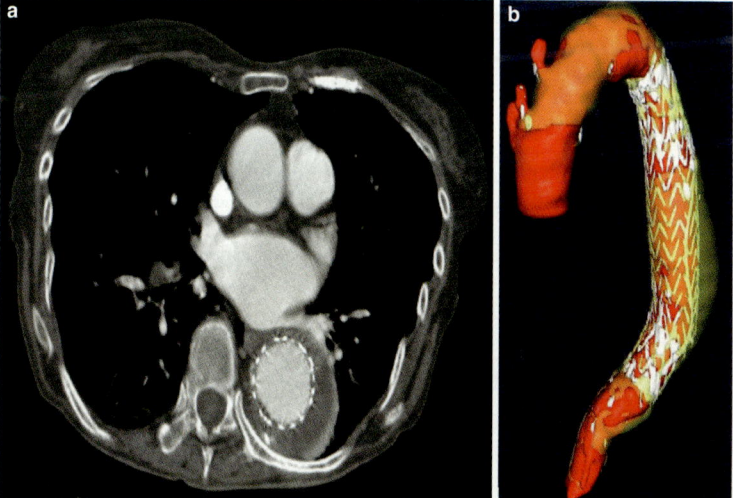

Fig. 32.8 (**a, b**) Post-operative CT scan demonstrating exclusion of the thoracic aneurysm with no identifiable endoleak

recovery room, extubated, and pulses palpable in both lower extremities. A postoperative CT scan demonstrated satisfactory exclusion of thoracic aneurysm with no endoleak (Fig. 32.8a, b).

32.5 Discussion

A retroperitoneal, ilio-femoral conduit is the most widely used bypass technique for access during endovascular repair of descending thoracic aortic aneurysms. Retroperitoneal conduits have been used in up to 22% of reported series.[4–6] In the phase II multicenter Gore TAG trial[4] access using retroperitoneal conduits was used in 15% of cases of endovascular repair of thoracic aortic aneurysms. Indications for use of retroperitoneal conduit include small vessel size, diseased access vessels, and tortuosity of access vessels. There currently does not exist a grading system to determine which patients would require a retroperitoneal conduit and, as such, clinical judgment along with careful pre-operative imaging of access vessels should be taken into account. Tunneling of the conduit from the abdominal wall to the groin through a separate incision is recommended in obese patients to allow for optimal working angles. We recommend that the conduit be tunneled through separate groin incisions and sewed to the femoral artery as an ilio-femoral bypass rather than oversewing the graft in patients with diseased iliac arteries who in future may need access for another procedure requiring sheath delivery.

References

1. Fairman RM, Velazquez O, Baum R, et al. Endovascular repair of aortic aneurysms (critical events and adjunctive procedures). *J Vasc Surg*. 2001;33:1226–1232.
2. Yano OJ, Faries PL, Morrissey N, Teodorescu V, Hollier LH, Marin ML. Ancillary techniques to facilitate endovascular repair of aortic aneurysms. *J Vasc Surg*. 2001;34:69–75.
3. Diethrich EB, Ramaiah VG, Kpodonu J, Rodriguez-Lopez JA. *Endovascular and Hybrid Management of the Thoracic Aorta. A Case Based Approach.* 1st ed. West Sussex: Wiley-Blackwell; 2008.
4. Makaroun MS, Dillavou ED, Kee ST, et al. Endovascular treatment of thoracic aortic aneurysms (results of the phase II multicenter trial of the GORE TAG thoracic endoprosthesis). *J Vasc Surg*. 2005;41:1–9.
5. Fairman RM, Velazquez O, Baum R, et al. Endovascular repair of aortic aneurysms (critical events and adjunctive procedures). *J Vasc Surg*. 2001;33:1226–1232.
6. Wellons ED, Milner R, Solis M, Levitt A, Rosenthal D. Stent-graft repair of traumatic thoracic aortic disruptions. *J Vasc Surg*. 2004;40:1095–1100.

Part IX
Endografting for Thoracic Aortic Dissections

Chapter 33
Endovascular Management of Acute Type B Dissection

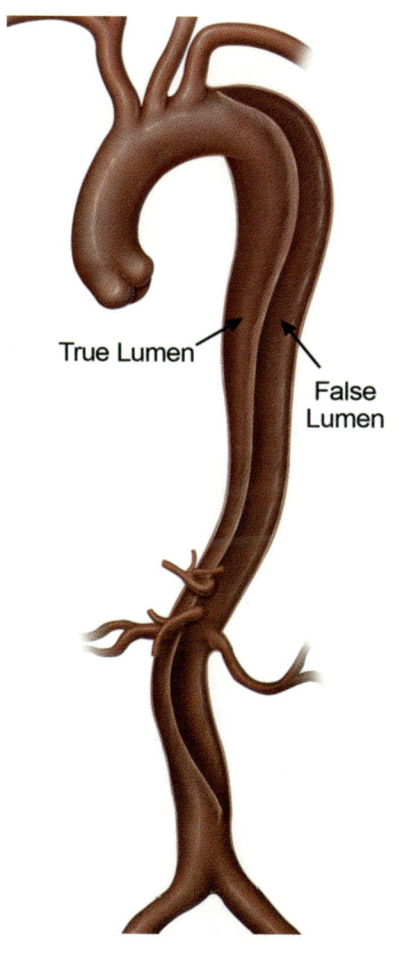

True Lumen

False Lumen

J. Kpodonu, *Manual of Thoracic Endoaortic Surgery*,
DOI 10.1007/978-1-84996-296-4_33, © Springer-Verlag London Limited 2010

The current indications for intervention in acute type B dissections involve rupture or signs of impending rupture, rapid diameter progression, malperfusion of abdominal or peripheral vessels, persisting pain, and uncontrollable hypertension. The effectiveness of surgical or endovascular repair for aortic dissection is dependent on closure of the entry tear, re-expansion of the true lumen, and the depressurization of the false lumen. The surgical mortality rate in complicated, acute dissections remains 14–31%, with a remarkable increase in patients with end-organ ischemia.[1–8] Closure of the primary entry tear by endovascular repair may lead to thrombosis of the false lumen with remodeling of the true lumen in both the acute and chronic settings (Fig. 33.3). Furthermore, lowering the pressure in the false lumen may restore perfusion in any compromised aortic branch vessels.

33.1 Current Trials

Clearly, there are a number of significant issues concerning the natural history and treatment of type B aortic dissection that require resolution by carefully planned and executed clinical trials. A number of trials are sponsored by industry partners; we describe a selection of these trials.

33.1.1 VIRTUE

The VIRTUE study is a prospective single-arm clinical registry designed to evaluate the Valiant Thoracic Stent Graft (Medtronic CardioVascular, Endovascular Innovations, Santa Rosa, CA) in the treatment of acute, subacute, and chronic type B dissections. The study is sponsored by Medtronic, and the principal investigator is Professor Matt Thompson. The study plans to recruit 100 patients with type B dissection, treated with the Valiant Thoracic Stent Graft from 18 European centers.

The primary endpoint is procedure-, device-, or disease-related mortality at 12 months, but more importantly, patients will be evaluated by serial imaging up to 36 months after the procedure; the results of CT imaging will be evaluated by a core lab. This study will provide reliable data regarding the morphology of the aorta after endovascular treatment and, in particular, may help define the results of endovascular therapy in subacute and chronic cases. Similar registry data are being acquired by both Bolton Medical (Sunrise, FL) and LeMaitre Vascular, Inc. (Burlington, MA).

33.1.2 ADSORB

The ADSORB study is a randomized trial of patients with acute uncomplicated type B dissection, and the principal investigator is Professor J. Brunkwall. The study will recruit 270 patients from 30 European sites and randomize them to endovascular repair using the TAG prosthesis (Gore & Associates, Flagstaff, AZ) or best medical therapy. Primary endpoints are focused on aortic morphology after treatment, and secondary endpoints include dissection and all-cause mortality; imaging will be interpreted by a core lab. In the light of recent data defining the outcome of uncomplicated dissection, randomizing this subgroup of patients might be considered controversial to some. However, like many randomized trials, the acquisition of data regarding the natural history of medically treated disease will be invaluable and will help define subgroups of patients with uncomplicated dissection who will benefit from treatment.

33.1.2.1   Zenith Dissection Endovascular System

The Zenith dissection system (Cook Medical, Bloomington, IN) combines a covered proximal endograft (TX2) with an uncovered, open mesh distal component (TZD). The Zenith system is proposed to facilitate remodeling of the aorta with effective closure of the entry site without coverage of a long length of aorta. The system has a number of potential advantages and is attractive in concept. A trial of 40 patients at six European and Australian sites is planned to evaluate the effectiveness of the system in treating acute type B aortic dissection. Endpoints for this study include survival at 30 days, as well as clinical utility, incidence and rate of adverse events, mortality, and factors related to morbidity at 12 months.

33.1.2.2   Endovascular Technique for Type B Dissections

Open retrograde cannulation of the common femoral artery is performed using an 18 G needle. A 9 Fr sheath is introduced into the common femoral artery and a 0.035 in. angled soft tip glide wire is advanced into the distal thoracic aorta, with care taken to make sure it is within the true lumen. Alternatively to be completely sure one is within the true lumen percutaneous access of the left brachial artery is performed and with the help of a 65 cm 5 Fr guiding sheath, the wire is advanced into the true lumen of the thoracic aorta. Percutaneous retrograde access of the contralateral femoral artery is similarly performed and a 5 Fr sheath was introduced. Heparin is given to achieve an activated clotting time of 200 s. In case of brachial access the brachio-femoral wire is snared through the groin with the help of a Goose neck snare. An oblique arch aortogram is performed using a 5 Fr pigtail angiographic catheter that is advanced through the percutaneous groin sheath. The aortogram performed demonstrates the dissection flap with compressed true lumen and possibly the entry point close to the subclavian artery (Fig. 33.1); evidence of extravasation of contrast would suggest acute thoracic aortic rupture. An intravascular ultrasound (IVUS) should be performed to identify the true lumen, false lumen, entry point of the dissection flap as well as studying the branched vessel flow pattern to decide on proper treatment plan (Fig. 33.2). The proximal neck and distal neck diameters and the length of aorta to be covered are measured in preparation for the selection of an endograft. Entry points identified at the level of the subclavian artery should be covered with an endoluminal graft. The IVUS probe is exchanged for a 260 cm stiff Lunderquist (Cook, Bloomington, IN) stiff wire. The open groin 9 Fr sheath

Fig. 33.1 Reconstructed CT
scan of a patient presenting
with acute onset of chest pain
which demonstrates a type B
dissection with entry point
distal to the left subclavian
artery

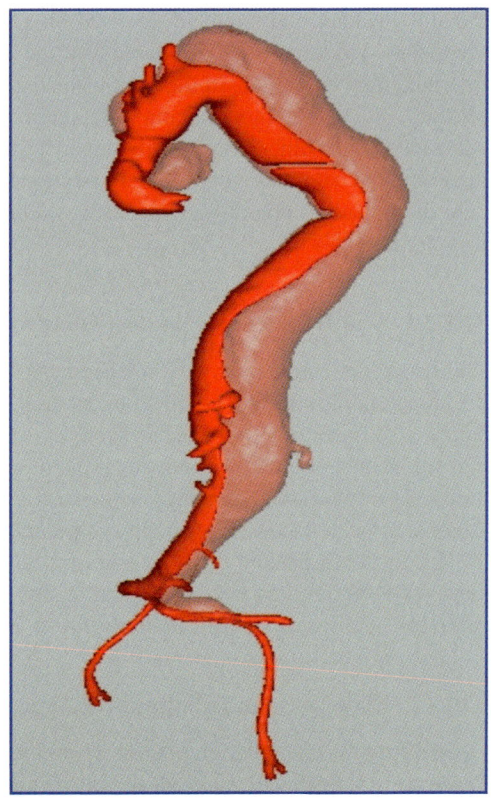

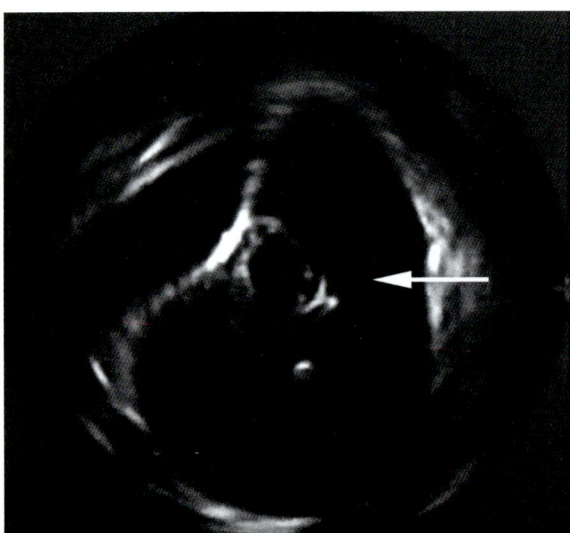

Fig. 33.2 Intravascular ultrasound demonstrates a collapsed true lumen with arrow demonstrating
expanded false lumen

Fig. 33.3 Deployment of
Cook Zenith endovascular
stent gradft system which
comprises a two-piece
covered stent graft and an
uncovered stent graft for true
lumen expansion and branch
vessel perfusion and sealing
off entry tear with
re-expansion of the true
lumen

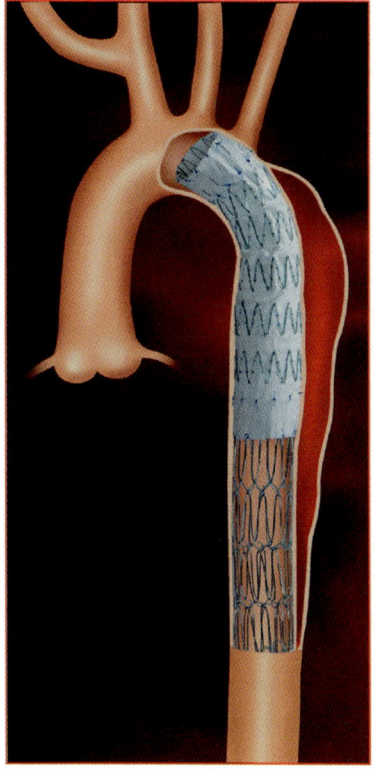

in the common femoral artery is exchanged for a device delivery sheath and the
endoluminal graft is advanced into the thoracic aorta and deployed under fluoroscopic and angiographic guidance to exclude the entry point and to re-expand the
collapsed true lumen. The deployment of the thoracic endograft should result in
collapse of the false lumen, expansion of the true lumen, and thrombosis of antegrade flow into the false lumen sac (Fig. 33.3). A completion aortogram (Fig. 33.4)
is performed to confirm exclusion of the dissecting flap, true lumen expansion, and
absence of antegrade flow in the false lumen. In cases where there is inadequate
distal true lumen expansion as noted on angiogram, the petticoat concept which
involves deploying an uncovered stent distal to the covered endograft to expand true
lumen in the distal and abdominal aorta while still ensuring flow to the branched
vessels is obtained. Adjunctive measures including branch vessel stenting and occasionally percutaneous fenestration techniques are required to restore true lumen flow
when malperfusion is present despite true lumen expansion from a thoracic stent
graft. Oncc results are satisfactory wires and sheaths are removed and the common femoral artery repaired and a closure device deployed to the percutaneously
accessed vessels. Post-operative CT scan should be performed prior to discharge
and periodically to ensure that satisfactory stabilization and remodeling of the aorta
occur (Fig. 33.5).

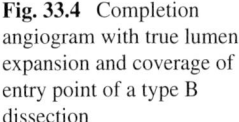

Fig. 33.4 Completion
angiogram with true lumen
expansion and coverage of
entry point of a type B
dissection

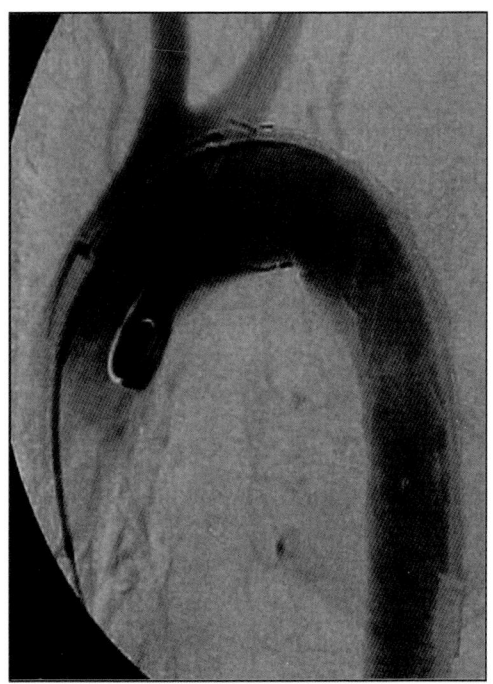

33.2 Discussion

Surgery for aortic dissection requires open thoracotomy, aortic cross-clamping, extracorporeal circulation, and graft interposition. There is a predictably high rate of complications associated with this surgery in these patients who are frequently poor candidates with an in-house mortality rate reported as high as 29.3% when intervention is required. The merits of early versus late intervention continue to be argued in the literature 40 years after the first publication of superior results with medical management. The continued debate on the appropriate treatment reflects the situation. Despite the minimal invasiveness of endoluminal graft for the treatment of type B dissections complications relating to respiratory, renal systems as well as hematomas, lymphocele, and pseudoaneurysms did arise. Results suggest that exclusion of the proximal entry point with endovascular prosthesis may stabilize the thoracic aorta and aid in the prevention of aneurysm expansion, malperfusion, and ultimately decreasing the incidence of thoracic aortic rupture when endoluminal grafts are used to treat acute type B dissections.

Prospective randomized, controlled studies would be required to definitively address the utility of this therapeutic modality in the prevention of aortic expansion and rupture in the setting of type B dissection as well as comparison to medical therapy. However, the myriad of presentations of thoracic aortic dissection

Fig. 33.5 Reconstructed CT
scan of the chest
demonstrates an endovascular
stent graft excluding the entry
point of an acute type B
dissection with true lumen
expansion

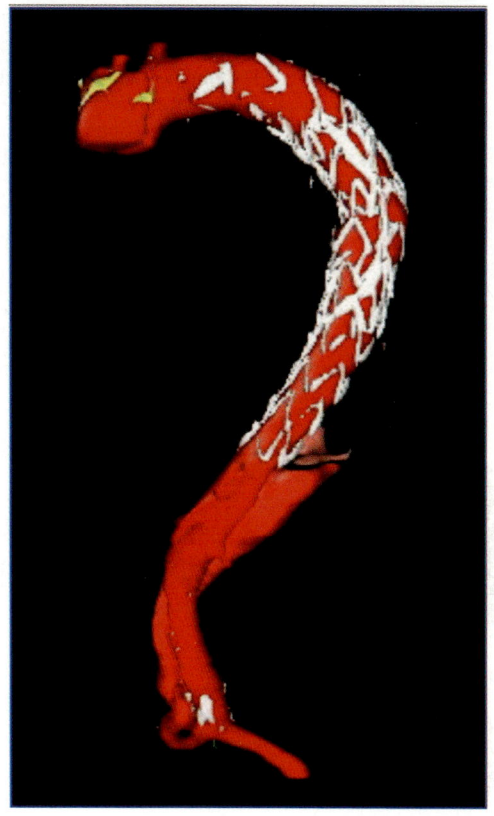

would make such an initiative difficult. There is certainly room for improvement
with regard to traditional therapeutic approaches to aortic dissection. The Gore
TAG thoracic endoprosthesis is the only commercial endograft available in the
US market. The current instructions for use of the device state that the device
is only approved for the use of the treatment of descending thoracic aneurysms.
The use of the Gore TAG thoracic endoprosthesis to treat dissections has been
mainly restricted to single-center studies at this time. Other novel devices currently under FDA investigation include a covered proximal part and an uncovered
distal part may further improve the paraplegia rate as we believe there would
be less segments of the descending thoracic aorta subject to a covered endoprosthesis. Our experience indicates that endografting of the thoracic aorta is a
beneficial adjunct in the management of this difficult disease entity and is associated with satisfactory short-term and mid-term results. We believe that long-term
follow-up of patients and current and future devices are necessary to further
define the role of thoracic endografting in the management of type B thoracic
dissection.

References

1. Sayed S, Thompson MM. Endovascular repair of the descending thoracic aorta: evidence for the change in clinical practice. *Vascular*. 2005;13:148–157.
2. Leurs LJ, Bell R, Degrieck Y, et al. Endovascular treatment of thoracic aortic diseases: combined experience from the EUROSTAR and United Kingdom thoracic endograft registries. *J Vasc Surg*. 2004;40:670–679; discussion 679–680.
3. Tsai TT, Fattori R, Trimarchi S, et al. Long-term survival in patients presenting with typeB acute aortic dissection: insights from the International Registry of Acute Dissection. *Circulation*. 2006;114:2226–2231.
4. Powell JT. How much evidence is needed for the introduction of new technologies into clinical practice in vascular surgery? *Eur J Vasc Endovasc Surg*. 2006;31:1–2.
5. Schoder M, Czerny M, Cejna M, et al. Endovascular repair of acute type B aortic dissection: long-term follow-up of true and false lumen diameter changes. *Ann Thorac Surg*. 2007;83:1059–1066.
6. Nienaber CA, Kische S, Zeller T, et al. Provisional extension to induce complete attachment after stent-graft placement in type B aortic dissection: the PETTICOAT concept. *J. Endovasc Ther*. 2006;13:738–746.
7. Nienaber CA, Zannetti S, Barbieri B, et al. INvestigation of STEnt grafts in patients with type B aortic dissection: design of the INSTEAD trial—a prospective, multicenter, European randomized trial. *Am Heart J*. 2005;149:592–599.
8. Diethrich EB, Ramaiah VG, Kpodonu J, Rodriguez JA. *Endovascular and Hybrid Management of the Thoracic Aorta. A Case Based Approach*. 1st ed. West Sussex: Wiley-Blackwell; 2008.

Chapter 34
Endovascular Management of Chronic Type B Thoracic Aortic Dissection

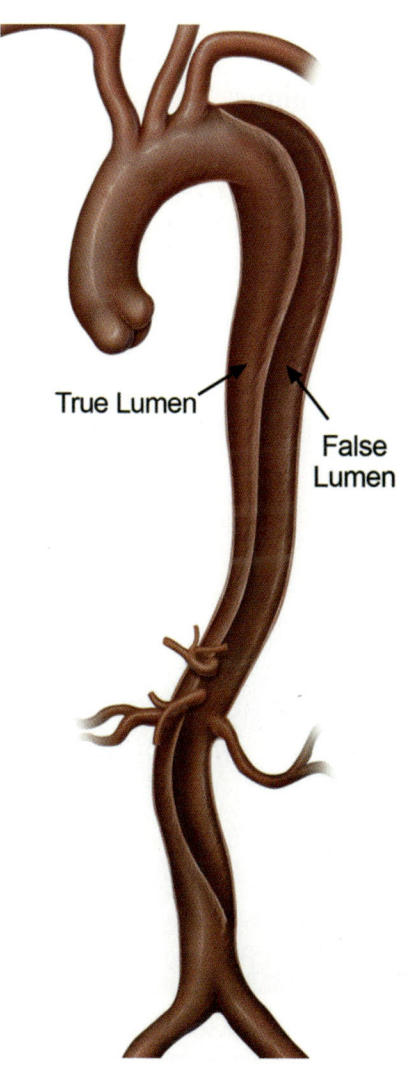

True Lumen

False Lumen

J. Kpodonu, *Manual of Thoracic Endoaortic Surgery*,
DOI 10.1007/978-1-84996-296-4_34, © Springer-Verlag London Limited 2010

The natural progression of chronic type B dissection is to dilate over time. In close to 85% of patients[1] with chronic type B dissection, there is partial to full patency of the false lumen with the risk of progressive dilatation to aneurismal formation in 35% of patients[2] with cause of late mortality related to rupture. Surgical aortic replacement is required in these patients to avoid aortic rupture and is still associated with a relatively high mortality of 4–17%.[3,4] Endoluminal graft treatment of chronic dissection is primarily aimed at covering the entry tear to prevent false lumen flow and subsequent aneurysmal dilatation of the thoracic aorta and for treatment of aneurismal dilatation of the false lumen to prevent aortic rupture. Remodeling of the aorta can occur at mid-term follow-up with shrinkage of false lumen and expansion of true lumen. The remodeling of the aorta is not as conspicuous as in acute aortic dissection.[5]

34.1 Endovascular Techniques

CT angiography (Fig. 34.1) and Intravascular ultrasound are helpful in determining location of entry tears, shape and diameter of landing zones, diameter and tortuosity of access vessels, and involvement of branched vessels. Hemodynamics between true and false lumen can be appreciated with aortography and intravascular ultrasound.

Access through the left brachial artery with a 5 Fr sheath is recommended when treating type B dissections to be sure you access the true lumen (Fig. 34.2). An

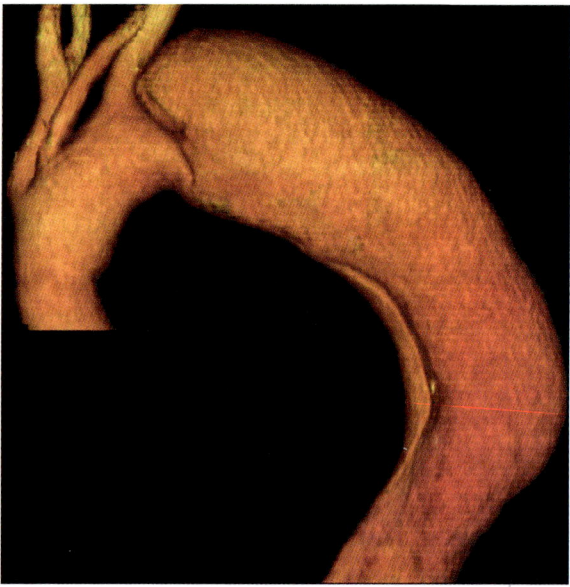

Fig. 34.1 Reconstructed CT scan of a patient with a chronic type B dissection demonstrating an entry point distal to the left subclavian artery, a compressed true lumen, and an aneurysmal false lumen

Fig. 34.2 Retrograde
percutaneous puncture of the
left brachial artery

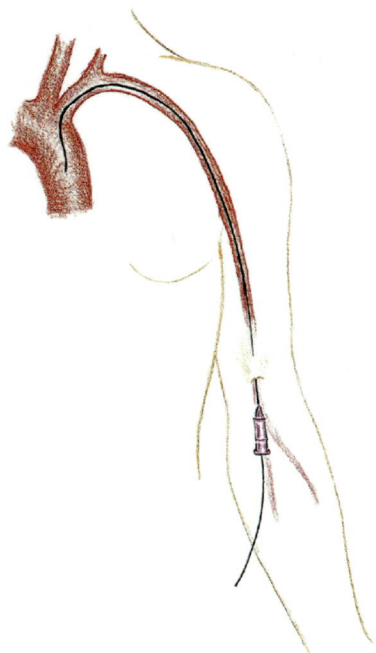

aortogram performed through an angiographic 5 Fr pigtail catheter is performed
to demonstrate the aneurysmal dissecting aneurysm with compressed true lumen
(Fig. 34.3). Intravascular ultrasound is also performed to determine the size of the
dissecting aneurysm, entry point of dissecting flap, and hemodynamics of the true
and false lumen flow. Through the 5 Fr brachial access, a 0.035 in. soft tip angled

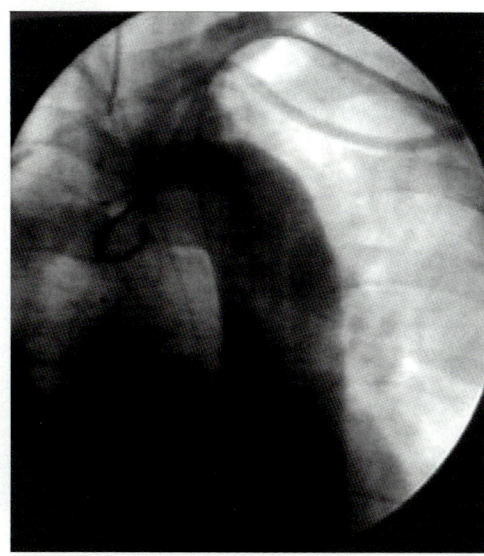

Fig. 34.3 Thoracic
aortogram performed through
the left brachial artery
demonstrates a type B
dissection with true and false
lumen flow separated by
dissecting sputum

glide wire is advanced from the left brachial artery into the thoracic arch with care to cannulate the true lumen under fluoroscopy; similarly a 0.035 in. soft tip glide wire is advanced through a 9 F sheath placed in the common femoral artery in a retrograde fashion. Care should be taken that at all times the wire is within the true lumen. A snare can be used to snare an extra-long brachial wire that is within the true lumen through the femoral access and used as a brachio-femoral wire[6,7] (Fig. 34.4). True lumen angiogram should be done to assess branch vessel perfusion. Any vessel which is compromised by a dissecting flap can be treated with a branch vessel stent graft if perfusion is true lumen dependent. Intravascular ultrasound (IVUS) probe is advanced through the 9 Fr groin sheath to confirm that the wire is within the true lumen; identify all the entry tears especially the proximal entry tear, the dissecting septum; assess branch vessel perfusion; and determine the proximal and distal neck diameters for the proper selection of an endoluminal stent graft system. The IVUS probe is used as an exchange catheter for exchanging the soft tip 0.035 in. glide wire to an extra stiff 260 cm Lundiquist wire (Cook, Bloomington, IN). An exchange of the 9 Fr sheath for the device delivery sheath is performed and the endoluminal stent graft chosen is deployed under fluoroscopic guidance and angiographic road map visualization to the exact area making sure the entry point of the dissection flap is excluded to seal off antegrade flow to the false lumen. Balloon angioplasty of the proximal and distal ends of the endograft is sometimes necessary for optimal apposition to the aortic wall although not recommended for acute type B dissection. Presence of infra-renal aneurismal dilatation or aneurysm can also be treated with an endoluminal stent graft after studying luminal flows with an angiogram and IVUS (Fig. 34.5). A completion angiogram is performed to demonstrate complete exclusion of the false dissecting aneurysm and exclusion of entry point. All

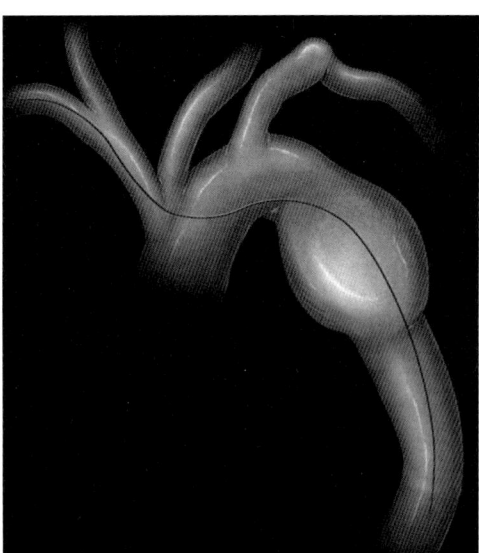

Fig. 34.4 Brachio-femoral wire used to ensure true lumen cannulation is achieved

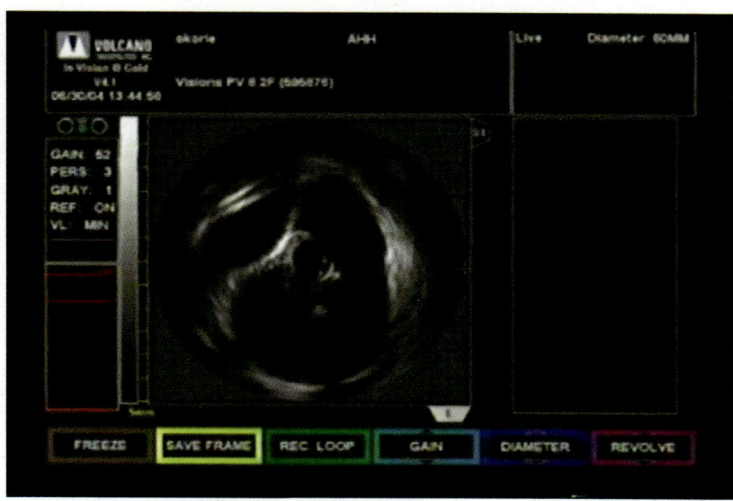

Fig. 34.5 Intravascular ultrasound in a patient with a type B dissection to demonstrate true (smaller lumen), dissecting septum and the larger false lumen

wires and sheaths are removed and the common femoral artery is primarily repaired. The brachial sheath is removed and a closure device or manual pressure is applied to establish hemostasis. A post-operative CT scan is performed prior to discharge to demonstrate satisfactory exclusion of dissecting aneurysm with no identifiable endoleak (Fig. 34.6).

34.2 Discussion

Aneurysms that are the sequelae of chronic dissection tend to be more extensive and occur in younger patients compared with degenerative aneurysms. Treatment with effective β-blockade is an essential feature of long-term therapy and follow-up. The rationale of such therapy is based on the recognition that patients with aortic dissection have a systemic illness that places their entire aorta at risk for further dissection, aneurysm, or rupture. Guidelines recommend progressive upward titration of β-blockade to achieve a blood pressure <125/80 in usual patients and <120 mmHg in those with Marfan syndrome. In addition, aggressive β-blockade has been shown to retard the growth of the aortic root in these patients and may have a similar effect on the thoracoabdominal aorta.

Serial imaging is the cornerstone of long-term follow-up, in managing patients with type B dissections. Axial imaging modalities as well as 64-slice CT imaging should encompass the entire aorta. The rational for endografting is to exclude the entry tear and induce false lumen thrombosis to prevent the aortic pressure from acting on the aortic wall. Location of entry tear, shape and size of the landing zone, and diameter and tortuosity of access route should be obtained by CT scan,

Fig. 34.6 Post-operative reconstructed CT scan of the chest performed demonstrates satisfactory exclusion of the entry point in a chronic type B dissection with improved true luminal gain and thrombosis of the antegrade false lumen flow

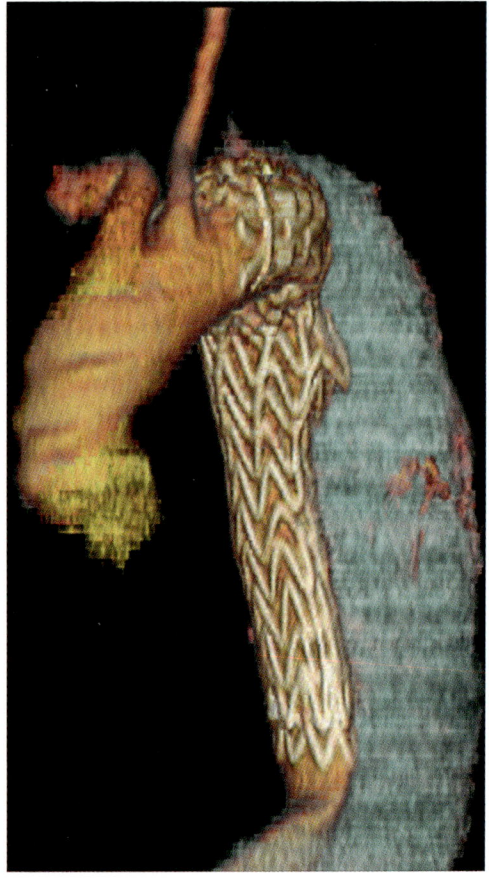

intravascular ultrasound, or angiogram. Sufficient proximal neck length 1.5–2.0 cm must be available to allow sealing off the entry tear. True lumen must be large enough to allow delivery of a device since in chronic dissection the intimal flap is fibrotic and not easily distensible. Due to the non-distensibilty of the true lumen in chronic dissection stent grafts have to be able to adapt to the shape of the true lumen, which in most circumstances is not circular. Stent grafts with hooks should not be used in dissection due to the possibility of the hooks causing a new intimal tear. Migration is less of an issue since most dissections have a tapering true lumen; hence tapered graft would be more suitable for the treatment of chronic dissection. Complications of endograft therapy include post-implantation syndrome which is characterized by fever and leukocytosis. Paraplegia develops in about 5% of patients undergoing endografting, which is less than open surgical repair. Left arm ischemia can occur when the left subclavian artery is covered by the stent graft to exclude intimal tears close to the left subclavian artery. Two clinical trials to date The EUROSTAR/United Kingdom registry report[8] and The Investigation of

Stent grafts in patients with type B aortic dissection (INSTEAD) trial[9] have been set up to address the use of endoluminal graft therapy in the management of thoracic aortic dissections. The EUROSTAR/United Kingdom registry report[8] is the largest compendium of patients treated with thoracic aortic stent grafts to date. In the combined registry, 131 patients with aortic dissection (5% proximal, 81% distal, 14% not classified) were treated with stent grafts and 57% had symptoms of rupture, aortic expansion, or side branch occlusion. Although no meaningful long-term data are available, primary technical success was achieved in 89%, and 30-day mortality was 8.4%.[4,5] Paraplegia occurred in 0.8% of those treated, and survival at 1 year after treatment was reported in 90% of 67 patients who had such follow-up. The Investigation of Stent grafts in patients with type B aortic dissection (INSTEAD) trial, currently recruiting patients in Europe with an expected completion in 2006, is the first randomized trial investigating the role of stent graft treatment of uncomplicated type B aortic dissection compared with best medical therapy alone. Inclusion criteria are patients with distal chronic (2–52 weeks from the onset of symptoms) dissections without evidence of malperfusion syndrome. Thus, the INSTEAD trial 1 addresses whether patients with chronic, uncomplicated, distal aortic dissection treated with an endovascular stent graft have an improved initial outcome and freedom from late dissection complications. In designing the trial, 80 patients treated by the primary author with stent graft repair of type B aortic dissection were retrospectively compared with 80 patients managed medically. Two-year survival was 67.5% in the medically treated group and 94.9% in the group managed with endovascular stent graft treatment.

Currently in the United States, no thoracic endograft devices are specifically approved for the commercial treatment of a descending aortic dissection. These devices are commonly being used in "off-label" procedures for this purpose. To determine the role of endoluminal grafts in the treatment of dissections, both device manufacturers and academic centers are now conducting sanctioned studies to objectively look at the patient outcomes for such a procedure. Looking into the future, endoluminal grafts with designed side branches that allow for arterial blood flow for critical vessels while covering a diseased area will usher in the next generation of endovascular technologies. The initial experience with endovascular technology in chronic dissections combined with evolving device designs will play an increasingly more important role in the future for dissection management.

References

1. Yamaguchi T, Naito H, Ohta M, et al. False lumens in type III aortic dissections: progress CT study. *Radiology*. 1985;156:757–760.
2. Kato M, Bai H, Sato K, et al. Determined surgical indications for acute type B dissection based on enlargement of aortic diameter during the chronic phase. *Circulation*. 1995;92(Suppl. II):107–112.
3. Miller DC, Mitchell RS, Oyer PE, Stinson EB, Jamieson SW, Shumway NE. Independent determinants of operative mortality for patients with aortic dissections. *Circulation*. 1984;70(Suppl. 1):1153–1164.

4. Svensson LG, Crawford ES, Hess KR, Coselli JS, Safi HJ. Dissection of the aorta and dissecting aortic aneurysms. *Circulation*. 1990;82(Suppl. IV):24–28.

5. Hollier LH, Symmonds JB, Pairolero PC, Cherry KJ, Hallett JW, Gloviczki P. Thoracoabdominal aortic aneurysm repair. Analysis of postoperative morbidity. *Arch Surg*. 1988;123:871–875.

6. Kpodonu J, Rodriguez-Lopez JA, Ramaiah VG, Diethrich EB. Use of the right brachio-femoral wire approach to manage a thoracic aortic aneurysm in an extremely angulated and tortuous aorta with an endoluminal stent graft. *Interact Cardiovasc Thorac Surg*. 2008;7(2):269–271.

7. Diethrich EB, Ramaiah VG, Kpodonu J, Rodriguez JA. *Figures Courtesy Endovascular and Hybrid Management of the Thoracic Aorta. A Case Based Approach*. 1st ed. West Sussex: Wiley-Blackwell; 2008.

8. Leurs L, Bell R, Degrieck Y, et al. Endovascular treatment of thoracic aortic diseases (combined experience from the EUROSTAR and United Kingdom thoracic endograft registries). *J Vasc Surg*. 2004;40:670–680.

9. Nienaber CA, Zannetti S, Barbieri B, Kische S, Schareck W, Rehders TC. INSTEAD study collaborators. Investigation of Stent grafts in patients with type B aortic dissection (design of the INSTEAD trial – a prospective, multicenter, European randomized trial). *Am Heart J*. 2005;149:592–599.

Chapter 35
Retrograde Type A Dissection After Endovascular Management of Type B Dissection

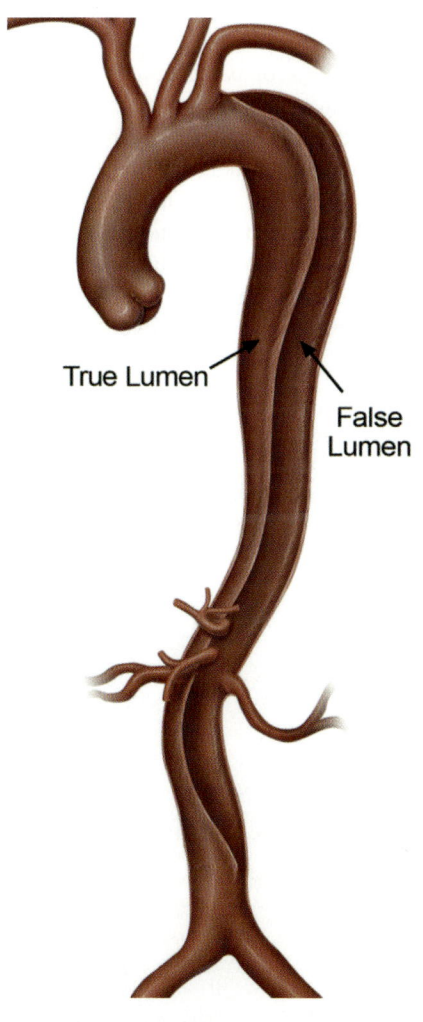

True Lumen

False Lumen

J. Kpodonu, *Manual of Thoracic Endoaortic Surgery*,
DOI 10.1007/978-1-84996-296-4_35, © Springer-Verlag London Limited 2010

Thoracic endografting has recently been approved by the Federal Drug Administration in the United States for the treatment of thoracic aortic aneurysms. The first thoracic stent graft for the treatment of thoracic aortic aneurysm (TAA) was reported by Dake et al.[1] Kato[2] described the use of stent graft to treat dissecting aneurysms at about the same time. Stanford type B dissections are managed conservatively with meticulous control of blood pressure and pain medication for uncomplicated cases. As much as 43% of acute type B dissections treated medically will progress to aortic enlargement with close to 30% dilated to 6 cm or greater within a mean 59 months.[3] Surgical treatment of acute type B dissection is reserved for patients with a complicated course, such as frank or impending rupture, branch vessel occlusion with visceral and/or leg ischemia, or refractory hypertension or pain. Despite significant improvement in anesthesia, surgical techniques, and post-operative care, the mortality rate in emergent surgical repair of type B aortic dissections is between 29 and 50%.[4,5] Frequent complications are respiratory failure 51%,[6] renal failure 17%,[7] or paraplegia 7–24%[6,7]; other notable complications include severe bleeding, stroke, cardiac events, or sepsis. Closure of the entry tear of a type B dissection is essential to reduce aortic diameter and promote both de-pressurization and shrinkage of the false lumen, which could lead to thrombosis, fibrous transformation, and subsequent remodeling and stabilization of the aorta.[8–10] Retrograde type A dissection following stent graft placement for the treatment of type B dissection is a rare but fatal complication associated with a high mortality.[11–17] Once ascending aortic dissection occurs, emergent surgical treatment should be performed as soon as possible.[18]

35.1 Case Scenario

A 53-year-old male with past medical history significant for hypertension and coronary artery disease developed sudden severe crushing chest pain associated with a

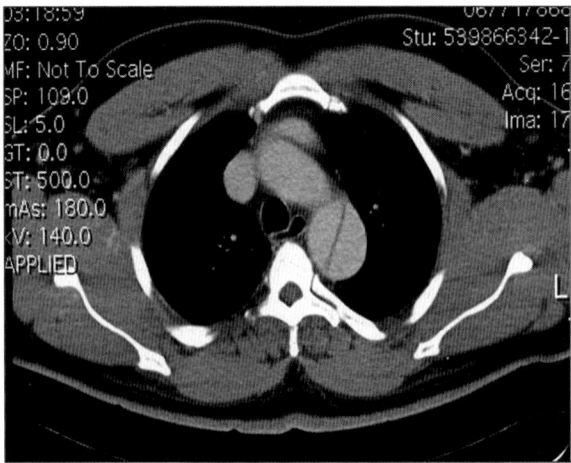

Fig. 35.1 CT scan demonstrates a type B dissection[19]

hypertensive crisis as well as monocular blindness and compromised renal function. Aggressive management of his pain and blood pressure was undertaken and a CT scan of his chest performed revealed an acute type B dissection (Fig. 35.1).

Medical management was instituted to control the blood pressure and pain; however due to difficulty controlling both his pain and blood pressure with intravenous antihypertensive medications as well as malperfusion evidenced by his compromised renal function, he was felt to be a good candidate for endoluminal graft therapy.

35.2 Technical Details of Endoluminal Graft Deployment

Open retrograde cannulation of the right common femoral artery using an 18 G Cook needle was performed; a 9 Fr sheath was introduced over a 0.035 in. soft tip glide wire. Percutaneous retrograde access of the left common femoral artery was similarly performed and a 5 Fr sheath was introduced. An oblique thoracic aortogram was performed using a pigtail from the 5 Fr sheath (Fig. 35.2a) which demonstrated a bovine arch with a collapsed true lumen with the intimal flap distal just juxta distal to the left subclavian artery. An intravascular ultrasound was also performed through the 9 Fr sheath to identify true lumen, false lumen, and entry point of the dissection at the level of the left subclavian. A 9 Fr sheath in the right common femoral artery was exchanged for a 24 Fr Gore sheath. A Gore device 37 mm × 20 cm was deployed at the level of the mid-descending thoracic aorta followed by a 40 mm × 20 cm distal to innominate artery to exclude the entry point. Partial occlusion of the innominate artery required deployment of an express stent 7 mm × 38 mm through a retrograde right brachial approach. The thoracic endograft

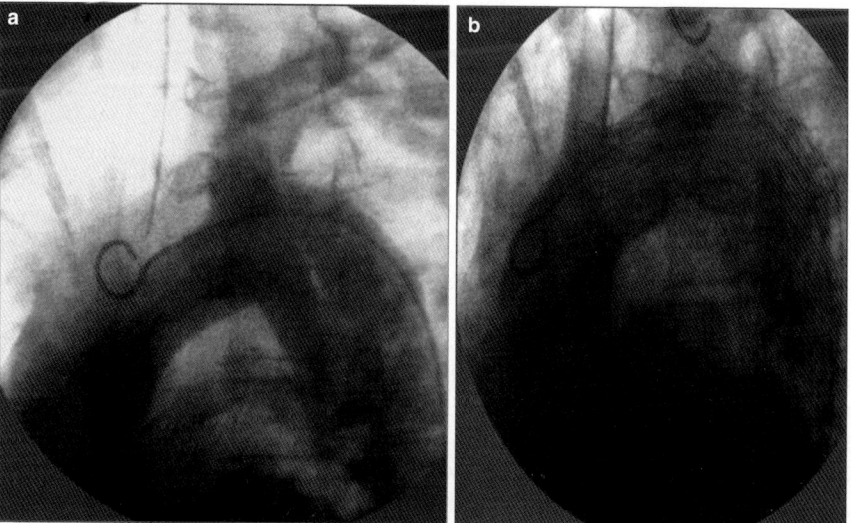

Fig. 35.2 (a) Angiogram demonstrates a type B dissection.[19] (b) Completion angiogram demonstrates adequate deployment of endoluminal graft with no endoleak[19]

deployed resulted in collapse of the false lumen and an expansion of the true lumen on completion aortogram with no endoleak noted and brisk flow to the innominate vessel (Fig. 35.2b). Wires and sheaths were removed and the right common femoral artery was repaired and a closure device deployed to the left common femoral artery.

Post-operative CT scans demonstrate thrombosis of false lumen and exclusion of entry point at left subclavian artery with no endoleak.

35.3 Post-operative Surveillance (Retrograde Type A Dissection)

The patient was discharged from the hospital in satisfactory condition and presented 1 month later to the emergency room with an acute episode of chest pain; he was taken to the catheterization lab and angiogram revealed a retrograde type B dissection. CT scan performed showed a retrograde type A dissection (Fig. 35.3 a–c). He was taken to the operating room where replacement of the ascending aorta with a 32 mm Hemashield Dacron graft was done (Fig. 35.4). He was subsequently discharged from the hospital in satisfactory condition.[19]

35.4 Discussion

Acute retrograde type A dissection after endovascular stent graft repair is a fatal complication following stent graft treatment of thoracic aortic pathologies. The incidence tends to be more common in the use of stent graft deployment to treat Stanford type B dissection. Dissections that originate in the descending aorta and extend in a retrograde direction into the ascending aorta may lead to aortic valve regurgitation, cerebrovascular ischemia, pericardial tamponade, and obstruction of the coronary artery. Open surgery is the treatment of choice in an effort to avert these life-threatening complications. Possible etiologies for this rare but fatal complication of thoracic stent grafting can be classified as procedure related, device related, and natural progression of disease.

Formation of a new intimal tear leading to a dissection or a pseudoaneurysm may occur at the margin of a stent graft.[20,21] The delay between stent graft implantation and identification of a complicating intimal tear or dissection can vary from immediately post-operative deployment of stent graft to months after the procedure.[22,23] In a report by Won et al. retrograde type A dissection was diagnosed at 1–5 months post-procedure (mean 3.2 months).

Procedure-related complications of retrograde type A dissection following stent graft placement arise from wires and sheath manipulation in the aortic arch during the endovascular procedure that may cause localized intimal tears in the extremely fragile and easily injured intimal flap and aortic wall. Wire and sheath handling or balloon dilatation during the endovascular procedure may have caused intimal injuries during the endovascular procedure and extend in a retrograde manner during the following days, weeks, or months.

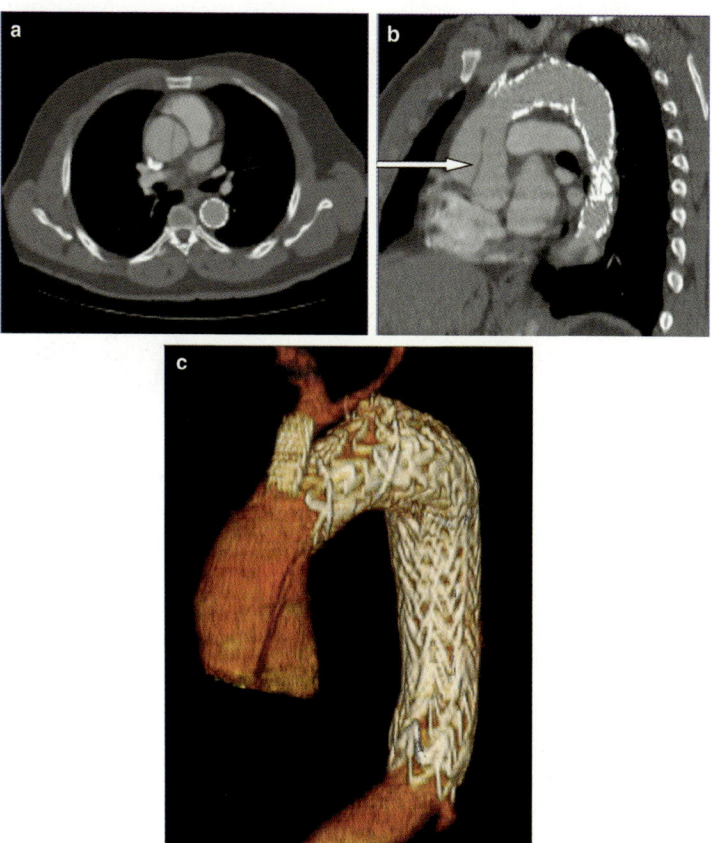

Fig. 35.3 (**a**) Axial CT scan demonstrates endoluminal graft exclusion of a type B dissection with a new intimal tear in the ascending aorta (type A dissection). (**b**) Sagittal CT 1 cuts demonstrate a type A dissection (*white arrow*). (**c**) Sixty-four slice CT scan demonstrates a bovine arch with endoluminal graft excluding a type B dissection distal to innominate artery with a new intimal tear in the ascending aorta

Device-related complications arise from semi-rigid designed grafts not able to adapt perfectly to the aortic curve in an angulated aortic arch which may require several balloon dilation for conformation to the aorta resulting in intimal tears which may progress to a frank dissection. Stent grafts with bare spring used for anchoring at their proximal ends can create new intimal tears especially in the fragile dissected aorta. Stent grafts require repeated balloon dilations to conform to the curved geometry of the aortic arch and to form a tight seal. In addition, routine stent graft oversizing may contribute to intimal injuries despite exact measurements Oversizing of stent grafts >10% results in a higher radial force against the aortic wall, with potential intimal injury and tears occurring if oversizing is >20% of indication for use (IFU) recommendations

Fig. 35.4 Replacement of ascending aorta with a 32 Hemashield graft

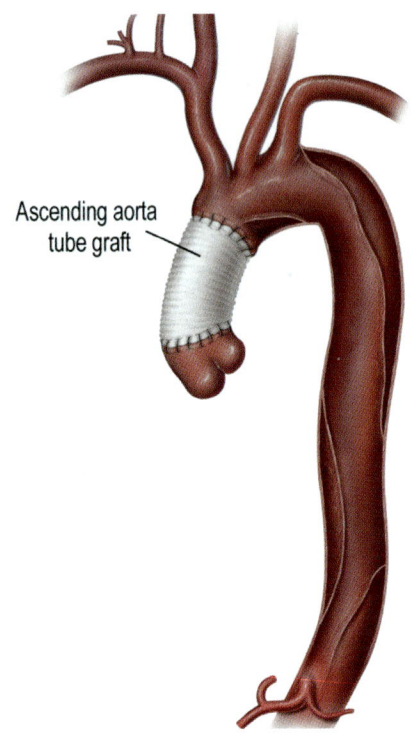

Ascending aorta
tube graft

Progression of disease could result in the formation of new intimal injuries and dissections at sites unrelated to the stent graft procedure. Congenital weakness of the aortic wall must also be considered in patients who have no obvious cause for a dissection. Stent graft implantation in such patients must be performed very cautiously. We suspect that the fragility of the aortic wall caused by this pathology finally results in a retrograde type A dissection, which is triggered by the stent graft procedure. We recommend that the use of stent graft in patients with Marfan should be discouraged because of the fragility of the aortic wall.

Persistent blood flow into the false lumen at the end of the procedure might also be a positive predictor for retrograde type A dissection. The influence of the different stent grafts on intimal injury is questionable. Retrograde type A dissection has been reported in patients who were treated with a Talent endoprosthesis with a free flow design on the proximal cage, resulting in death. The cause may be related to the limited flexibility of the currently available devices that produce forced wall stress at the outer curvature leading to intimal injuries.[24–26] Although forced and repeated balloon dilation is an important factor that contributed to intimal injuries, careful balloon dilation is recommended since the self-expanding action of the stent grafts also results in continuous expansion of the true lumen over time.

Despite the minimal invasive nature of stent graft implantation, sometimes fatal complications may arise from its deployment with retrograde ascending aortic dissection one of the most severe one. Between 1998 and 2007 we have treated a total of 512 patients with a thoracic aortic stent graft for various aortic pathologies. The Gore TAG excluder device was used in 400 patients, with eight patients developing a retrograde type A dissection (2.0%); there were three males and five females with the diagnosis made at a median of 116 days. Fifty percent of the patients were identified during the perioperative period. Retrograde type A dissection was diagnosed within the perioperative period in three patients with 100% mortality.[27] Of the eight patients who developed a retrograde type A dissection one patient was previously treated for a thoracic aortic aneurysm, one patient for a penetrating aortic ulcer and six patients for a type B dissection (75%). There were 97 patients treated for type B dissection during that time period resulting in a 6/97 (6.2%) incidence of a retrograde type dissection in that group category. The mortality rate for a retrograde type A dissection was 5/8 (62.5%) mostly as a result of complications with three deaths within the perioperative period. The three surviving patients were diagnosed at 1, 7, and 19 months, respectively, and all had an ascending aorta replacement with a tube graft. Table 35.1 represents data on our initial seven patients. Possible etiologies for retrograde type A dissection that we knew of were possibly related to oversizing more than 20% the indication for use. The larger the stent graft, the greater the radial force it gives to the aortic wall resulting in good apposition to the aortic wall. Occasionally oversizing has resulted in intimal injuries especially in fragile aortas. In the treatment of two patients oversizing of the aorta was responsible for retrograde type A dissection with one patient receiving an endograft that had been oversized by 27.4%. Incomplete seal of the entry tear of a type B dissection occurred in one patient, with progression of disease of the aorta responsible in one patient diagnosed at 19 months prior to stent graft placement for a type B dissection.

Other possible etiologies could have been related to balloon dilatation of endografts to achieve good wall apposition resulting in aortic intimal injury and the tips of the guidewire and the delivery system could cause damage to the aortic intima. In our report we did not use any stent grafts with uncovered struts which have been known to cause intimal injuries at the proximal and distal fixation points.

Retrograde type A dissection, a potentially lethal complication following endovascular stent graft repair of thoracic aortic pathologies may present as an acute or delayed presentation. Better patient selection, precise stent graft deployment,

Table 35.1 Initial seven patients who developed a retrograde type A dissection following stent graft therapy for various thoracic aortic pathologies

#	Age	Sex	Etiology	Graft used % oversize	Time to discovery	Result
1	83	F	Dissection	11.1	POD#1	Death
2	78	F	Dissection	8.1	POD#10	Death
3	53	M	Dissection	21.2	1 month	Tube graft
4	78	F	Aneurysm	27.6	7 months	Tube graft
5	67	M	Dissection	21.2	19 months	Tube graft
6	60	M	Dissection	19.4	21 months	Death
7	74	F	Dissection	17.2	30 months	Death

careful wire and sheath manipulation in the arch of the aorta, coverage of a large part of the descending aorta in the straight portion as opposed to the angled or curved part of the aorta, and avoidance of aggressive ballooning of stent grafts in the treatment of type B dissection can reduce the incidence of retrograde type A dissection. The inflexibility of stent grafts and pulsatile forces of the aorta have as much adverse effects as acutely dissected intima. The development of stent grafts with smoother edges, flexible bodies, and avoidance of stents with barbs at proximal ends that could create new intimal tears could further help decrease this fatal complication of endoluminal stent graft use especially in the treatment of type B dissections.

References

1. Dake MD, Miller DC, Semba CP, et al. Transluminal placement of endovascular stent-grafts for the treatment of descending thoracic aortic aneurysms. *N Engl J Med.* 1994;331:1729–1734.
2. Kato N, Hirano T, Takeda K, et al. Treatment of aortic dissections with a percutaneous intravascular endoprosthesis: comparison of covered and bare stents. *J Vasc Interv Radiol.* 1994;5:805–812.
3. Marui A, Mochizuki T, Mitsui N, et al. Toward the best treatment for uncomplicated patients with type B acute aortic dissection: a consideration for sound surgical indication. *Circulation.* 1999;100:II275–II280.
4. Miller DC, Mitchell RS, Oyer PE, et al. Independent determinants of operative mortality for patients with aortic dissections. *Circulation.* 1984;70:I153– I164.
5. Cambria RP, Brewster DC, Gertler J, et al. Vascular complications associated with spontaneous aortic dissection. *J Vasc Surg.* 1988;7:199–209.
6. Crawford ES, Hess KR, Cohen ES, et al. Ruptured aneurysm of the descending thoracic and thoracoabdominal aorta. Analysis according to size and treatment. *Ann Surg.*1991; 213:417–426.
7. Velazquez OC, Bavaria JE, Pochettino A, et al. Emergency repair of thoracoabdominal aortic aneurysms with immediate presentation. *J Vasc Surg.* 1999;30:996–1003.
8. Nienaber CA, Fattori R, Lund G, et al. Nonsurgical reconstruction of thoracic aortic dissection by stent-graft placement. *N Engl J Med.* 1999;340:1539–1545.
9. Czermak BV, Waldenberger P, Fraedrich G, et al. Treatment of Stanford type B aortic dissection with stent-grafts: preliminary results. *Radiology.* 2000;217:544–550.
10. Czermak BV, Mallouhi A, Perkmann R, et al. Serial CT volume and thrombus length measurements after endovascular repair of Stanford type B aortic dissection. *J Endovasc Ther.* 2004;11:1–12.
11. Totaro M, Miraldi F, Fanelli F, et al. Emergency surgery for retrograde extension of type B dissection after endovascular stent graft repair. *Eur J Cardiothorac Surg.*2001;20:1057–1058.
12. Fanelli F, Salvatori FM, Marcelli G, et al. Type A aortic dissection developing during endovascular repair of an acute type B dissection. *J Endovasc Ther.* 2003;10:254–259.
13. Nienaber CA, Eagle KA. Aortic dissection: new frontiers in diagnosis and management. Part II: therapeutic management and follow-up. *Circulation.* 2003; 108:772–778.
14. Pasic M, Bergs P, Knollmann F, et al. Delayed retrograde aortic dissection after endovascular stenting of the descending thoracic aorta. *J Vasc Surg.* 2002; 36:184–186.
15. Grabenwoger M, Fleck T, Ehrlich M, et al. Secondary surgical interventions after endovascular stent-grafting of the thoracic aorta. *Eur J Cardiothorac Surg.* 2004;26:608–613.
16. Bethuyne N, Bove T, Van den Brande P, et al. Acute retrograde aortic dissection during endovascular repair of a thoracic aortic aneurysm. *Ann Thorac Surg.* 2003;75:1967–1969.

17. Misfeld M, Notzold A, Geist V, et al. Retrograde type A dissection after endovascular stent grafting of type B dissection [in German]. *Z Kardiol.* 2002;91:274–277.
18. Totaro M, Miraldi F, Fanelli F, Mazzesi G. Emergency surgery for retrograde extension of type B dissection after endovascular stent graft repair. *Eur J Cardiothorac Surg.* 2001;20:1057–1058.
19. Diethrich EB, Ramaiah VG, Kpodonu J, Rodriguez JA. *Figures Courtesy of Endovascular and Hybrid Management of the Thoracic Aorta. A Case Based Approach.* 1st ed. West Sussex: Wiley-Blackwell; 2008.
20. Kato N, Hirano T, Kawaguchi T, et al. Aneurysmal degeneration of the aorta after stent graft repair of acute aortic dissection. *J Vasc Surg.* 2001;34: 513–518.
21. Pamler RS, Kotsis T, Gorich J, Kapfer X, Orend KH, Plassmann LS. Complications after endovascular repair of type B aortic dissection. *J Endovasc Ther.* 2002;9:822–828.
22. Totaro M, Miraldi F, Fanelli F, et al. Emergency surgery for retrograde extension of type B dissection after endovascular stent graft repair. *Eur J Cardiothorac Surg.*2001;20:1057–1058.
23. Fanelli F, Salvatori FM, Marcelli G, et al. Type A aortic dissection during endovascular repair of an acute type B dissection. *J Endovasc Ther.* 2003;10:254–259.
24. Duebener LF, Lorenzen P, Richardt G, et al. Emergency endovascular stent-grafting for life-threatening acute type B aortic dissections. *Ann Thorac Surg.* 2004;78:1261–1267.
25. Fattori R, Napoli G, Lovato L, et al. Descending thoracic aortic diseases: stent-graft repair Radiology 2003;229:176–183.
26. Totaro M, Miraldi F, Fanelli F, Mazzesi G. Emergency surgery for retrograde extension of type B dissection after endovascular stent graft repair. *Eur J Cardiothorac Surg.* 2001;20:1057–1058.
27. Kpodonu J, Preventza O, Ramaiah VG, et al. Retrograde type A dissection after endovascular stenting of the descending thoracic aorta. Is the risk real? *Eur J Cardiothorac Surg.* 2008;33(6):1014–1018.

Part X
Endografting for Varied Thoracic Aortic Pathologies

Chapter 36
Aorto-bronchial Fistula

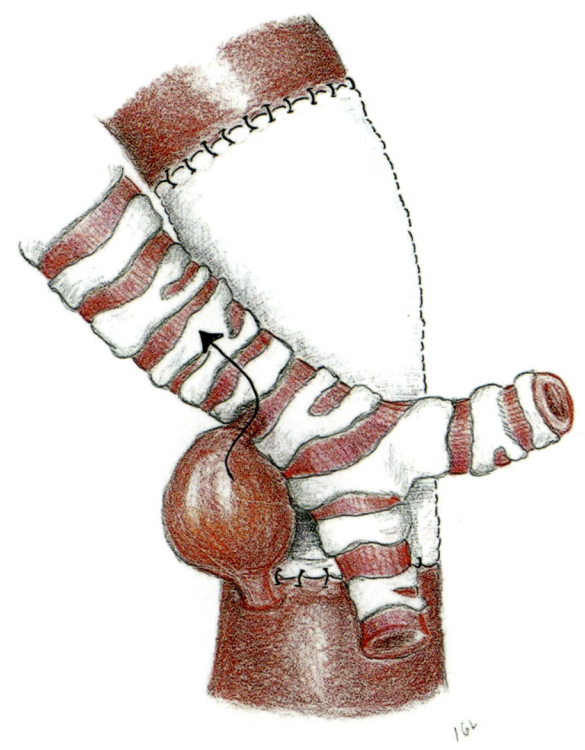

Aorto-bronchial fistula (ABF) is a rare, life-threatening complication associated with previous thoracic aortic surgery. Patients typically present with hemoptysis and its presence, once confirmed, mandates urgent repair. CT scans, aortography, bronchoscopy, and transesophageal echocardiography are the most common modalities used to make the diagnosis. Open surgery of aorto-bronchial fistulas is associated with respiratory insufficiency, stroke, paralysis, acute renal failure, myocardial

J. Kpodonu, *Manual of Thoracic Endoaortic Surgery*,
DOI 10.1007/978-1-84996-296-4_36, © Springer-Verlag London Limited 2010

infarction, cardiac failure, hemorrhage, secondary graft infection, and a mortality rate ranging from 25 to 41%.[1,2] Endovascular stent grafting provides a less invasive approach to exclude the fistulous tract as well as the pathological aorta with reduced morbidity and mortality.[3]

36.1 Endovascular Techniques

The diagnosis of aorto-bronchial fistula should be confirmed by appropriate imaging which includes transesophageal echocardiogram (Fig. 36.1), CT angiography (Fig. 36.2a,b), aortography (Fig. 36.3) bronchoscopy (Fig. 36.4), and intravascular ultrasound (Fig. 36.5) if the technology is available.[4] The procedure should be performed under general anesthesia with the airway protected with a double lumen endotrachial tube to protect the non-bleeding airway. Bilateral arterial lines are

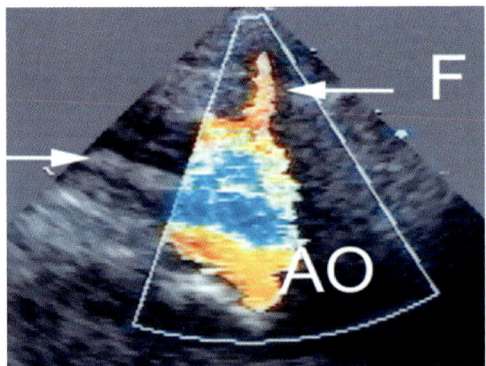

Fig. 36.1 Transesophageal echocardiogram performed in a patient with a fistulous tract (F) between the aorta (AO) and the bronchus

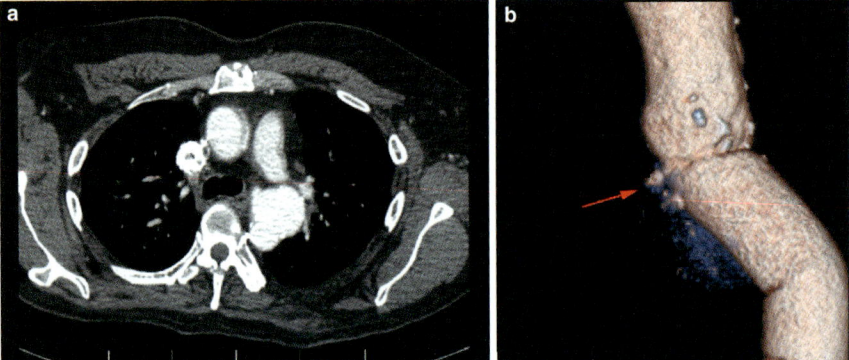

Fig. 36.2 (**a**, **b**) Axial CT scan performed in a patient with previous descending thoracic aorta repair who presented with hemoptysis which demonstrates a pseudoaneurysm of the descending thoracic aorta with disruption of anastomosis

Fig. 36.3 Thoracic
aortogram in a patient with an
aorto-brochial fistula. A
fistulous tract is demonstrated
between the aorta and the left
main stem bronchus

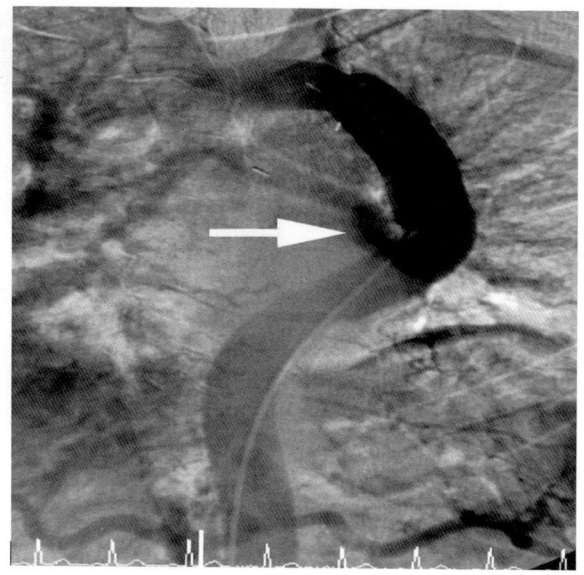

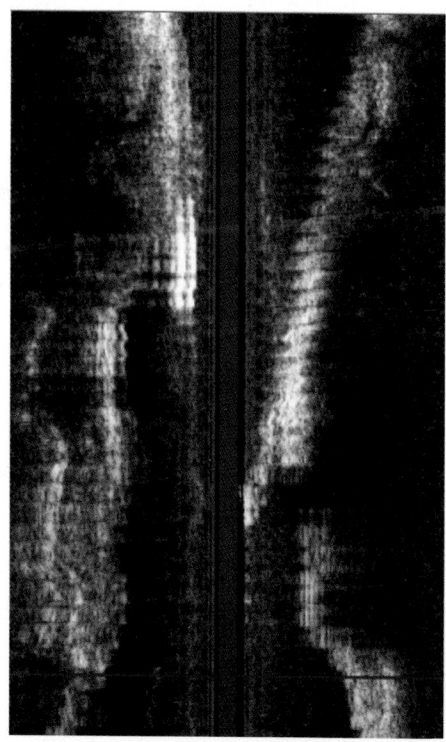

Fig. 36.4 Intravascular
ultrasound in a patient with a
pseudoaneurysm resulting
from disruption of the
proximal anastomosis of a
previous thoracic aortic
repair

Fig. 36.5 Bronchoscopy
performed in a patient with
previous descending thoracic
repair from a motor accident
who presented with
hemoptysis demonstrates
blood clot in the left main
stem bronchus

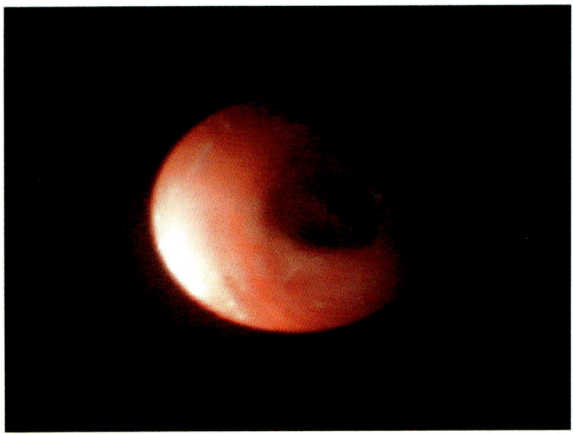

placed. Pre-operative imaging of the access arteries and the thoracic aorta should
be performed to ensure that the common femoral artery is of adequate caliber for
advancement of the delivery sheath as well to determine landing zones, diameter of neck and length of aorta to be excluded by the pathology. Intravascular
access is obtained through both common femoral arteries with a 9 Fr sheath. The
patient is given 5000 units of intravenous heparin for anticoagulation. An arterio-
graphic 5 Fr pigtail catheter is advanced through the common femoral artery groin
sheath. Aortography and intravascular ultrasonography are performed to measure
the dimensions of the thoracic aorta neck, length of aortic pathology to be excluded
by the endoluminal graft, and distances from the brachiocephalic and visceral vessels as well as to demonstrate the fistulous tract. An extra stiff angled wire must be
advanced into the arch aorta using an exchange catheter. Aortogram is performed in
a left anterior oblique view to demonstrate the arch vessels and in an anteroposte-
rior view to demonstrate the descending thoracic aorta and visceral branches. The
appropriate-sized delivery sheath is chosen and advanced into the descending thoracic aorta. An endoluminal graft of appropriate size and length is selected based
on pre-operative CT imaging, aortography, and intravascular ultrasound measurements and deployed under fluoroscopic guidance and on a road map angiogram
with the mean arterial pressure decreased to less than 60 mmHg with intravenous
antihypertensive therapy. Post-deployment balloon angioplasty is performed as necessary to fix the proximal and distal landing zones and any area of overlap in
which more than 1 endoluminal graft is deployed. Completion arteriography is performed to assess accurate placement and to demonstrate absence of endoleak. The
patient is kept in the intensive care unit overnight. A post-operative CT scan of the
chest (Fig. 36.6) is performed the next day to demonstrate that the graft is in good
position and no evidence of an endoleak. The patient is seen at 1 and 6 months
thereafter with a clinical examination and a follow-up CT scan should there be no
endoleak at discharge and much sooner should there be concerns of an endoleak or
a non-satisfactory deployment of the endoluminal graft.

Fig. 36.6 Reconstructed CT scan of the chest in a patient with aorto-bronchial fistula treated with an endovascular stent graft which demonstrates satisfactory position of the thoracic stent graft with no evidence of endoleak

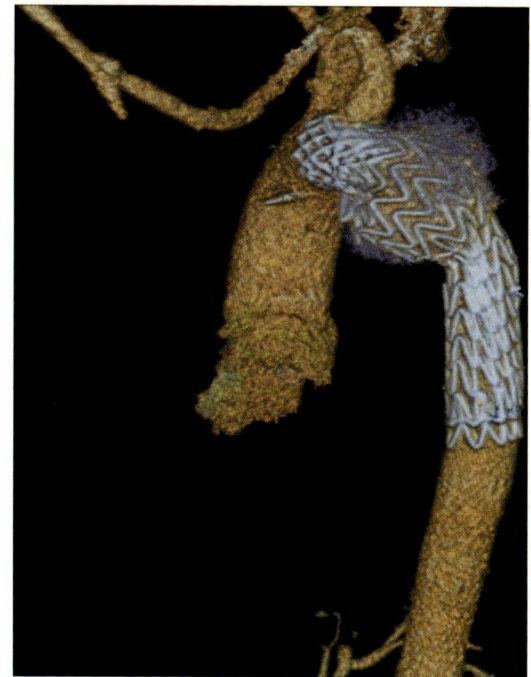

36.2 Discussion

The risk of open operation for ABF is high due to emergency conditions, difficult redo operations, and the possibility of infectious complications. In ABF, there is usually a communication between the previous aortic graft and the tracheobronchial tree. Conventional, open surgical correction involves a thoracotomy and carries a fairly high morbidity and mortality due to the difficulty of operative dissection. Although long-term results of endovascular repair are lacking, stent graft repair of ABF is our preferred treatment due to the avoidance of aortic cross-clamping, thoracotomy, extracorporeal circulation, as well as the potential hemodynamic instability that is inherent with an open repair.

References

1. Leobon B, Roux D, Mugniot A, et al. Endovascular treatment of thoracic aortic fistulas. *Ann Thorac Surg.* 2002;74:247–249.
2. Macintosh EL, Parrott JC, Unruh HW. Fistulas between the aorta and tracheobronchial tree. *Ann Thorac Surg.* 1991;51:515–519.
3. Svenson LG, Patel V, Robinson MF. Variables predictive of outcome in 832 patients undergoing repairs of the descending thoracic aorta. *Chest.* 1993;104:1248–1253.
4. Diethrich EB, Ramaiah VG, Kpodonu J, Rodriguez JA. *Endovascular and Hybrid Management of the Thoracic Aorta. A Case Based Approach.* 1st ed. West Sussex: Wiley-Blackwell; 2008.

Chapter 37
Endovascular Management of Penetrating Aortic Ulcer

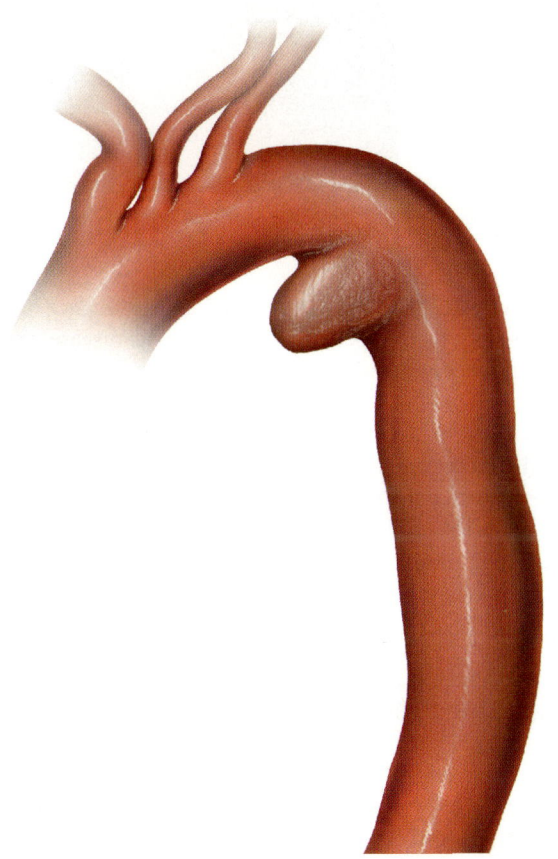

Penetrating aortic ulcers (PAU) of the thoracic aorta arise when atherosclerotic lesions rupture through the internal elastic lamina of the aortic wall with subsequent hematoma formation between the media and the adventitia. The ulcers are most often found in the distal descending thoracic aorta but can occur throughout the thoracic and abdominal aorta and have a characteristic appearance on chest

J. Kpodonu, *Manual of Thoracic Endoaortic Surgery*,
DOI 10.1007/978-1-84996-296-4_37, © Springer-Verlag London Limited 2010

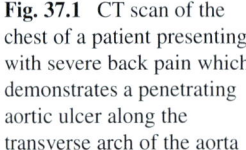

Fig. 37.1 CT scan of the chest of a patient presenting with severe back pain which demonstrates a penetrating aortic ulcer along the transverse arch of the aorta

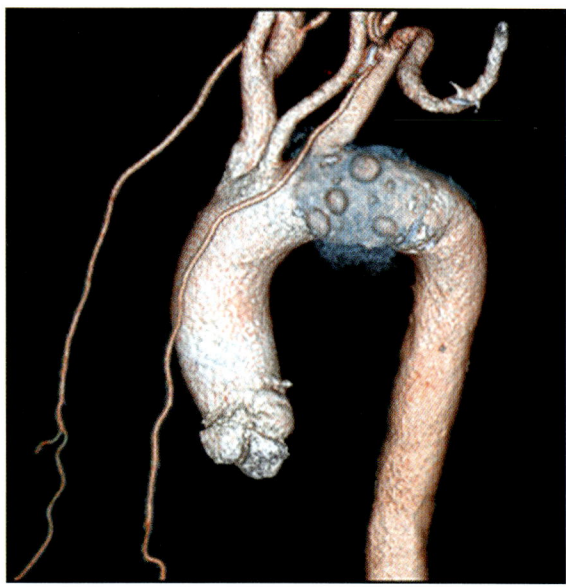

computed tomography (CT) (Fig. 37.1) and magnetic resonance imaging. PAUs may represent one pathology in the spectrum of acute aortic diseases but it may be associated with aortic dissection and aneurysm formation, although it is distinct from those conditions.

The natural history of asymptomatic thoracic aortic ulcers remains unknown, although when the ulcers are symptomatic, they can be associated with >50% risk of rupture. Patients with penetrating aortic ulcers often have cardiovascular-related co-morbidities and open surgical repair, especially in emergency circumstances, is associated with a high morbidity and mortality. Endovascular techniques do offer a less invasive approach in this group of patients with cardiovascular co-morbidities.

37.1 Endovascular Procedure

The principle of management of penetrating aortic ulcer is to exclude the symptomatic penetrating aortic ulcer with the shortest diameter endoluminal graft to prevent aortic rupture, dissection, or a pseudoaneurysm. The patient is usually elderly with multiple co-morbidities which make open surgical repair risky.

Under general anesthesia, open retrograde cannulation of the common femoral artery is performed and a 9 Fr introducer sheath is introduced. Percutaneous access of the contralateral common femoral artery is similarly performed and a 5 Fr introducer sheath introduced. The patient is subsequently heparinized. An oblique thoracic arch aortogram is performed with a 5 Fr pigtail catheter advanced through the percutaneous groin sheath. The fluoroscopic C-arm should be positioned in

Fig. 37.2 Angiogram in a patient with severe back pain which demonstrates an aortic penetrating aortic ulcer in the descending thoracic aorta

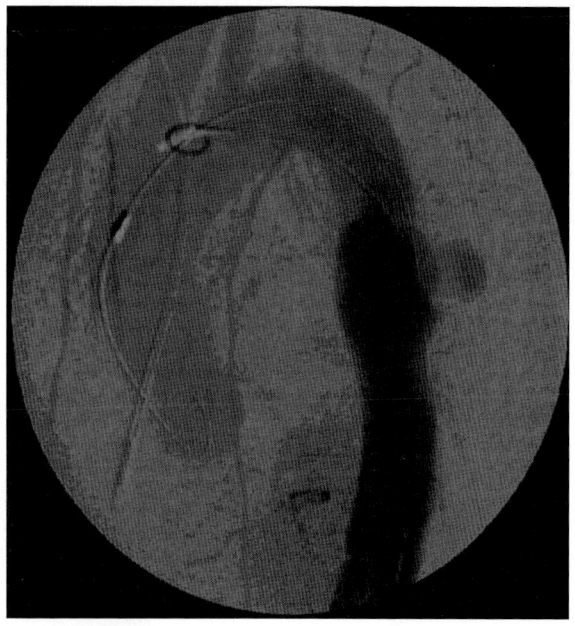

a left anterior oblique angle to demonstrate the arch vessels and the arch aorta. Pathologies of the descending thoracic aorta are best visualized with the C-arm in the anterior–posterior position. The angiogram once performed should demonstrate the penetrating aortic ulcer (Fig. 37.2). Intravascular ultrasound (IVUS) is

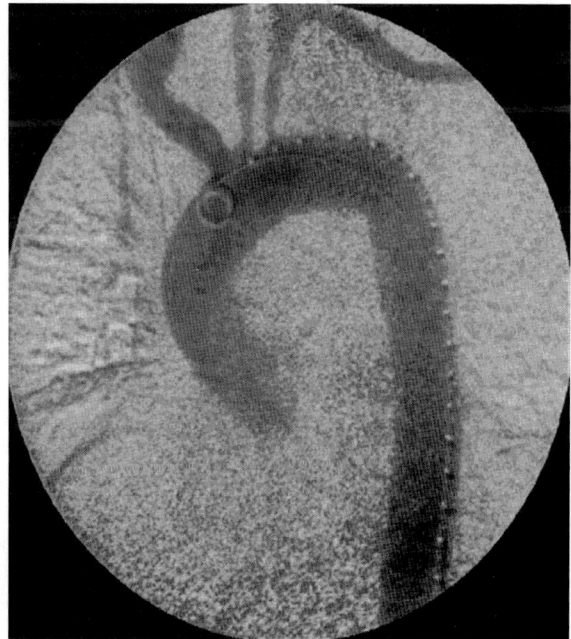

Fig. 37.3 Angiogram post-deployment of endoluminal graft demonstrates satisfactory exclusion of a penetrating aortic ulcer with no evidence of an endoleak

performed using a (Volcano therapeutics, Inc., Cordova, CA) 8.2 Fr probe through the 9 Fr groin sheath. The advantage of IVUS is to identify the penetrating aortic ulcer, site of possible pseudoaneurysm, dissection or rupture, determine proximal neck diameter/length of thoracic aorta to be covered and the distal neck diameter/length. Based on the CT scan measurements, IVUS measurements, and angiographic findings, a proper-sized endograft is chosen to exclude the penetrating aortic ulcer. A completion angiogram is performed and once satisfied with the deployment of the endograft (Fig. 37.3), all wires and sheaths are removed and the common femoral artery repaired. Manual pressure is used to compress the percutaneously accessed femoral artery. Post-operative CT scan should be performed prior to discharge to demonstrate satisfactory exclusion of the pathology (Fig. 37.4).

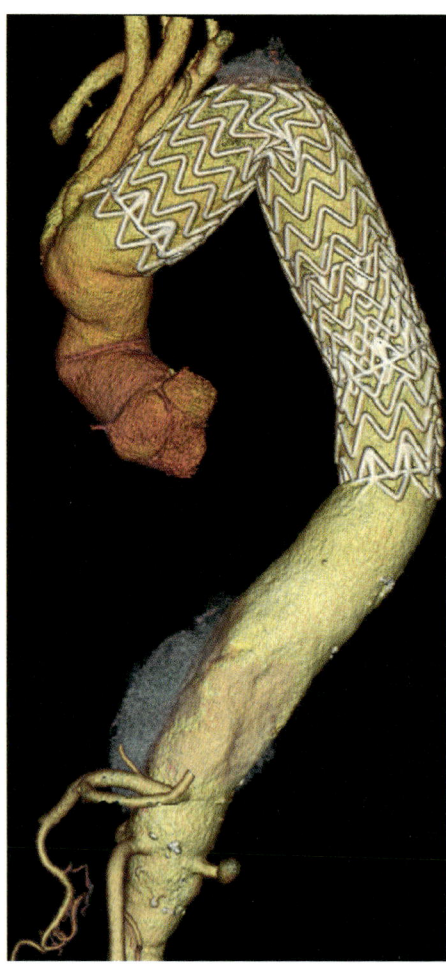

Fig. 37.4 Post-operative CT scan in a patient treated with an endoluminal graft for a penetrating aortic ulcer. The shortest length endoluminal graft is chosen to exclude the symptomatic penetrating aortic ulcer

37.2 Case Scenario

An 85-year-old frail man with a history of diabetes and hyperlipidemia presented with new onset back pain and a recent history of hoarseness. His cardiovascular workup was negative for coronary artery disease. His blood pressure was well

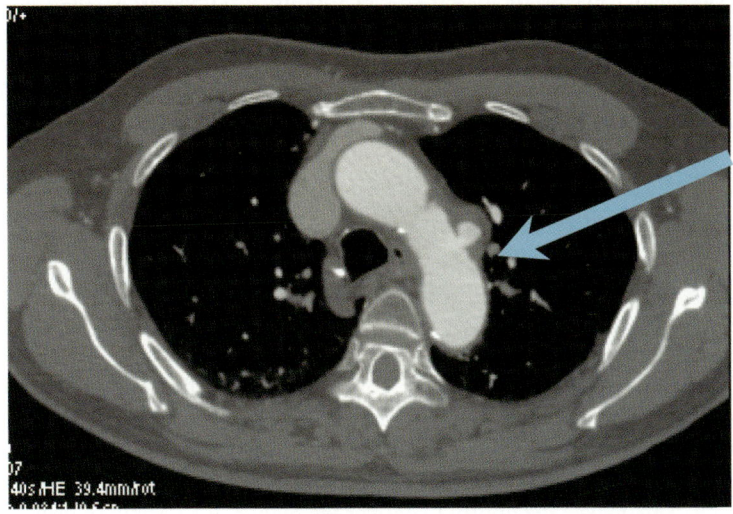

Fig. 37.5 A CT scan image showing the penetrating ulcer with surrounding hematoma

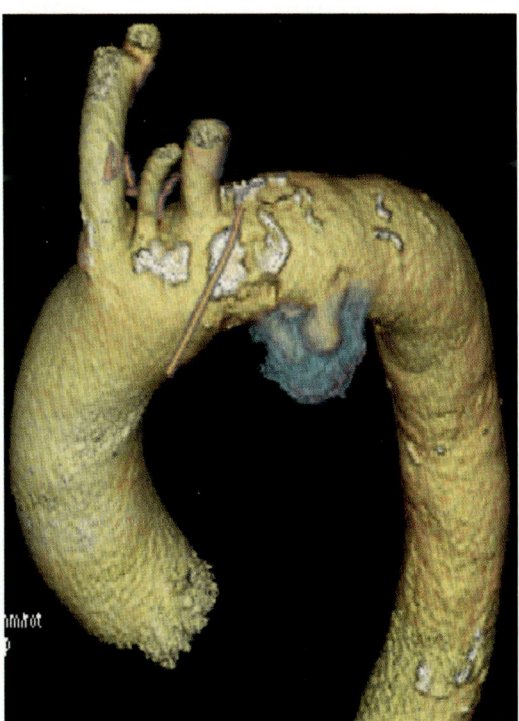

Fig. 37.6 A 3D model demonstrating the ulcer in relation to the supra-aortic arch vessels

controlled with a beta-blocker.[1] A CT scan performed demonstrated a penetrating aortic ulcer with a focal 2 cm pseudoaneurysm containing mural thrombus involving the lesser curve of the distal aortic arch (Figs. 37.5 and 37.6). The mass effect of the penetrating aortic ulcer and pseudoaneurysm on the recurrent laryngeal nerve could be responsible for the recent change in voice. The presence of back pain is often associated with the increased risk of rupture. Taking into account all of the symptoms and co-morbidities, there was a significant indication for endovascular management with an endoluminal graft. Endoluminal graft therapy for the management of symptomatic penetrating aortic ulcers is a less invasive approach which does not require cross-clamping of the aorta and a thoracic incision.

37.3 Endovascular Technique

Under general anesthesia, a cutdown incision was made in the right groin with percutaneous access obtained in the opposite groin. The patient was heparininzed for the entire duration of the procedure. A 5 Fr pigtail catheter was advanced through the left groin sheath into the thoracic aorta. An oblique thoracic arch aortogram was performed which demonstrated the penetrating aortic ulcer just distal to the left subclavian artery (Fig. 37.7). For cases involving the proximal thoracic aorta, the C-arm apparatus is usually angled 50–70° so that the views are perpendicular to the target arch. This makes the ability to deliver the device in an accurate fashion more achievable. Due to the ulcer coming off the lateral wall of the aorta, visualization

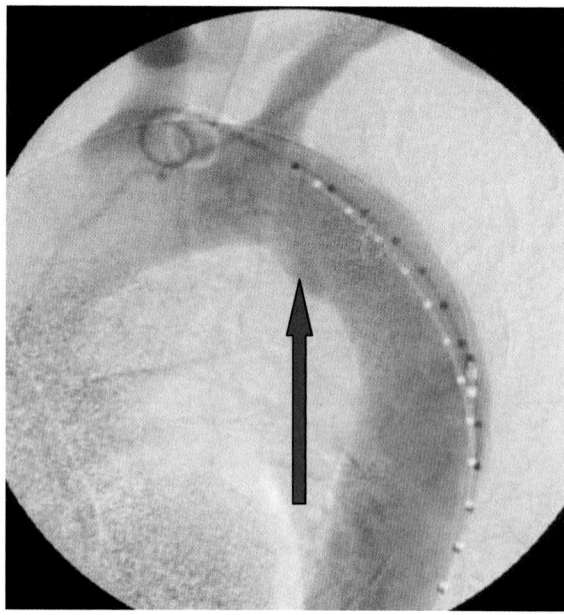

Fig. 37.7 Angiogram demonstrating a penetrating ulcer (*blue arrow*) on the lesser curvature of the aortic arch

using angiography would be difficult. An IVUS probe was introduced to evaluate the proximal neck to validate the measurements taken from the CT scan and confirm that a proximal neck of 2 cm was available to seat the graft properly. The CT measurements were confirmed and a treatment length of 8 cm was determined by a wire "pull-back" method. The IVUS probe was exchanged for a Lunderquist (Cook Inc, Bloomington) wire. Based on the measurements, a 37 mm × 10 cm Gore TAG (W.L. Gore & Associates, Flagstaff, AZ) graft was chosen to be deployed to exclude the aortic pathology.

The right 9 Fr sheath was exchanged for a 24 Fr sheath and the Gore 37 mm × 10 cm device was advanced through the Gore sheath. An anterior–posterior thoracic aortogram was performed and a road map obtained with a guiding needle placed at the proximal and distal landing zones. After ensuring the mean blood pressure was lower than 90 mmHg, a Gore TAG 37 mm × 10 cm graft was deployed successfully excluding the ulcer. The 24 Fr sheath was exchanged to a 14 Fr sheath and a 40 mm Coda balloon (Cook, Inc., Bloomington, IN) was advanced into the endoluminal graft. Balloon angioplasty of both the proximal and distal necks was performed to ensure proper aortic wall apposition of the endoluminal graft. A completion angiogram showed exclusion of the aortic penetrating ulcer with no endoleak (Fig. 37.8). All wires and sheaths were removed; the right common femoral artery was closed in a transverse fashion with restoration of flow. A vascular closure device was deployed to the left common femoral artery. Patient had bilateral palpable pulses at the end of the procedure was subsequently extubated and transferred to

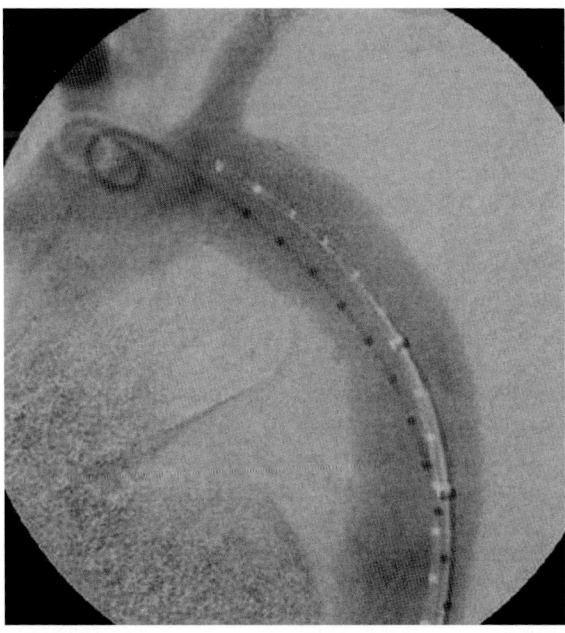

Fig. 37.8 A completion angiogram with exclusion of penetrating ulcer with an endograft

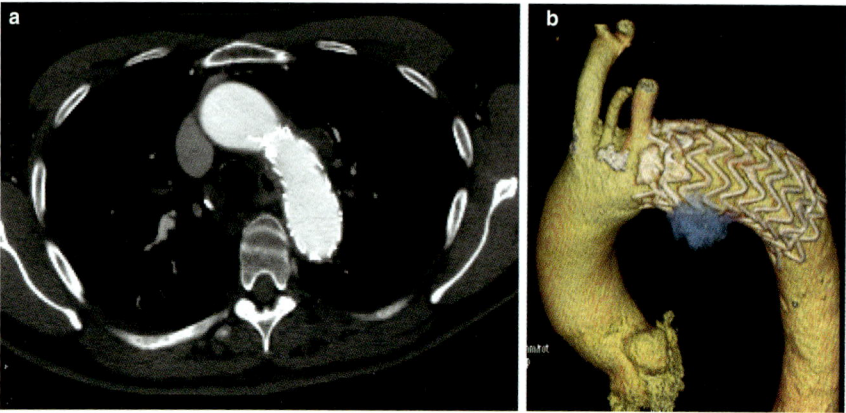

Fig. 37.9 (**a**) Axial CT scan demonstrating exclusion of penetrating aortic ulcer and thrombosed pseudoaneurysm sac. (**b**) A 64-slice 3D image showing a thrombosed penetrating ulcer

recovery room in satisfactory condition. A discharge CT scan demonstrated successful exclusion of the ulcer (Fig. 37.9). He was discharged from the hospital within three days and placed on a surveillance program that mirrors the recommendations from the manufacturer. At the 1-month follow-up, the patient's hoarseness was markedly improved, with the back pain resolved. His most recent annual examination notes an endoluminal graft in proper position with continued exclusion of his penetrating aortic ulcer.

37.4 Discussion

Penetrating aortic ulcers usually arise in atheromatous plaques located in the descending thoracic aorta that can burrow through the internal elastic lamina into the media. This can lead to a variable amount of intramural hematoma formation and may be complicated by aortic dissection and progressive aneurysmal dilatation.

Penetrating ulcers present perhaps one of the most appealing clinical indications for this stent graft technology.[2−4] Simple stent graft coverage of the penetrating ulcer can limit the progression of dissection and exclude areas of adventitial interruption allowing healing to occur. Even with successful stent graft implantation, retrograde aortic dissections and new ulcer formation have been noted in a significant percentage of patients. The incidence of these events demonstrates the diffuse and severe nature of this disease process and the need for serial evaluation following an endovascular procedure.

In a recent report of 21 patients who underwent endovascular treatment for PAU at The Arizona Heart Institute,[5] the average age was 73 ± 12 years. Patients presented with acute symptoms (<14 days; 16/21, 76.2%) and chronic symptoms (5/21, 23.8%). Successful delivery and deployment were achieved in all cases. The 30-day mortality was 0% with an overall mortality of 4.8% at 14 ± 18 months. No death was related to the device or procedure. There were no endoleaks detected in our case series and no incidents of paraplegia.

Based on our experience with the use of endoluminal grafts to treat PAU,[5,6] it is the opinion that patients with evidence of intimal tear, who are symptomatic, and not responding to medical management are ideal candidates for this type of surgery. This recommendation is dependent on the patient being properly assessed for arterial access, landing zone evaluation, desired length of the treatment area, and its location in respect to vital blood vessels.

References

1. Diethrich EB, Ramaiah VG, Kpodonu J, Rodriguez JA. *Figures Courtesy of Endovascular and Hybrid Management of the Thoracic Aorta. A Case Based Approach.* 1st ed. West Sussex: Wiley-Blackwell; 2008.
2. Demers P, Miller C, Mitchell RS, Kee ST, Chagonjian L, Dake M. Stent graft repair of penetrating atherosclerotic ulcers in the descending thoracic aorta. Mid-term results. *Ann Thorac Surg.* 2004;77:81–86.
3. Sailer J, Peloschek P, Rand T, Grabenwoger M, Thunher S, Lammer J. Endovascular treatment of aortic type B dissection and penetrating ulcer using commercially available stent grafts. *AM J Roentgenol.* 2001;177:1365–1369.
4. Schoder M, Grabenwoger M, Holzenbein T, et al. Endovascular stent graft repair of penetrating atherosclerotic ulcers of the descending aorta. *J Vasc Surg.* 2002;36:720–726.
5. Brinster DR, Wheatley GH, Williams J, Ramaiah VG, Diethrich EB, Rodriguez-Lopez JA. Are penetrating aortic ulcers best treated using an endovascular approach? *Ann Thorac Surg.* 2006;82:1688–1691.
6. Wheatley GH 3rd, Gurbuz AT, Rodriguez-Lopez JA, et al. Midterm outcome in 158 consecutive Gore TAG thoracic endoprostheses: single center experience. *Ann Thorac Surg.* 2006; 81(5):1570–1577; discussion 1577.

Chapter 38
Endovascular Approach to Coarctation of the Thoracic Aorta

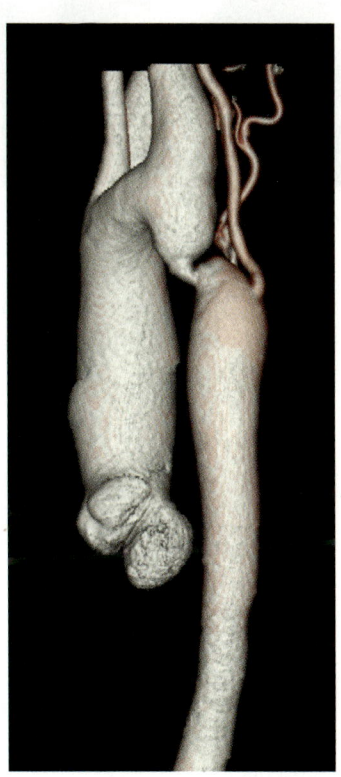

Primary coarctation of the aorta is defined as a congenital narrowing of the aorta characterized by stenosis of the juxta ductal aorta. Symptoms and signs include systemic hypertension and a differential blood pressure between the upper and lower extremities as well as occasional back and chest pain. A differential of more than 20 mmHg warrants further investigation in a symptomatic patient. Open surgical repair has been considered the "gold standard" for this aortic defect. Endovascular

J. Kpodonu, *Manual of Thoracic Endoaortic Surgery*,
DOI 10.1007/978-1-84996-296-4_38, © Springer-Verlag London Limited 2010

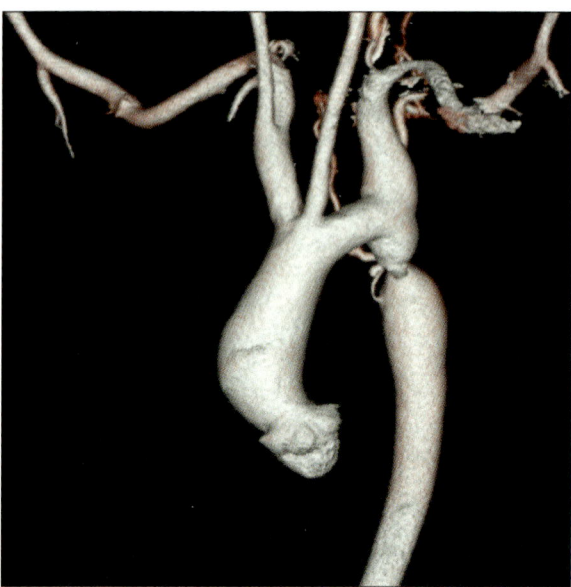

Fig. 38.1 64 slice CT scan of the chest demonstrates a severe coarctation of the thoracic aorta

techniques are currently being applied to treat coarctation of the aorta. CT angiography (Fig. 38.1) is a reliable diagnostic tool to confirm an adult onset coarctation of the aorta.

38.1 Endovascular Techniques

Bilateral arterial lines are placed in both upper extremities to determine the pressure gradient between both arms. Open retrograde cannulation of the common femoral artery is performed in the usual fashion with an 18 G needle and a 9 Fr sheath is introduced. An 0.035 in. angled glide wire is advanced into the distal aorta. Occasionally one has to use a guiding catheter to navigate the tight area of coarctation to advance the glide wire into the distal arch of the aorta. Percutaneous access of the contralateral common femoral artery is similarly performed and a 5 Fr sheath introduced. The patient is subsequently given 5000 units of heparin. A 5 Fr pigtail catheter is advanced into the arch of the aorta and a thoracic aortic angiogram is performed with the fluoroscopic arm angled in a left anterior oblique angle to visualize the arch aorta (Fig. 38.2). Intravascular ultrasound (IVUS) (Fig. 38.3) is useful to determine the exact diameter of the area of coarctation, the proximal diameter of the pre-stenotic thoracic aorta, the post-stenotic dilatation diameter of the thoracic aorta, and the length of aorta to be treated. IVUS is performed for confirmation of the pathology by exchanging the angiographic pigtail catheter for an IVUS probe. Once all the data is acquired an exchange of the 9 Fr sheath to a 65 cm 14 Fr

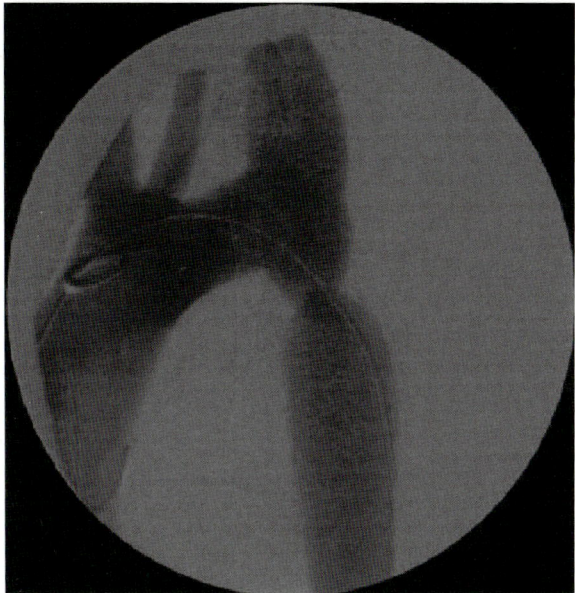

Fig. 38.2 An angiogram of a patient with a severe coarctation of the thoracic aorta

Keller-Timmermans (Cook, Bloomington, IN) sheath is performed. An appropriately sized balloon is selected for balloon angioplasty of the area of coarctation to improve luminal gain and to decrease the gradient between both arms to ideally less than 20 mmHg difference. A post-balloon angioplasty angiogram is performed to demonstrate any increase in the luminal diameter of the area of coarctation as well as to rule out any dissection or rupture of the thoracic aorta. An appropriately sized Palmaz stent (Fig. 38.4) is selected and mounted on an appropriately sized balloon. The balloon most often used is a 16 mm Maxi LD balloon (Boston Scientific, Nantucket, MA). The stent is deployed to the area of coarctation as demarcated on

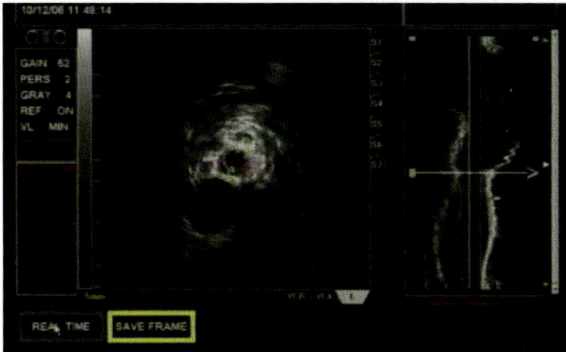

Fig. 38.3 IVUS demonstrates the area of coarctation with post-stenotic dilatation

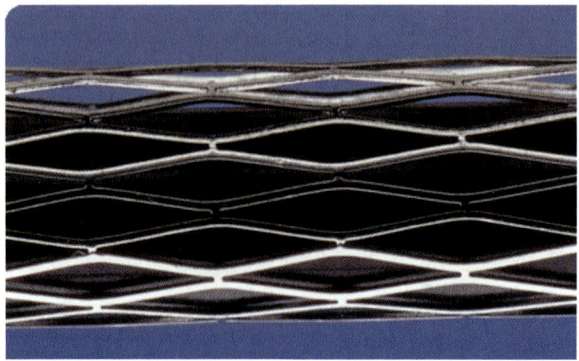

Fig. 38.4 Palmaz XL 4010 stent

a road map angiogram. A repeat angiogram should be performed to demonstrate any increased luminal gain. Post-deployment stent balloon angioplasty is usually performed with a 25 mm × 4 cm Maxi LD balloon (Boston Scientific, Nantucket, MA) with flaring of the proximal and distal ends of the stent for fixation to the aortic wall. Post-stent gradients are again confirmed and a desirable gradient of less than 10 mmHg at the completion of the procedure is judged to be excellent. Post-stent IVUS (Fig. 38.5) is performed to confirm satisfactory position of the stent as well as to determine the new diameter of the post-stented thoracic aorta. A completion angiogram is performed at the end of the procedure (Fig. 38.6). All wires

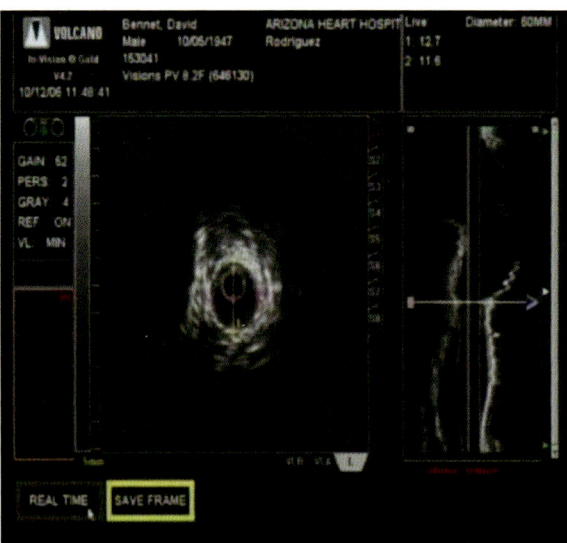

Fig. 38.5 IVUS post-stent deployment demonstrating increased luminal gain

Fig. 38.6 Completion angiogram post-stent placement for coarctation of the aorta with increase in luminal gain

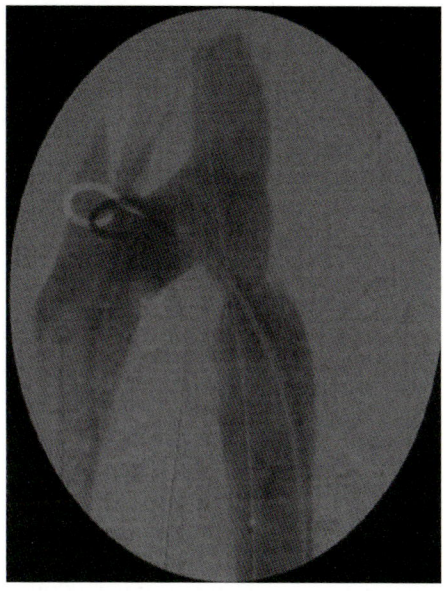

and sheaths are removed and the common femoral artery repaired with restoration of blood; the incision is closed. A closure device or manual pressure is used to achieve hemostasis once the 5 Fr sheath is pulled from the contralateral limb. A CT scan (Fig. 38.7a, b) is performed prior to discharge and periodically with follow up pressure gradients.

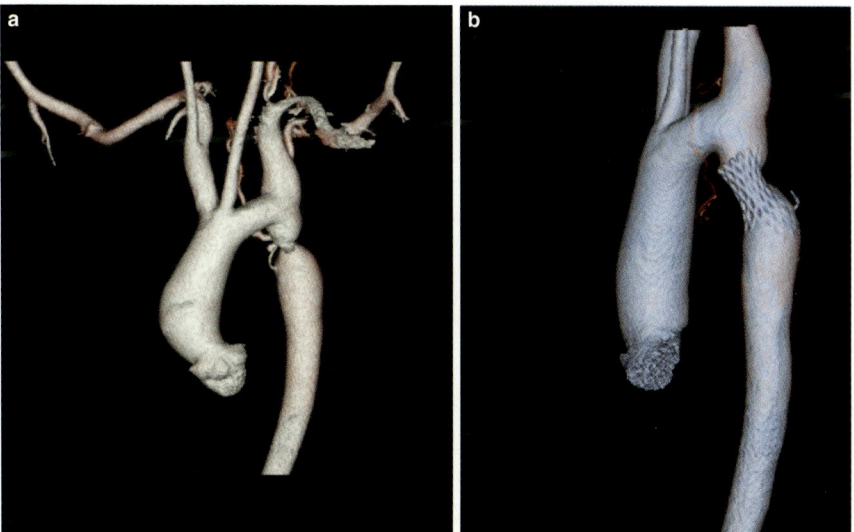

Fig. 38.7 (**a, b**) Pre- and post-procedure CT with 3D reconstruction models. The presence of a Palmaz stent and a relief in the severity of the coarctation can be seen in the Post-image

38.2 Discussion

Over a 9-year period at our institution, we treated 22 patients (17 males and 5 females) with coarctation, with 9 patients treated for primary coarctation and 13 patients for recurrent coarctation and pseudoaneurysm post-surgical repair of coarctation.[1,2] A review of the first six patients showed that five patients were symptomatic from cardiac-related causes and all patients had a cardiac-related history (Table 38.1). Gradients recorded across the area of coarctation were as high as 70 mmHg. Technical success was achieved in all patients with a decrease in post-stent gradients below 20 mmHg in all patients, with two of those patients showing no gradients at all. To date, the first patient in this series is approximately 9 years out from the procedure and has no documented coarctation-related symptoms.

The endovascular management of adult primary aortic coarctation has recently been accepted as a minimally invasive alternative to the open surgical approach. In order to make endovascular management even more attractive, changes need to be made in stent design and sizing to better accommodate to the typical coarctation presentation. Current device designs are often too long in length, have little or no taper between proximal and distal ends, and lack the ability to conform to a very tortuous aorta. As with any endovascular treatment, there is little

Table 38.1 Summary of our first six patients treated with a primary coarctation

Number	Age	Indication	History	Treatment	Results (pressure gradient)
1	52	Lt. UE tingling	CHF, Afib	BA/Palmaz 4010/BA	Initial: 60 mm Post: no gradient
2	29	No symptoms	Sys + pulm HTN, severe AI, ARF, chronic hematuria	BA/Palmaz 4010/BA	Initial: 60 mm Post: 20 mm
3	48	Increasing chest pain	MI, NIDDM, HTN, arrhythmia, colitis	BA/Palmas 4010/BA	Initial: 60 mm Post: no gradient
4	49	Exercise intolerance	HTN, DM, obesity, cardiomyopathy, claudication	BA/Palmaz 4010/BA	Initial: 70 mm Post: 5 mm
5	40	Increasing dyspnea	HTN	BA/Palmaz 4010/BA	No hemodynamic significance
6	59	Chest pain	CAD, PTCA	BA/Palmaz 4010/BA	Post: less than 10 mm

Lt, left; *UE*, upper extremity; *CHF*, congestive heart failure; *Afib*, atrial fibrillation; *sys*, systemic; *pum*, pulmonary; *HTN*, hypertension; *AI*, aortic insufficiency; *ARF*, acute renal failure; *DM*, diabetes mellitus; *CAD*, coronary artery disease; *PTCA*, percutaneous transluminal coronary angiography; *BA*, balloon angioplasty

long-term data available and additional studies would be required to determine the ultimate efficacy of endovascular management of primary adult coarctation of the aorta.

References

1. Diethrich EB, Ramaiah VG, Kpodonu J, Rodriguez JA. *Figures Courtesy of Endovascular and Hybrid Management of the Thoracic Aorta. A Case Based Approach.* 1st ed. West Sussex: Wiley-Blackwell; 2008.
2. Shennib H, Rodriguez-Lopez J, Ramaiah V, Wheatley G, Kpodonu J, Williams J, Olson D, Diethrich EB. Endovascular management of adult coarctation and its complications: intermediate results in a cohort of 22 patients. *Eur J Cardiothorac Surg.* 2010 Feb;37(2):322–327.

Chapter 39
Endovascular Management of Traumatic Aortic Disruption

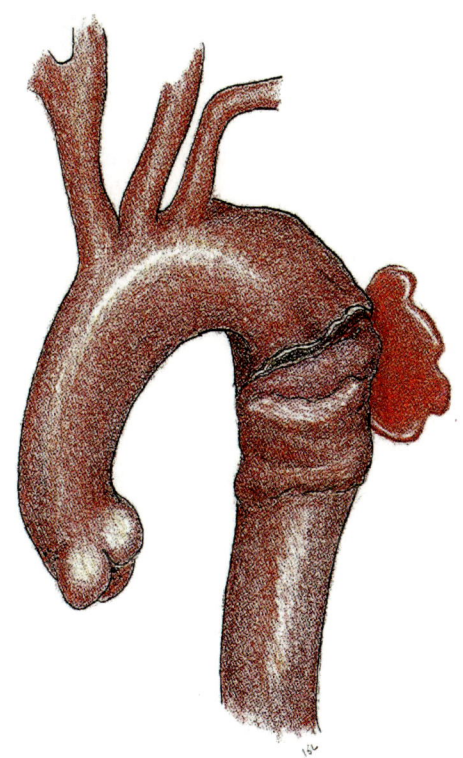

39.1 Introduction

Endovascular management of traumatic thoracic aortic disruption mostly from motor vehicle accidents (Fig. 39.1) offers a minimal invasive approach to managing critically ill patients while avoiding aortic cross-clamping and extra-corporeal circulation.[1] Younger patients are particularly challenging because their

J. Kpodonu, *Manual of Thoracic Endoaortic Surgery*,
DOI 10.1007/978-1-84996-296-4_39, © Springer-Verlag London Limited 2010

Fig. 39.1 Trauma patient
presenting with multiple
injuries including traumatic
disruption of the thoracic
aorta

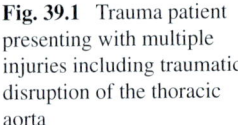

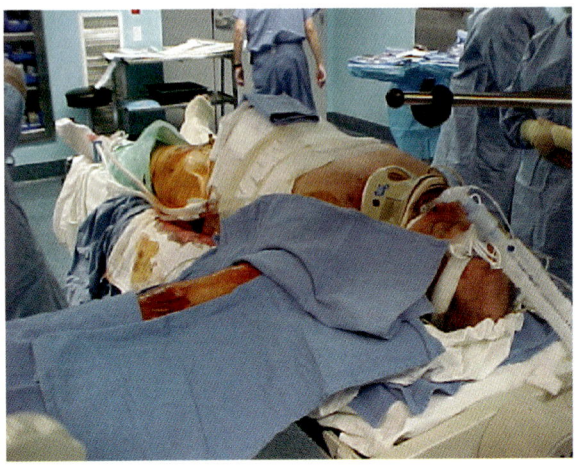

Fig. 39.1 Trauma patient presenting with multiple injuries including traumatic disruption of the thoracic aorta

thoracic aorta is often small, narrow with tighter radius angle of the thoracic arch. Other critical issues include small iliac vessels which may be problematic for delivery of the endograft. The smallest thoracic endograft currently available commercially in the United States is the 26 mm diameter Gore TAG device. Attempts to place this device in aorta 23 mm in diameter can create a situation of significant oversizing which have been associated with numerous instances of device collapse.[2]

The use of customized off-the-shelf abdominal components like iliac extender cuffs and aortic cuffs permits management of the small thoracic aorta in traumatic transactions without the need for graft oversizing. One shortcoming of the abdominal cuffs is obviously their short length, requiring the use of multiple devices and creating the potential for device separation and potential endoleak. This could be a particular problem in situations involving a large defect. Another issue with respect to the abdominal cuffs is the relatively short delivery system requiring deployment of the endoluminal graft on the back table with custom assembly of the abdominal components in longer delivery sheaths able to reach the thoracic aortic arch.

Device collapse has been reported in cases of graft oversizing in the small thoracic aorta and also when endoluminal grafts are deployed in horizontal arches. Deployment of endografts in horizontal arches subjects the device to extreme tangential forces that cause collapse with a fair degree of predictability. Options for treatment of device collapse include explantation with open repair or insertion of a second stent graft device or balloon-expandable stent within the collapsed device.[2,3] Most transactions do occur at or near the aortic isthmus which may require coverage of the left subclavian artery to achieve adequate proximal fixation. Coverage of the left subclavian artery is fairly well tolerated but occasionally symptoms of left hand ischemia may result which may require an elective left carotid artery to left subclavian bypass. Elective left carotid to left subclavian bypass operations should be performed prior to coverage of the left subclavian in patients with an internal mammary bypass graft to the left anterior descending artery and patients with a dominant left vertebral artery.

With advances in graft technology devices designed specifically to address the small thoracic and the horizontal aorta will decrease the incidence of graft oversizing and collapse associated with current commercially available endografts. A broader range of diameters and lengths as well as more flexible endografts should be designed to fully appose to the inner curve of the thoracic aorta. Until such grafts are available the treatment of patients with traumatic transaction should be individualized and patients should be enrolled in study protocols with routine clinical and imaging surveillance.

39.2 Endovascular Techniques

Procedure is generally performed under general anesthesia. Open retrograde cannulation of the right common femoral artery is performed with an 18 G Cook needle and a 0.035 in. soft tip glide wire is passed in the aorta and exchanged for a 6 Fr sheath after 5000 units of heparin was given. Percutaneous access of the left common femoral artery is similarly performed and a 9 Fr sheath introduced. Oblique thoracic arch aortogram performed through the left sheath via a pigtail catheter to

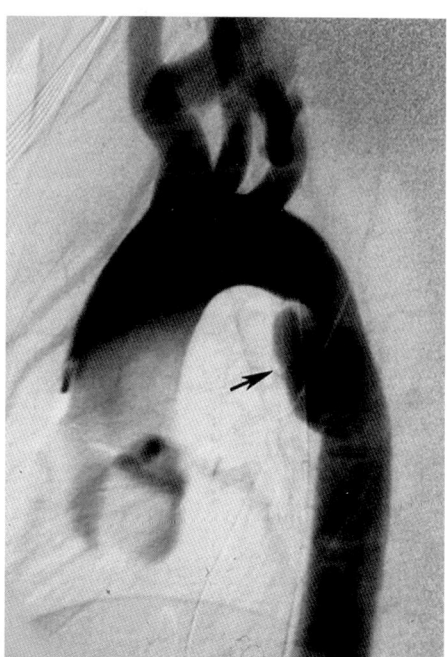

Fig. 39.2 Periaortic hematoma identified on arch angiogram

Fig. 39.3 IVUS
demonstrates a traumatic
disruption of intima

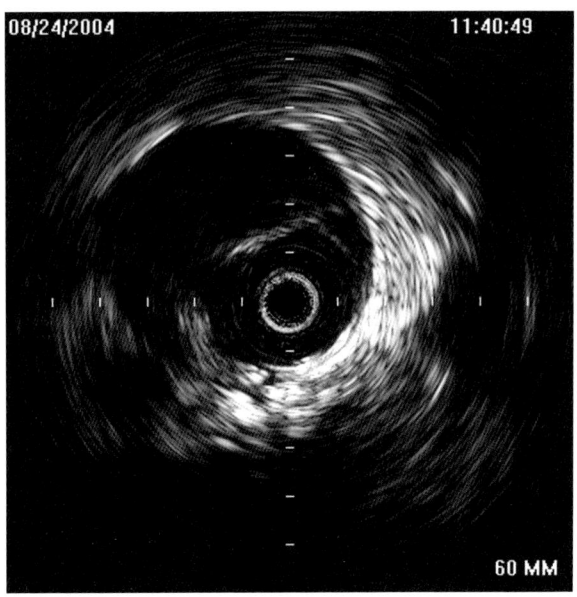

delineate the arch and the descending thoracic aorta may demonstrate the aortic disruption or a periaortic hematoma (Fig. 39.2). Intravascular ultrasound (Fig. 39.3) is performed by passing the probe through the right groin sheath. The area of transection is identified close to the left subclavian artery. The proximal and distal neck diameters and length of aorta to be covered are determined. Based on the measurements an appropriately sized endoluminal graft is chosen for deployment. The right groin 9 Fr sheath is exchanged for a device sheath and the endoluminal graft advanced and deployed over an extra stiff wire after marking the exact proximal and distal landing zones on our road map angiogram. A Gore tri-fold balloon or a Cook Coda balloon can be used to perform post-deployment balloon angioplasty of the proximal and distal segments of the graft for good aortic fixation. A completion angiogram is performed to demonstrate exclusion of the area of transection with no endoleak. All wires and sheaths are removed; the right common femoral artery is closed in a transverse fashion with restoration of flow. A vascular closure device is deployed to the left common femoral artery which was percutaneously accessed. Post-operative CT scan should be performed to demonstrate adequate exclusion of area of traumatic disruption (Fig. 39.4). In young patients oversizing of the endoluminal graft in a small angulated aorta and a short arch radius may lead to a bird beaking effect in which the endograft protrudes through the arch aorta with no apposition of the graft to the lesser curvature of the arch aorta (Fig. 39.5). Potential complications may include endoleak, graft migration, stent fracture, graft collapse (Fig. 39.6), and aortic occlusion.

Fig. 39.4 Post-operative CT
scan with satisfactory
exclusion of traumatic
disruption of the thoracic
aorta

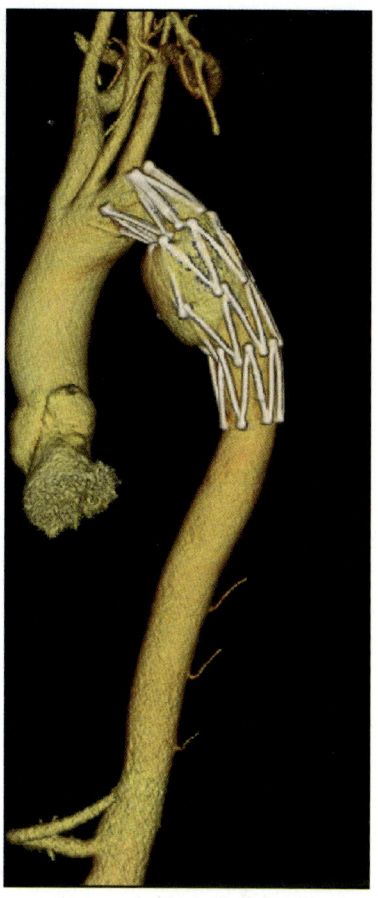

Fig. 39.5 Angiogram
demonstrating a bird beak
effect

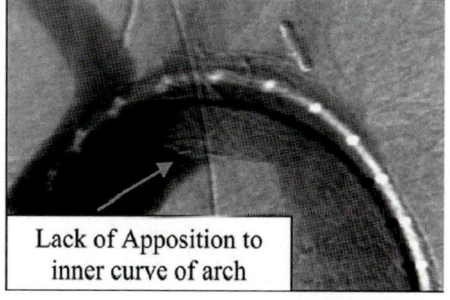

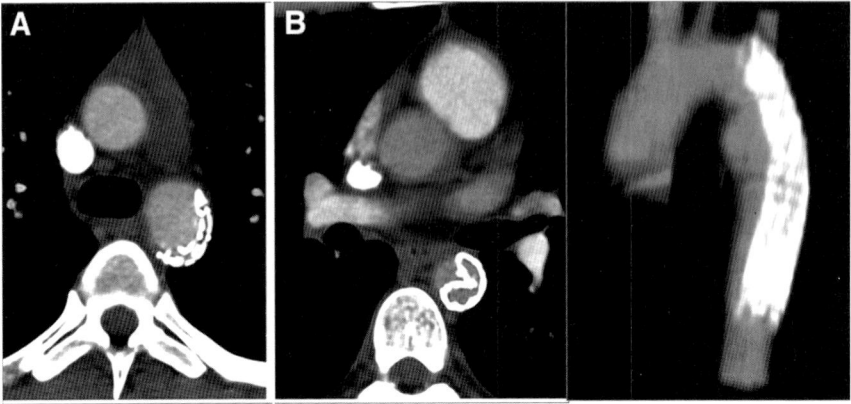

Fig. 39.6 CT scan of a patient with graft collapse as a result of graft oversize

39.3 Discussion

Endovascular management of traumatic aortic transaction confers an advantage over open surgical repair by avoiding thoracotomy, cross-clamping, single lung ventilation, reduced blood loss, heparinization, and reduced ischemic events relating spinal chord, viscera, and kidneys.[4-7] The endoluminal graft can be deployed with minimal operative intervention via the common femoral artery. Not all patients has adequate aortic morphology to undergo repair with potential shortcomings which include endoleaks, endograft migration and device infection caused by fistula formation. The endoluminal graft can be deployed with minimal operative intervention via the common femoral artery. Potential shortcomings include endoleaks. Endograft migration, device infection caused by fistula formation and not all patients has adequate aortic morphology to undergo repair. With advances in graft technology devices designed specifically to address the small thoracic and the horizontal aorta will decrease the incidence of graft oversizing and collapse associated with current commercially available endografts. A broader range of diameters and lengths as well as more flexible endografts should be designed to fully appose to the inner curve of the thoracic aorta. Until such grafts are available the treatment of patients with traumatic transaction should be individualized and patients should be enrolled in study protocols with routine clinical and imaging surveillance.

References

1. Szwerc MF, Benckart DH, Lin JC, Johnnides CG, Magovern JA, Magovern GJ. Recent clinical experience with left heart bypasses using a centrifugal pump for repair of traumatic aortic transection. *Ann Surg.* 1999;230:484–490; discussion 490–492.
2. Idu MM, Reekers JA, Balm R, Ponsen KJ, de Mol BA, Legemate DA. Collapse of a stent-graft following treatment of a traumatic thoracic aortic rupture. *J Endovasc Ther.* 2005;12: 503–507.

3. Steinbauer MG, Stehr A, Pfister K, Herold T, Zorger N, Topel I. Endovascular repair of proximal endograft collapse after treatment for thoracic aortic disease. *J Vasc Surg.* 2006;43:609–612.

4. Fujikawa T, Yukioka T, Ishimaru S, et al. Endovascular stent grafting for the treatment of blunt thoracic aortic injury. *J Trauma.* 2001;50:223–229.

5. Lachat M, Pfammatter T, Witzke H, et al. Acute traumatic aortic rupture: early stent graft repair. *Eur J Cardiothorac Surg.* 2003;21:959–963.

6. Lawlor DK, Ott M, Forbes TL, Kribs S, Harris KA, De Rose G. Endovascular management of traumatic thoracic injuries. *Can J Surg.* 2005;48(4):293–297.

7. Thompson CS, Rodriguez JA, Ramaiah VG, et al. Acute traumatic rupture of the thoracic aorta treated with endoluminal stent grafts. *J Trauma.* 2002;52:1173–1177.

Chapter 40
Thoracic Aortic Endografting for Traumatic Transection

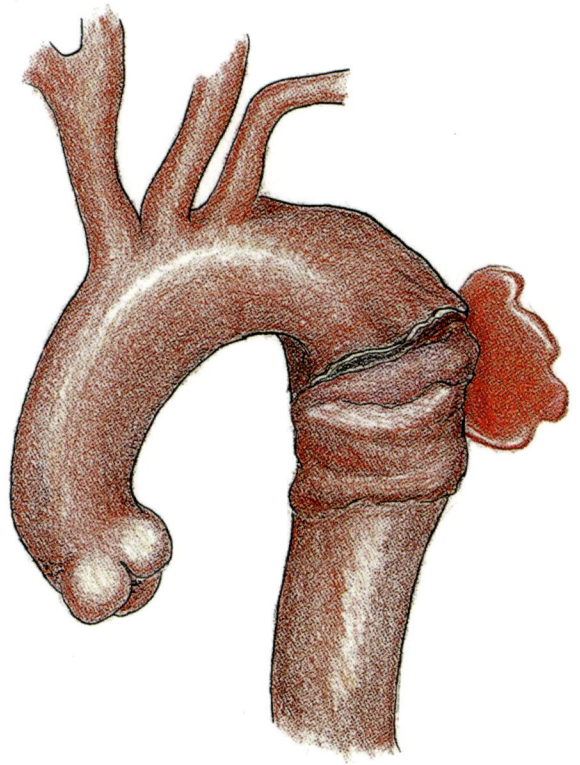

Most traumatic transections occur at the isthmus of the thoracic aorta. The thoracic aorta in the trauma patient is often normal and has a smaller aortic radius of aortic curvature in contrast to older patients with aortic aneurysms or various aortic pathologies that have wider aortic curvature. Aortic disruption often occurs close to the aortic isthmus requiring coverage of the subclavian artery to achieve a satisfactory proximal neck for fixation. A short endograft should be chosen to

J. Kpodonu, *Manual of Thoracic Endoaortic Surgery*,
DOI 10.1007/978-1-84996-296-4_40, © Springer-Verlag London Limited 2010

cover the area of injury and also to cover as few intercostals decreasing the risk of paraplegia. Endovascular technique used to treat thoracic aortic transection should take that into account. Consideration must also be given to small iliac vessels for access which may require retroperitoneal exposure to deliver the endoluminal grafts. Endovascular repair of young patients with traumatic aortic disruption poses a surgical challenge because of lack of commercially available thoracic endografts to treat the small thoracic aorta requiring sometimes customization with off-the-shelf abdominal endoluminal components to treat the small thoracic aorta. Complications of bird beaking with proximal collapse of the endograft are more common in traumatic patients due to oversizing which results from using commercially available endografts in small thoracic aorta.

40.1 Endovascular Techniques

Open exposure of the right common femoral artery is performed with the introduction an 18 G Cook needle and 0.035 in. soft tip angled glide wire into the arch aorta. A 9 Fr groin sheath is placed and heparin given although in traumatic transections patient may be coagulopathic and may require a substantially lower dose of heparin. Monitoring of the activated clotting time may be useful to determine a given dose. Percutaneous access of the left common femoral artery is similarly performed and a 6 Fr sheath introduced. An angiographic catheter is advanced meticulously into the arch aorta over a 0.035 in. guidewire through the left femoral sheath and an oblique thoracic arch aortogram is performed (Fig. 40.1) to delineate the arch, the descending thoracic aorta and aneurysm.[3] Intravascular ultrasound (Fig. 40.2) is performed when appropriate through the right groin sheath. The area of transection identified on angiogram can be confirmed with intravascular ultrasound by noting the intimal disruption (Fig. 40.2). Sizing of the thoracic aorta can also be achieved accurately with intravascular ultrasound if a good-quality CT scan of the chest is not available. Once the exact diameter and length of the endograft are chosen a 260 cm Lunderquist double-curve wire (Cook Inc., Bloomington, IN) is advanced into the arch aorta using an exchange catheter. The 9 Fr groin sheath should now be exchanged for the device delivery sheath and under a road map angiogram the device is deployed at the area of transection. Selective balloon angioplasty would depend on the device used and to the discretion of the physician. Intravascular ultrasound (Fig. 40.3) is performed to demonstrate correct placement of stent graft with adequate stent apposition to the thoracic aorta. A completion angiogram (Fig. 40.4) is performed to confirm adequate deployment of the graft and lack of endoleak. All wires and sheaths should be removed and the right common femoral artery repaired in a transverse fashion with restoration of flow. A closure device (Fig. 40.5) can be deployed to restore hemostasis after removal of sheath in the left groin. Postoperative CT imaging (Fig. 40.6) is performed for graft surveillance at 1 month, 6 months, and yearly provided post-procedure scan shows no endoleak or stent malposition.

Fig. 40.1 Angiogram of a
patient with a traumatic
transection

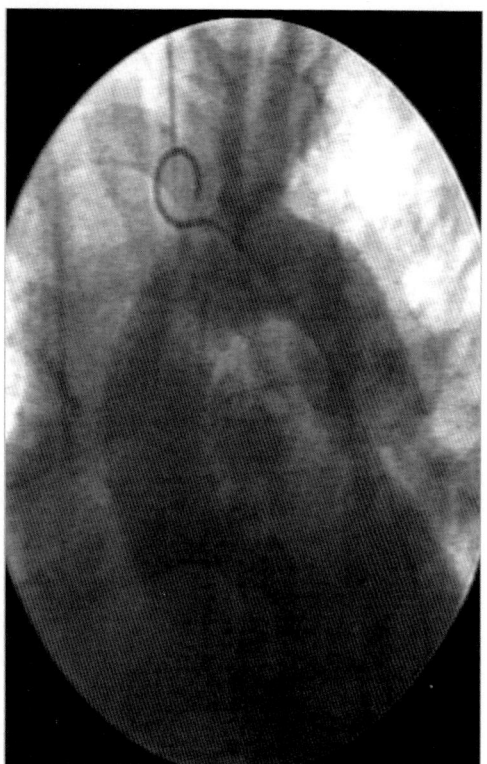

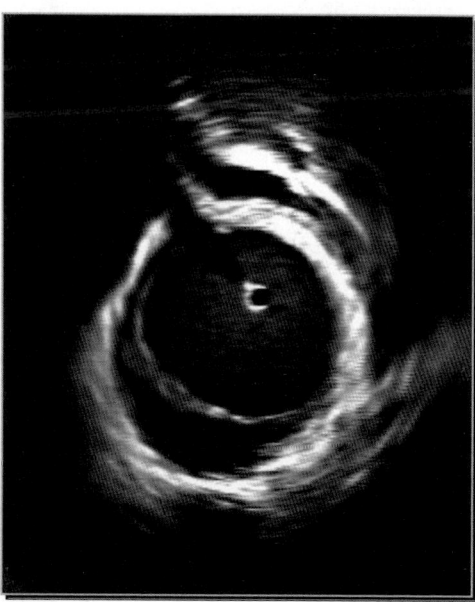

Fig. 40.2 Intravascular
ultrasound image of a patient
with traumatic transection of
the thoracic aorta with intimal
disruption

Fig. 40.3 Intravascular ultrasound post-repair of a traumatic transection with full apposition of stent graft to the thoracic aortic wall

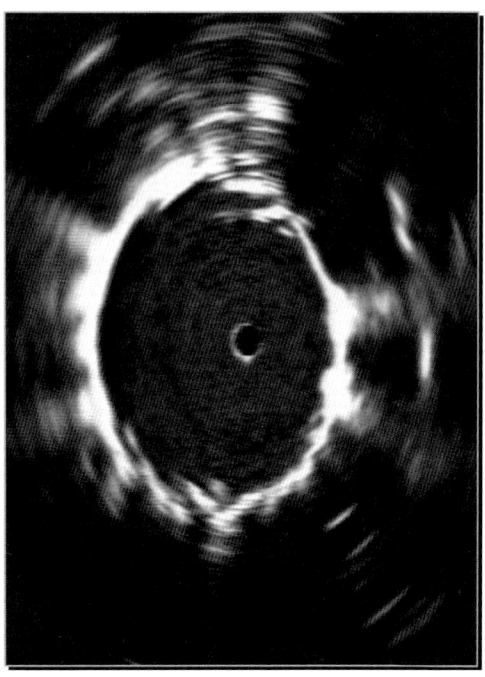

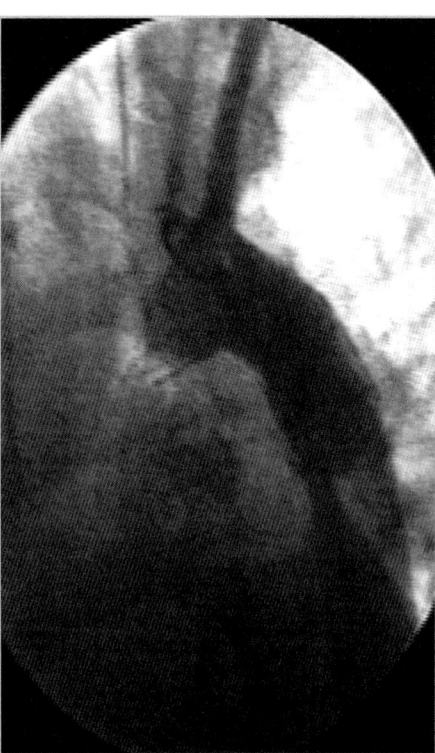

Fig. 40.4 Angiogram of a patient post-repair of traumatic transection with a stent graft

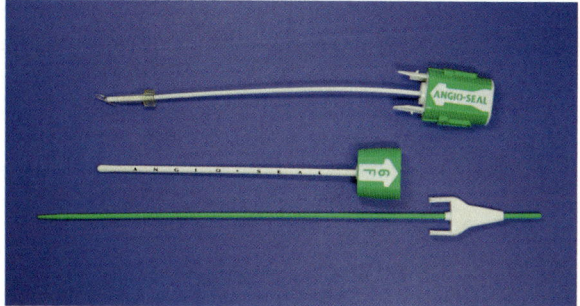

Fig. 40.5 Angioseal closure device used to achieve groin hemostasis

Fig. 40.6 CT scan image post-repair of a transection of the thoracic aorta

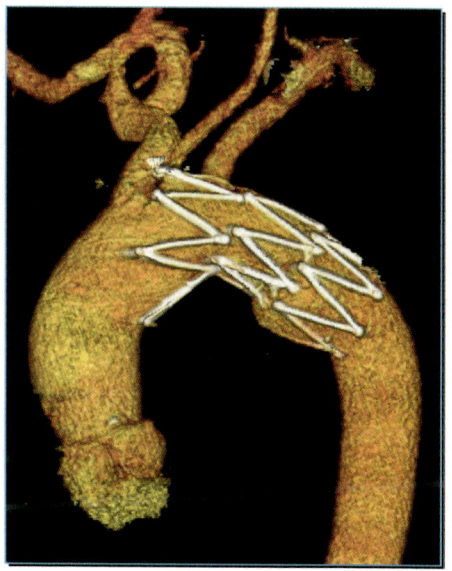

40.2 Discussion

No case of paraplegia has been reported to date with endovascular management of traumatic aortic transection. Rousseau et al.[1] reported a mortality and paraplegia rate of 21 and 7% for 35 patients who had open surgical repair for the management of blunt thoracic injury and a 0% mortality and paraplegia rate for 29 patients managed using endografts at a mean follow-up of 46 months (range 13–90 months).[2] Younger patients have a tapering luminal aortic diameter as well as a higher aortic pulsatile compliance than elderly patients. The smallest available commercially available endoluminal graft 22 mm in a thoracic aorta less than 19 mm may result in gross oversizing which may result in suboptimal conformability along the inner curve of the aortic arch which can lead to device fracture, endoleaks, migration, and device collapse which have been estimated to be about 3% in the traumatic aortic disruptions.

Endoluminal graft for the management of disruption of the thoracic provides a minimal invasive way to treat such lethal injuries with acceptable morbidity and mortality. Device refinements such as a more flexible shaft to accommodate the aortic curvature may be needed in young patients who have a sharp aortic angulation juxta distal to the subclavian artery reducing the need for coverage of left subclavian artery. Sometimes abdominal endoluminal grafts cuffs or iliac limbs may need to be custom assembled as thoracic endoluminal grafts to accommodate the small aortic diameter.

References

1. Rousseau H, Dambrin C, Marcheix B, et al. Acute traumatic aortic rupture: a comparison of surgical or stent graft repair. *J Thorac Surg*. 2005;129:1050–1055.
2. Verhoye JP, Bertrand DL, Kakon C, Heautot JF. Classification and design algorithm of post traumatic chronic lesions of the isthmus and the descending thoracic aorta. In: Rousseau H, Verhoye JP, Heautot JF, eds. *Thoracic Aortic Diseases*. Berlin: Springer; 2006:345–349.
3. Diethrich EB, Ramaiah VG, Kpodonu J, Rodriguez-Lopez JA. *Figures Courtesy of Endovascular and Hybrid Management of the Thoracic Aorta. A Case Based Approach*. 1st ed. West Sussex: Wiley-Blackwell; 2008.

Chapter 41
Hybrid Management of the Thoracic Aorta: Extending Proximal Landing Zones

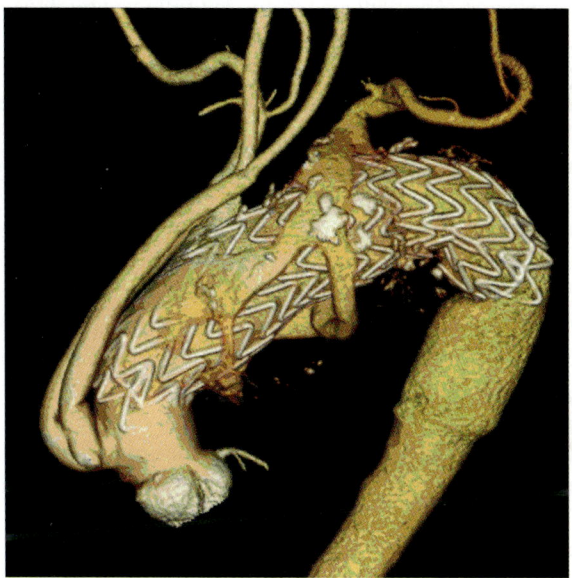

Adequate proximal fixation depends on a length of seal zone (minimum 1.5–2 cm) proximal to the adjacent aortic pathology, radius inner curve, aortic diameter, and graft oversizing (10–20%). Proximal extension of the landing zone to achieve good fixation occasionally requires that the supra-aortic vessels be debranched prior to deployment of a thoracic endoluminal graft. Various extra-thoracic and intra-thoracic debranching procedures combined with an endovascular stent graft are possible to extend the proximal zone without requiring cardiopulmonary bypass and circulatory arrest.

J. Kpodonu, *Manual of Thoracic Endoaortic Surgery*,
DOI 10.1007/978-1-84996-296-4_41, © Springer-Verlag London Limited 2010

41.1 Transposition of Left Subclavian to Left Carotid Artery Bypass/Left Subclavian to Left Carotid Artery Bypass Graft with Deployment of Endoluminal Graft[1,2]

The left carotid to left subclavian bypass or transposition of the left subclavian artery to the left carotid artery is indicated for patients with a dominant left vertebral artery system, patients with patent internal mammary bypass grafts and in those who experience left upper extremity ischemic symptoms following thoracic endografting with coverage of the left subclavian artery (Fig. 41.1a). Transposition of the left subclavian artery to left carotid bypass operation with thoracic endografting can be applied to patients with aneurysms or pseudoaneurysms close to or involving the ostium of the left subclavian artery requiring proximal extension of landing zone for deployment of an endoluminal graft. The procedure is performed by making a left-sided supra-clavicular incision. The platysma is divided followed by division of the clavicular head of the sternocleidomastoid medially to reveal the carotid sheath. The carotid sheath is identified and incised to expose the common carotid artery and the vagus nerve, which are protected. Next the omohyoid muscle is divided and the scalene fat pad identified and mobilized from lateral to medial to identify the phrenic nerve overlying the scalenus anterior muscle. The phrenic nerve is preserved and the scalenus anterior muscle divided to expose the left subclavian artery. The left subclavian artery is mobilized as far proximally to the ostium making sure to preserve the left vertebral artery and the internal mammary artery. Administration of 5000 units of heparin is performed followed by division of the left subclavian artery between clamps and oversews the proximal left subclavian artery. The distal end of the left subclavian artery is sewn directly to the left carotid artery in an end-to-side fashion (Fig. 41.1b) followed by deployment of an endoluminal graft (Fig. 41.1c). A 10 mm Gore-Tex graft (W.L. Gore & Associates, Flagstaff, AZ) can be sewn directly to the left subclavian artery to achieve a desired length in an end-to-end fashion after administering 5000 units of heparin and then sewn in an end-to-side fashion to the left carotid artery (Fig. 41.1d). A bypass graft can also be sewn to the left subclavian artery without transposition. The graft is tunneled beneath the internal jugular vein and after controlling the left common carotid an arteriotomy is made in the carotid artery and the graft sewn in an end-to-side fashion with 5-0 prolene. De-airing maneuvers are performed prior to unclamping the artery to restore flow. The neck incisions are closed. Exclusion of the thoracic aortic pathology can then be performed in the usual manner with an endoluminal graft (Fig. 41.1e).

41.2 Carotid to Carotid Bypass with Deployment of Endoluminal Graft[1,2]

This procedure is performed in patients with arch aneurysms distal to the innominate artery (Fig. 41.2a). In this procedure a carotid–carotid bypass is performed with deployment of a thoracic endograft. In performing a left carotid–right carotid bypass

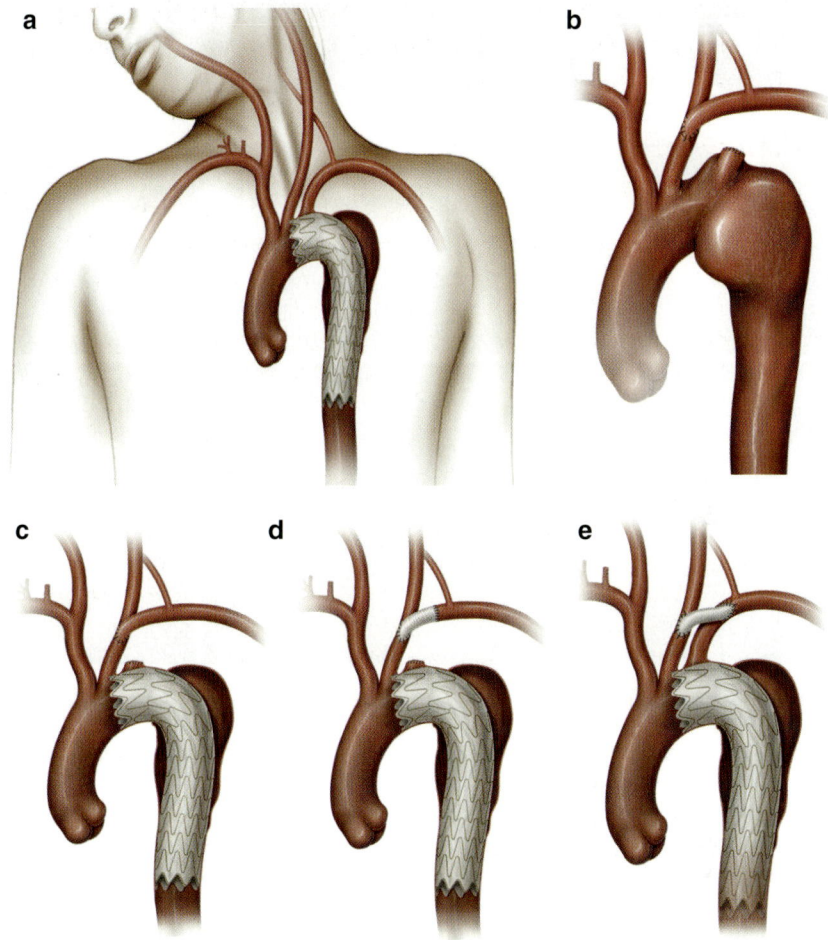

Fig. 41.1 (**a**) Endoluminal graft placement with coverage of the left subclavian artery. (**b**) Carotid subclavian artery transposition with deployment of a thoracic aortic stent graft (**c**). (**d**) Carotid subclavian transposition and carotid subclavian bypass (**e**) with deployment of thoracic endograft

hybrid operation, bilateral low-neck incisions are made parallel to the sternocleido-mastoid muscle (Fig. 41.2b, c). Adequate mobilization of the common carotid artery is achieved so that a low-lying bypass graft could be tunneled beneath the sternal notch for cosmetic reasons. An 8 mm Dacron Hemashield graft (Boston Scientific Corporation, Natick, MA) is tunneled beneath the sternal notch and 5000 units of heparin given to the patient followed by proximal and distal cross-clamps to the right common carotid artery and construction of end-to-side anastomosis using a 5-0 polypropylene suture. Cross-clamps are removed, the graft is unclamped, and flow re-established to the right common carotid artery. The left common carotid artery is similarly mobilized up to its origin, proximal and distal cross-clamps

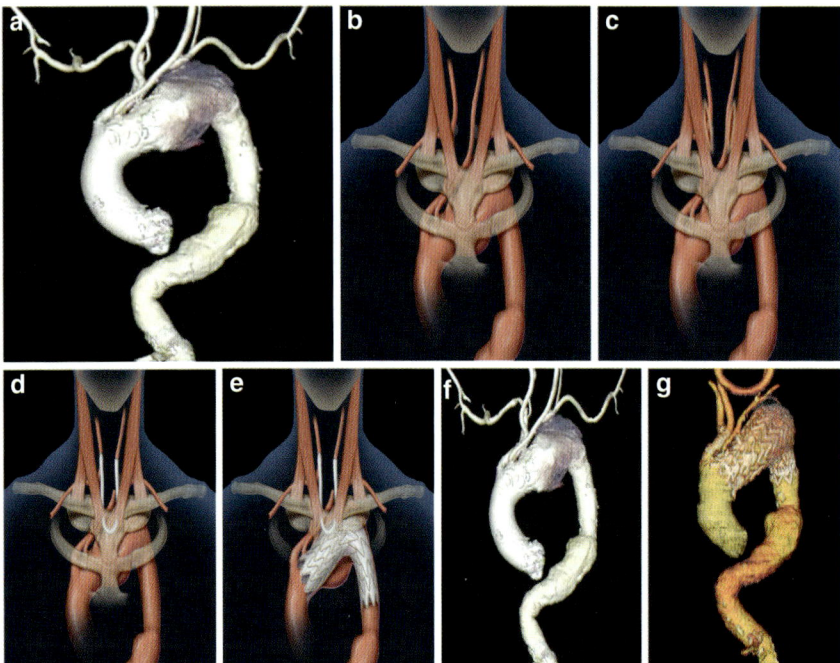

Fig. 41.2 (**a**) A 3D reconstruction of a 64-silce CT scan depicts the location of the arch aneurysm in relation to the arch vessels. (**b–e**) Illustration of a carotid–carotid bypass construction with deployment of a thoracic endograft. A 3D reconstruction of the chest showing an anterior view of the pre- (**a**) and post-repair procedure (**f**)

are applied, the artery is then transected close to the proximal clamp, and the distal end of the left common carotid artery is anastomosed to a 8 mm Dacron Hemashield (Boston Scientific Corporation, Natick, MA) graft as an end-to-end anastomosis. The proximal left common carotid artery is oversewn with a 4-0 transfixing suture. The cross-clamps are removed and flow subsequently established to the left common carotid artery through the newly created carotid–carotid bypass (Fig. 41.2d).

Once the bypass is performed the endoluminal graft is then deployed in the standard fashion as described (Fig. 41.2e). Post-operative CT scan is performed prior to discharge (Fig. 41.2f) to confirm exclusion of distal aneurysm and absence of endoleak. We have used this technique to treat distal arch pathologies in elderly and high-risk patients not suitable for extracorporeal circulation and hypothermic circulatory arrest.

Thoracic debranching with deployment of an endoluminal graft which requires a thoracotomy can also be performed to treat distal arch aortic pathologies including atherosclerotic arch aneurysms and traumatic pseudoaneurysms. This technique requires performing a right minithoracotomy in the third intercostal space, the advantage being the avoidance of cardiopulmonary bypass and circulatory arrest.

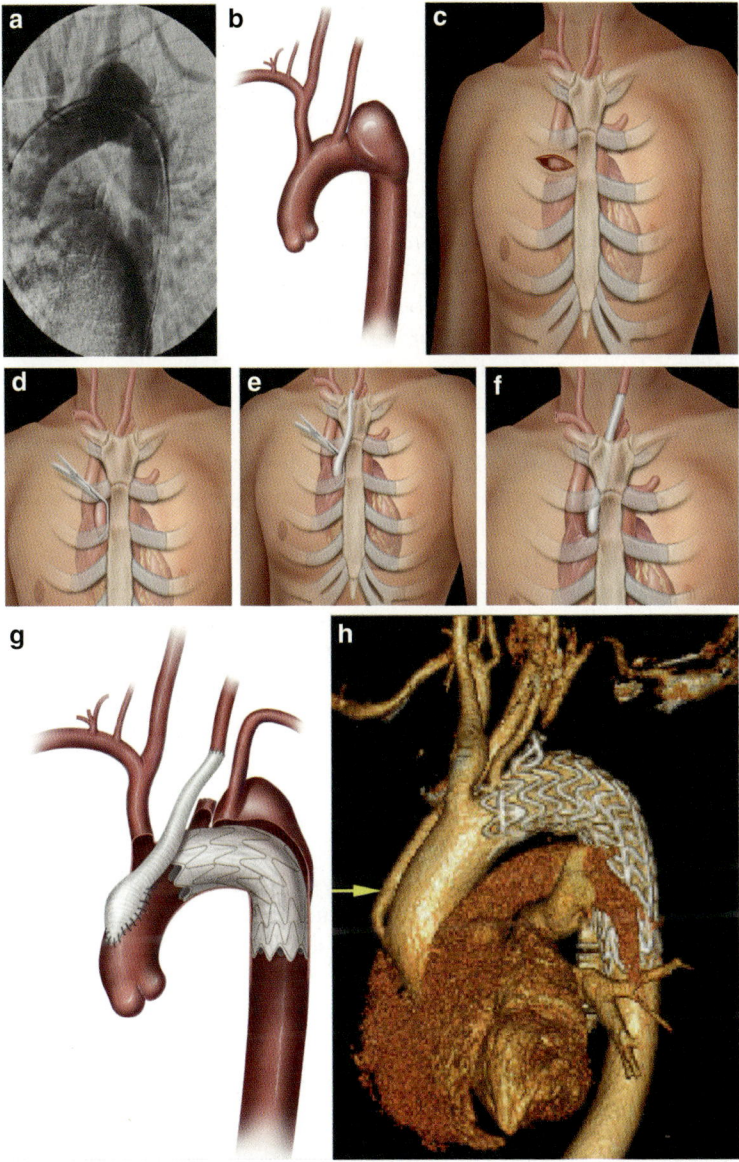

Fig. 41.3 (**a**) Angiogram and an Illustration demonstrate an arch aneurysm distal to left carotid artery (**b**). (**c**) Access is through an anterior minithoracotomy incision. (**d**) A partial cross-clamp is applied to the ascending aorta, and the aorta-to-left carotid bypass constructed with a 10 mm conduit (**e**). (**f**) Illustration demonstrates aorta-to left common carotid bypass with deployment of an endoluminal graft to exclude the arch aneurysm. (**g**) An artist's rendition of the complete procedure and a 2-year follow-up CT scan reconstruction. (**h**) A patent bypass graft (*yellow arrow*) with satisfactory exclusion of the pseudoaneurysm

41.3 Aorto to Left Carotid Bypass with Deployment of an Endoluminal Graft[1,2]

This technique can be used for distal arch aneurysm (Fig. 41.3a, b) that requires coverage of the left carotid artery ostium to achieve adequate proximal fixation with an endoluminal graft.

Using this hybrid technique requires a right anterior transverse thoracotomy incision be made over the right third intercostal space to expose the ascending aorta (Fig. 41.3c). Similarly a left neck incision is made, division of the platysma achieved, and the sternocleidomastoid muscle retracted laterally to expose the carotid sheath. The left common carotid artery is identified; we then administer 5000 units of heparin and subsequently apply a side biting clamp on the aorta (Fig. 41.3d) and anastomose the proximal end of an 8 mm Hemashield (Boston Scientific Corporation, Natick, MA) graft to the aorta (Fig. 41.3e); the clamp is released and the graft flushed. The graft is then clamped and tunneled up to the left neck (Fig. 41.3e); we then clamp the left common carotid artery proximally and distally; an arteriotomy is performed; and an end-to-side anastomosis is effected in standard fashion using running 5-0 prolene suture (Fig. 41.3f); pulses in the graft and distal left carotid artery are verified. The neck and the anterior thoracotomy incision are then closed. Deployment of an endoluminal graft as previously described is then performed under fluoroscopic guidance (Fig. 41.3g). Post-operative CT scan is performed to demonstrate exclusion of aneurysm by endoluminal graft and absence of endoleak (Fig. 41.3h).

41.4 Thoracic Debranching Hybrid Procedure[1,2]

This hybrid procedure is useful for arch aneurysms (Fig. 41.4a) in high-risk patients that cannot tolerate cardiopulmonary bypass and hypothermic circulatory arrest.

The procedure is performed using a classic median or partial median sternotomy (Fig. 41.4b). It is important to have sufficient cephalad exposure for adequate dissection of the brachiocephalic, left common carotid and left subclavian arteries for

---

Fig. 41.4 (a) CT scan in a patient with an arch aneurysm. (b) Illustration of a median sternotomy incision for replacement of ascending aorta. (c) Illustration of 16 mm × 8 mm woven Dacron graft with a 10 mm side limb sutured for antegrade deployment of endoluminal graft (d). (e) Illustration of the bifurcated conduit graft anastomosed to the ascending aorta; (f) the common carotid and innominate arteries are transected and anastomosed in end to end to the limbs of the bifurcated graft. (g) Advancement of a guidewire through the 10 mm conduit with (h) snaring of the conduit wire through the femoral sheath with a snare (Microvena). (i) A thoracic endograft sheath used for deployment of graft through the antegrade-sewn 10 mm conduit. (j) Advancement of a thoracic sheath followed by a (k) thoracic stent graft through the antegrade conduit with (l) deployment of endograft to exclude aneurysm. (m) Post-operative 64-slice CT scan examination demonstrating the rerouting of the supra-aortic trunks and exclusion of arch aneurysm

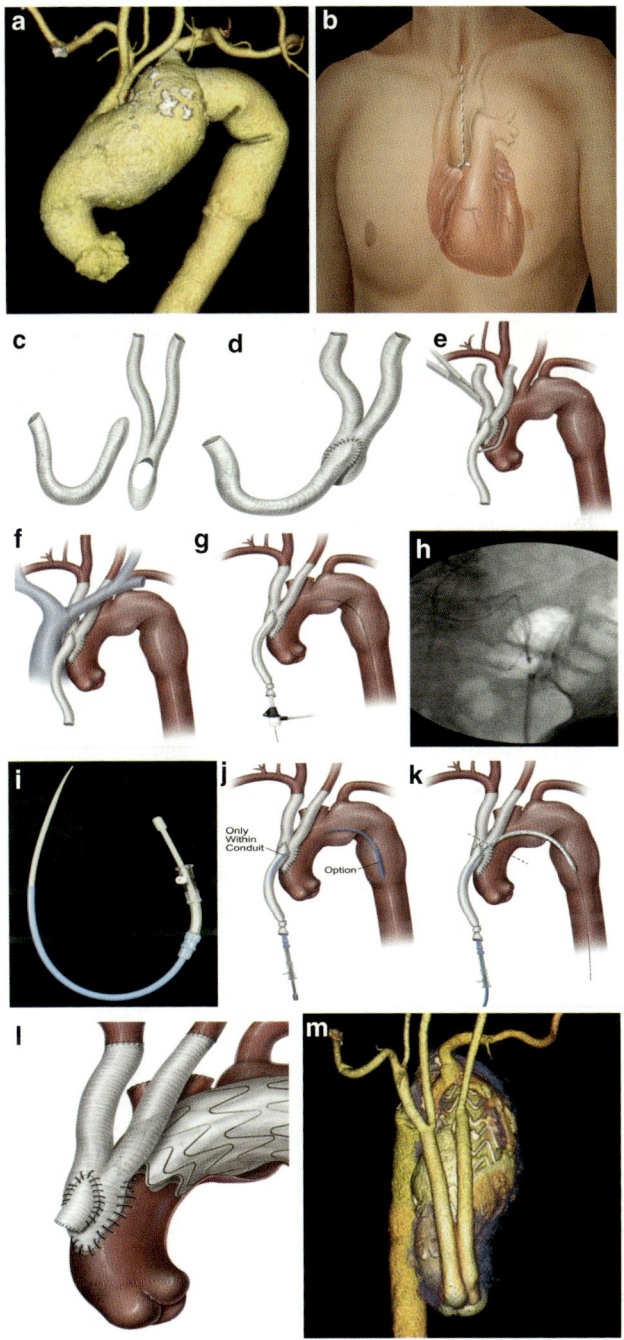

Fig. 41.4 (continued)

debranching. The supra-aortic vessels are exposed above and below the innominate vein. It is important to mobilize the innominate vein from the confluence of the left internal jugular vein and the left subclavian vein to the superior vena cava for adequate exposure for vascular anastomosis and tunneling of the graft limbs. The graft should be tunneled beneath the innominate vein in order to avoid postoperative compression of the vein. This occurred early in our series in one patient who subsequently required thrombolysis. The most common debranching procedure includes only the two proximal arteries; however, the left subclavian artery could also be reached through the exposure unless it has a more distal origin that would make the anastomosis difficult. From the practical standpoint most patients are able to tolerate coverage of the left subclavian artery at the time of endografting without any sequelae. Patients who have or will need a patent left internal mammary artery for coronary revascularization or incomplete right vertebral communication to the basilar system, where occlusion of the left vertebral would compromise posterior circulation, require a left subclavian artery revascularization. This procedure can be performed after endografting if the patient exhibits symptoms of left-hand ischemia. Once preparation of the arch vessels is completed the patient is given 5000 units of heparin sulfate. Depending on the size of the arch vessels and the diameter of the ascending aorta, a bifurcated graft most commonly 14 × 7 mm or 16 × 8 mm is prepared with a 10 mm conduit anastomosed to the main body (Fig. 41.4c, d). The combined graft is anastomosed to the ascending aorta over a partial occlusion clamp (Fig. 41.4e). The systemic pressure is controlled to permit application of the clamp during the anastomosis. The left common carotid artery is clamped proximally and distally, transected, and the stump oversewn. The distal anastomosis is completed and flow is restored. The procedure is repeated for debranching of the brachiocephalic artery (Fig. 41.4f). The debranching procedure is completed by placing a marker on the bifurcated graft to identify the intended location for the proximal end of the endovascular stent graft. This can also be accomplished using clips, a circumferential wire, or more preferably the radiopaque marker from a surgical sponge. Attention is then turned to the antegrade delivery of the endoluminal graft. A 9 Fr sheath is attached to the 10 mm limb conduit (Fig. 41.4g). A similar sheath is inserted into either the right or the left common femoral arteries. A 0.035 in. angled glide wire is passed through the proximal sheath to the external iliac artery where it is captured and brought out through the femoral sheath by a snare wire (Microvena, White Bear Lake, MN) (Fig. 41.4h). This technique establishes a conduit to the femoral wire for antegrade endoluminal graft delivery; by pulling on each end of the wire, the passage of the endoluminal graft is enhanced and there is better control for exact landing of the graft. This is particularly useful when tortuosity of the vessels exits or in situations where the aortic arch has complex configurations. The conduit's 9 Fr sheath is substituted for a Gore 24 Fr delivery sheath (Fig. 41.4i). The sheath is passed through the conduit, with the option of either crossing the arch with the sheath or limiting the position to the distal end of the conduit (Fig. 41.4j); the latter is more common, particularly since the conduit–femoral wire makes delivery of the Gore TAG device easier in most cases. The endoluminal graft is positioned at the proximal marker and deployed (Fig. 41.4k). In addition to using the exteriorized wire, we routinely access the contralateral common femoral artery for placement of an angiographic catheter in the arch. We find this useful not only for graft deployment but also for completion arteriography and determination of the need for post-deployment balloon angioplasty. We do not routinely post-dilate unless an endoleak is observed or the graft does not appear to be adequately opposed to the thoracic aorta. The procedure is concluded by wire and sheaths removal and transition and closure of the conduit (Fig. 41.4l). Post-operative CT scan (Fig. 41.4m) is performed to demonstrate satisfactory exclusion of aneurysm with absence of endoleak.

An illustration of the bifurcated graft and the conduit sutured to the tube graft used to reconstruct the ascending aorta with transposition of arch vessels and antegrade advancement of endoluminal graft for deployment.

The sheath is withdrawn, and the endoluminal graft is delivered across the aortic arch and into the high descending thoracic aorta with retrograde placement of a second endoluminal graft from the left common femoral artery over the conduit-to-femoral wire.

41.5 Discussion

Thoracic aneurysms with a diameter >5 cm are associated with a 2-year patient survival of less than 30%.[3] Most patients, if untreated, die from aneurysm rupture. The significant morbidity and mortality associated with open surgical repair of thoracic aneurysms has resulted in an increasing use of a less invasive and safer treatment using endovascular therapy. Endovascular treatment of thoracic arch aneurysms is associated with fewer procedural-related complications, a shorter convalescence, and minimal neurological sequelae.[4]

Open graft replacement of arch aneurysms requires cardiopulmonary bypass, various degrees of hypothermia, and circulatory arrest, which increases the morbidity of the procedure. The use of a hybrid approach to treat aortic arch aneurysms can be satisfactorily performed with a lower morbidity and mortality than the traditional open surgical approach. This method gives high-risk patients another option for treatment should they be declined for open surgery due to significant co-morbidities or they want a less invasive approach. Variations of reconstruction of common carotid and subclavian arteries can be performed to provide adequate landing zones for the treatment of TAA.[5] These variations in technique allow for a customized approach in terms of rerouting the arch vessels to achieve only the necessary length of healthy, normal aorta needed to seat an endoluminal graft properly.

References

1. Kpodonu J, Diethrich EB. Hybrid interventions for the treatment of the complex aortic arch. *Perspect Vasc Surg Endovasc Ther.* 2007;19(2):174–184.

2. Diethrich EB, Ramaiah VG, Kpodonu J, Rodriguez JA. *Endovascular and Hybrid Management of the Thoracic Aorta. A Case Based Approach.* 1st ed. West Sussex: Wiley-Blackwell; 2008.
3. Crawford ES, Denatale RW. Thoracoabdominal aortic aneurysm: Observations regarding the natural course of the disease. *J Vasc Surg.* 1986;3:578–582.
4. Makaroun MS, Dillavou ED, Kee ST, et al. Endovascular treatment of thoracic aortic aneurysms: results of phase II multicenter trial of the Gore TAG thoracic endoprosthesis. *J Vasc Surg.* 2005;41:1–9.
5. Criado FJ, Clark NS, Arnatan MF. Stent graft repair in the aortic arch and descending thoracic aorta: 4 year experience. *J Vasc Surg.* 2002; 36:1121–128.

Chapter 42
Complications of Thoracic Aortic Endografting

42.1 Endoleaks

Endoleaks are defined as blood flow outside the lumen of the stent graft but within the aneurysm sac. The endoleak rate after endovascular thoracic aortic aneurysm repair ranges from 5 to 25%. Eighty percent of endoleaks are classified as type I and III endoleaks. Type II endoleaks are less frequent. Risk factors for developing thoracic aortic endoleaks include an aortic implantation zone of less than 2 cm from the left subclavian artery (LSA) and existence of an entry tear at the lesser curvature of the arch aorta. Type III endoleaks occur when there is structural failure with the

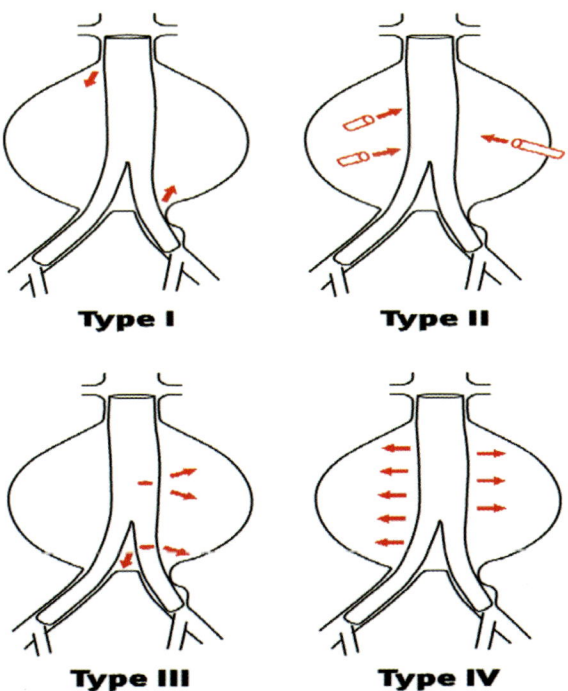

J. Kpodonu, *Manual of Thoracic Endoaortic Surgery,*
DOI 10.1007/978-1-84996-296-4_42, © Springer-Verlag London Limited 2010

stent graft including holes in stent graft fabric, stent graft fractures, and junctional separations that occur with modular devices. Type IV endoleaks are detected at time of implantation when patients are fully anticoagulated and are caused by stent graft porosity and usually resolve by reversal of anticoagulation. Type V endoleak refers to expansion of an aneurysm sac without the presence of an identifiable endoleak. Cause may include an undiagnosed endoleak, ultrafiltration, or thrombus which provides an ineffective barrier to pressure transmission.

42.2 Post-operative Image Surveillance for Endoleaks

Goal of post-operative image surveillance is to evaluate for aneurysm expansion or shrinkage, detect stent graft migration or fracture, and detect endoleaks. Thin section triple-phase CTA images obtained before, during, and after contrast administration is a highly accurate study. The time resolved nature of the triple-phase imaging gives important information as to when contrast enters or exits the aorta. Finding of a collection of contrast outside the stent graft lumen and inside the aneurysm sac defines an endoleak. Other useful imaging studies include IVUS and MRA which can both be used in patients with renal failure or iodine contrast allergy.

42.3 Type 1 Endoleak

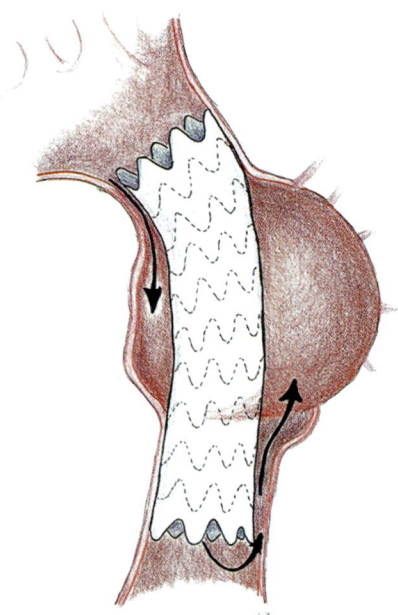

Type 1 endoleaks have flow that originates from either the proximal or the distal stent graft attachment site. Separation between the stent graft and the native arterial wall creates a direct communication with the systemic arterial circulation. Development of a type I endoleak after thoracic aortic aneurysm repair is associated with aneurysmal sac expansion and a potential rupture of the sac. Endoleaks are detected commonly intra-operatively using angiography (Fig. 42.1) or electively using CT angiography (Fig. 42.2).

Fig. 42.1 Digital subtraction angiography demonstrates a type 1 endoleak

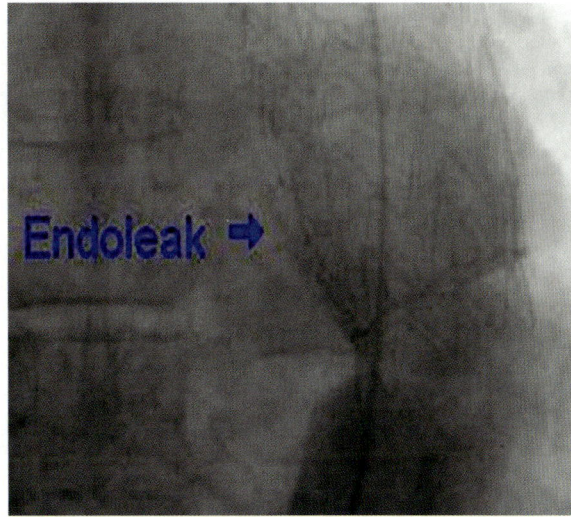

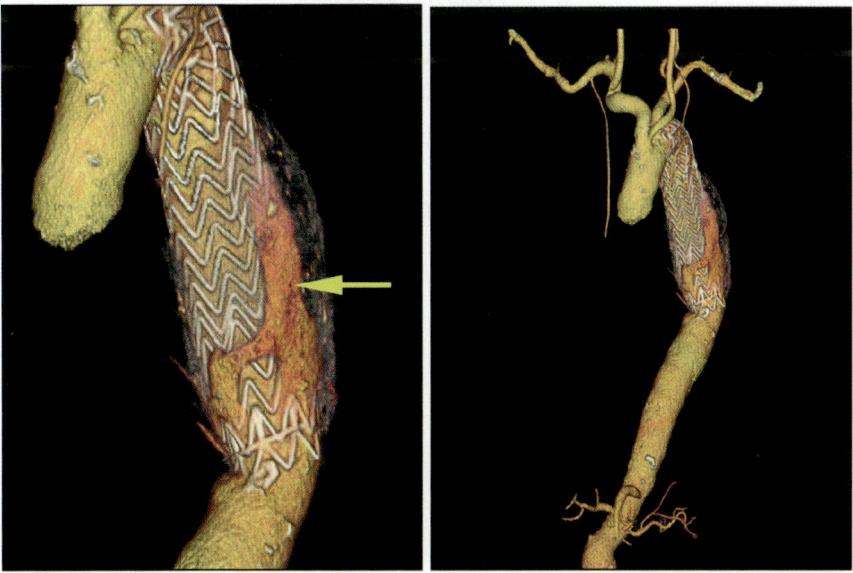

Fig. 42.2 Sixty-four slice CT scan demonstrates a distal type 1 endoleak post-stent graft

42.3.1 Management of a Type I Endoleak

42.3.1.1 Balloon Angioplasty

Balloon angioplasty is the first line of treatment of a type I endoleak. The use of a noncompliant balloon to balloon angioplasty the end of the endoluminal graft ensures appropriate apposition of the graft to the aortic wall (Fig. 42.3).

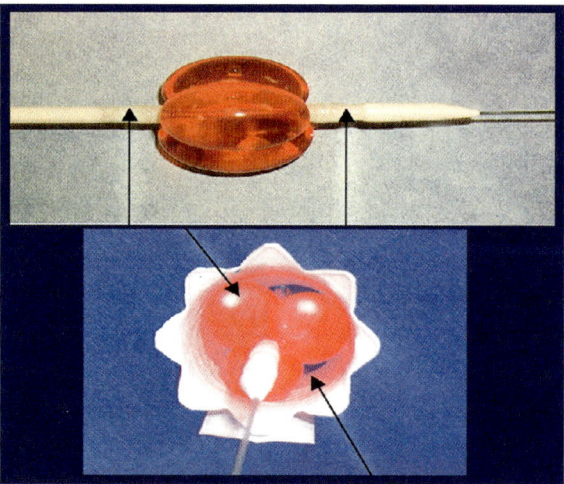

Fig. 42.3 W.L. Gore tri-lobed balloon used for balloon angioplasty of endograft for management of type 1 endoleak

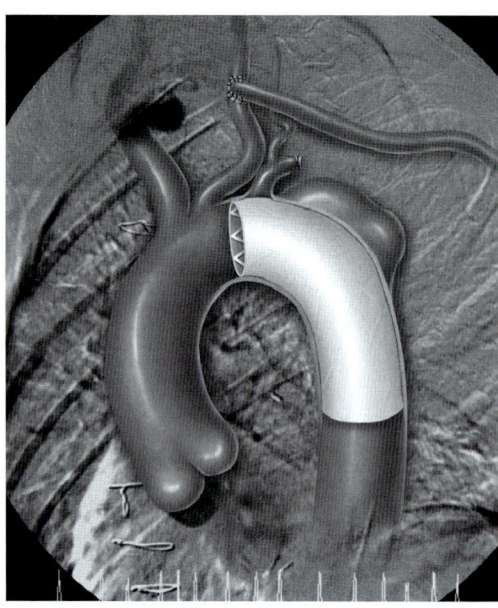

Fig. 42.4 Transposition of left subclavian artery with extension of the proximal landing zone >2.0 cm to prevent a type I endoleak

42.3.1.2 Placement of a Proximal or Distal Cuff

Placement of an endoluminal graft cuff to extend the proximal or distal landing with or without balloon angioplasty. Presence of a short proximal landing zone may require a left carotid to left subclavian artery or a transposition of left subclavian artery to left carotid artery (Fig. 42.4) in addition to deployment of a proximal cuff to extend the proximal landing zone for appropriate seal and resolution of endoleak.

42.3.1.3 Coil Embolization

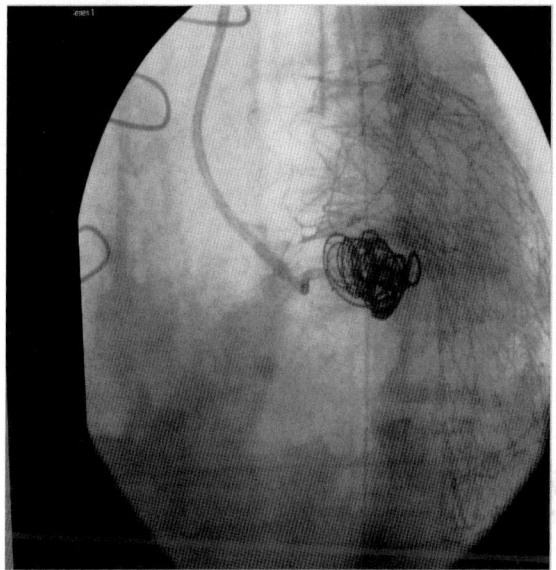

Fig. 42.5 Embolization coils can be used to thrombose flow feeding the aneurysm sac by assessing the aneurysm sac with the help of a guiding catheter

42.3.1.4 Open Conversion

Failure to resolve type I endoleak by an endovascular approach with an increase in aneurysm sac size is an indication for open conversion with removal of endoluminal graft and a repair using a tube graft (Fig. 42.6).

42.3.2 Management of a Distal Type 1 Endoleak

Management of a distal type I endoleak can also be managed by balloon angioplasty and extension of distal landing zone with a cuff. Presence of a short distal landing

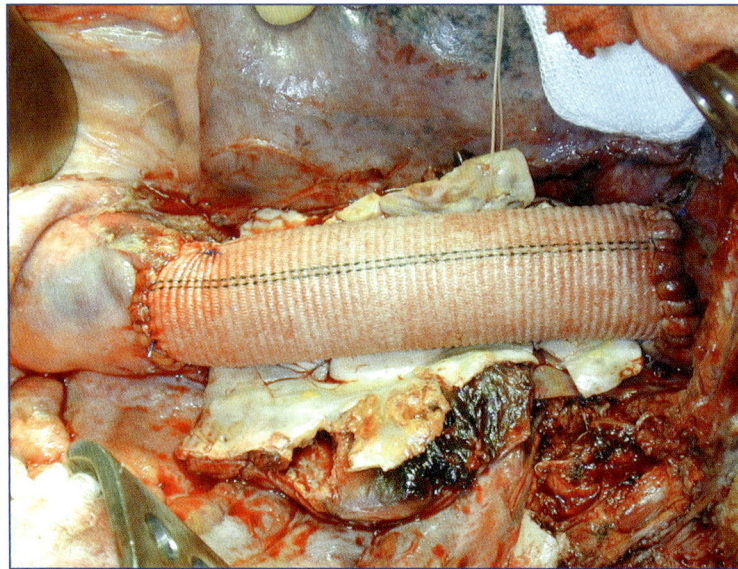

Fig. 42.6 Management of type 1 endoleak by open conversion with replacement of the descending thoracic aorta

zone (<2.0 cm) requires coverage of the celiac trunk or a celiac/superior mesenteric bypass to lengthen the distal landing zone.

42.3.3 Retrograde Type I Endoleak Associated with the Treatment of Type B Aortic Dissections

Retrograde type 1 endoleak post-endoluminal graft for type B dissections mostly represents some form of false lumen flow and the majority develops progressive thrombosis with time. Presence of a retrograde type I endoleak in the absence of any incremental increase in the false lumen sac size can be managed conservatively.

42.4 Type II Endoleaks

Type II endoleaks can result from retrograde flow from a covered artery (i.e., left subclavian artery) into the aneurysm sac or from bloodflow travelling through branches from the nonstented portion of the aorta, as well as through anastomotic connections into vessels with a direct communication with the aneurysm sac, usually from an intercostal or covered subclavian artery (Fig. 42.7). Most type II endoleaks will thrombose.

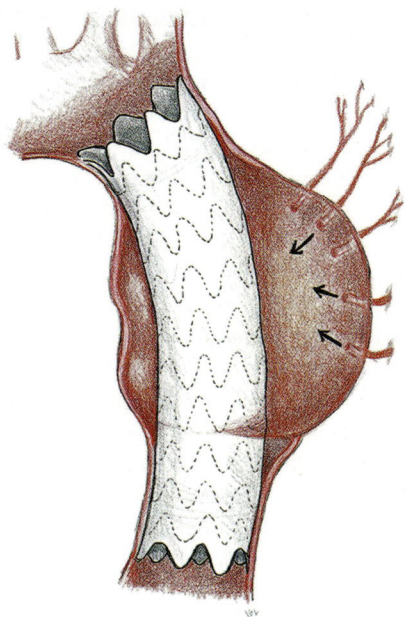

Small percentage of type II endoleaks transmit sufficient pressure to cause sac enlargement. Management includes 1. coil embolization of subclavian artery – by retrograde approach (Fig. 42.5); 2. coil embolization of aneurysm sac; 3. injection of thrombin in sac; and 4. thoracoscopic ligation of intercostal artery.

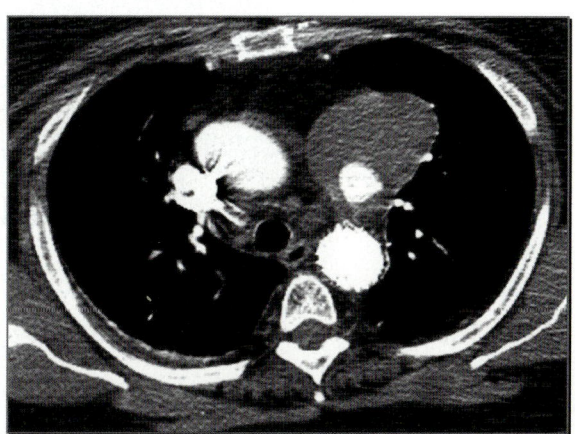

Fig. 42.7 CT scan demonstrates a type II endoleak

42.4.1 Management of Type II Endoleak by Coil Embolization

The technique of coil embolization to manage a type II endoleak involves placing bilateral radial arterial lines to confirm no gradient between both arms. The patient is subsequently placed under general anesthesia. A left percutaneous retrograde approach is used to cannulate the left brachial artery with a 35 cm 6 Fr sheath. Heparin is given to achieve an activated time greater than 200 s. A 5 Fr pigtail catheter is advanced over a 180 cm angled soft tip glide wire through the left brachial sheath and a selective left subclavian artery arch angiogram is performed to confirm the type II endoleak (Fig. 42.8). A Bereinstein catheter is exchanged for the 5 Fr angiographic pigtail catheter and a couple of 15 mm × 15 cm Cook (Bloomington, IN) embolization coils are deployed in the ostium of the left subclavian artery with care not to coil embolize the left vertebral artery in the process. Upon embolization, there should be noticeable drop in the left radial arterial line pressure with flattening of the pressure wave form. A completion angiogram performed post-embolization is performed to confirm satisfactory repair of the type II endoleak from the left subclavian artery origin (Fig. 42.9). A post-operative CT scan is performed to confirm satisfactory results (Fig. 42.10).

Fig. 42.8 Selective left subclavian artery angiogram demonstrates type II endoleak

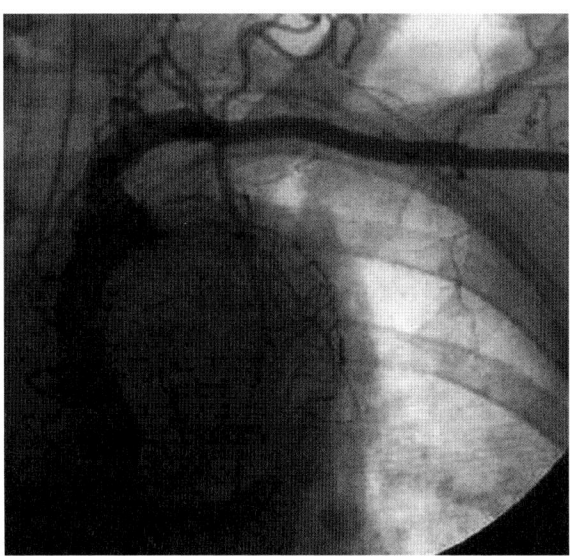

42.4.2 Management of a Type II Endoleak by Injection of Thrombin in Sac

Similarly an angiographic catheter is used to perform an angiogram to confirm the type II endoleak. A guiding catheter is used to go behind the thoracic endograft to

Fig. 42.9 Angiogram
post-coil embolization of left
subclavian artery with
resolution of type II endoleak

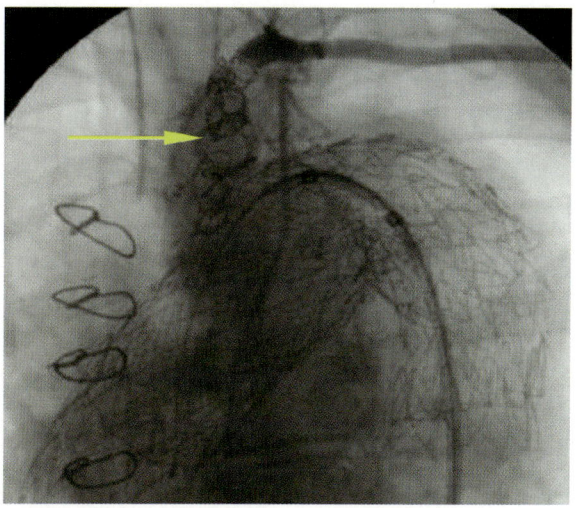

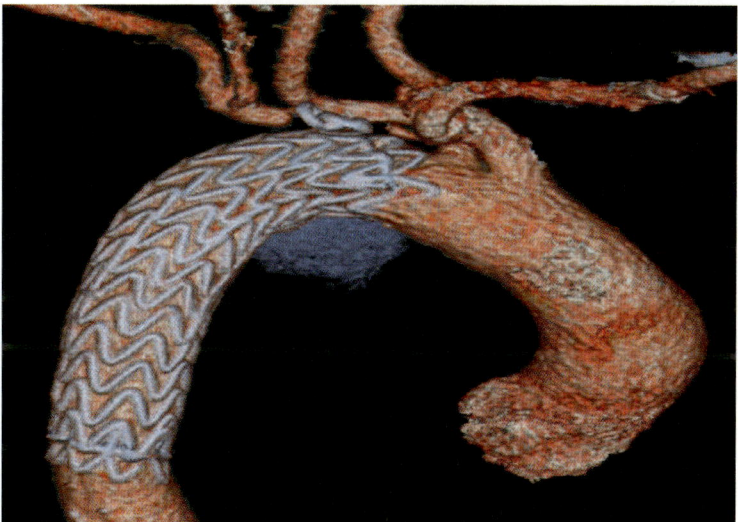

Fig. 42.10 Post-operative CT scan with coils demonstrated in left subclavian artery with resolution of type II endoleak

access the aneurysm sac. Thrombin can subsequently be injected into the sac. Dose of thrombin varies from 1 ml (500 IU to 3 ml 1500 IU).

42.4.3 *Thoracoscopic Ligation of Intercostal Artery*

Thoracoscopic ligation of the intercostal vessel feeding the aneurysm sac can be performed to interrupt flow to the aneurysm sac when endovascular approach fails.

42.5 Type III Endoleak

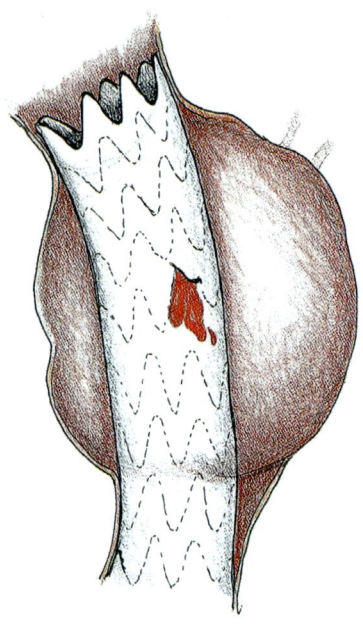

Type III endoleaks, whether from disconnecting parts or fabric damage, are associated with an increased risk of aneurysm rupture. Most type III endoleaks appear during medium-term follow-up and are thought to be caused by late endograft disintegration. Treatment consists of placement of extra piece of graft component (Fig. 42.11).

42.5.1 Stent-Related Maldeployment

Failure to land the endograft in the correct location usually requires placement of an additional device, either an additional endograft or a cuff. A supply of these should be available for use if required to prevent procedural failure. Maldeployment is avoided by avoiding hurrying during deployment. Perform check angiograms during deployment. Perform check angiograms in the appropriate obliquity.

Fig. 42.11 Components of endoluminal graft available to treat endoleaks as a result of late endograft disintegration from a type III endoleak

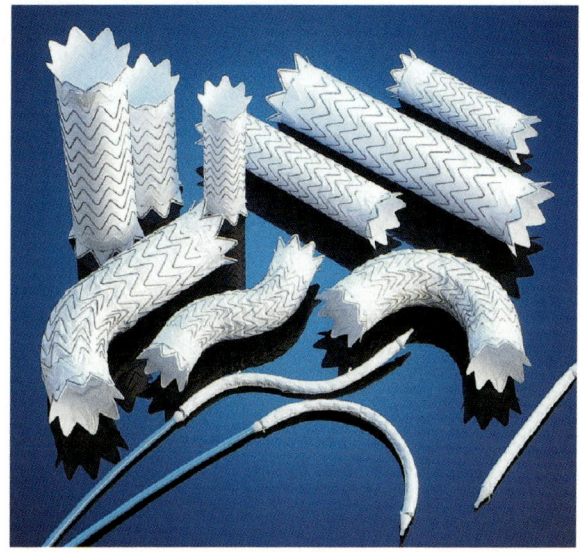

42.6 Complications Related to Vascular Access

This may consist of iliac artery rupture because of trauma caused by the large endograft delivery system. This is best treated by insertion of a covered stent. A supply of these should always be kept in stock.

42.6.1 General Complications

Stroke: Increased by excessive manipulations in the aortic arch. Increased by covering the left subclavian artery without bypass. Increased in the presence of atheroma in the aortic arch.

Paraplegia: Increased by endografting long lengths of thoracic aorta especially in patients with previous abdominal aortic repair. Paraplegia can be avoided by placement of a spinal drain when appropriate and by also increasing mean perfusion pressure above normal after endograft is deployed. Recommended mean arterial pressures should be above 80 mmHg.

Fever: may occur as a result of thrombosis of aneurysmal sac or the false lumen.

Reference

1. Diethrich EB, Ramaiah VG, Kpodonu J, Rodriguez JA. *Figures Courtesy of Endovascular and Hybrid Management of the Thoracic Aorta. A Case Based Approach*. 1st ed. West Sussex: Wiley-Blackwell; 2008.

Part XI
Future Technology

Chapter 43
Endovascular Management of Ascending Aortic Pathologies

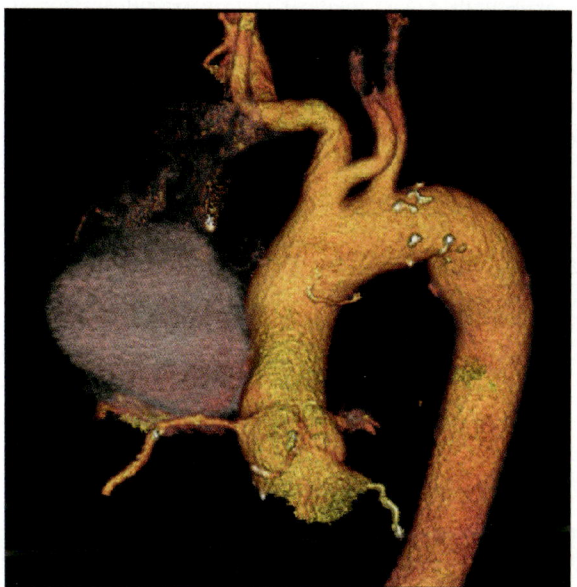

43.1 Introduction

Ascending aorta pseudoaneurysms are rare and occur infrequently from traumatic causes, infectious causes, anastomotic dehiscence of suture lines, and cannulation sites from previous aortic surgery.[1] Pseudoaneurysms of the ascending aorta are occasionally picked up on routine imaging for other causes. Computed tomography and angiography are the most common forms of diagnosis. A recent magnetic resonance imaging study found a pseudoaneurysm incidence of 13% associated with ascending aortic replacement.[2] Pseudoaneurysms of the ascending aorta are prone to rupture with fatal complications including death from pericardial tamponade, free rupture into the mediastinum, compressive symptoms of dyspnea, vocal cord

J. Kpodonu, *Manual of Thoracic Endoaortic Surgery*,
DOI 10.1007/978-1-84996-296-4_43, © Springer-Verlag London Limited 2010

paresis, or paralysis and pain. Indications for repair include compressive symptoms relating to the size of aneurysm and a maximum diameter of greater than 5.0 cm. The standard treatment involves replacing the diseased portion of the aorta with a Dacron patch that can sometimes require cardiopulmonary bypass. A redo median sternotomy offers a higher surgical risk to the patient and may be associated with a higher morbidity and mortality. A complete endovascular repair of ascending aortic pseudoaneurysms is an attractive option that can be offered in high surgical risk patients with suitable indications and amenable anatomy.

43.2 Case Scenario

A 74-year-old male with a past medical history significant for atrial fibrillation and pacemaker insertion was referred to our clinic to explore his options of an endovascular repair of his condition.[3,4] After the pacemaker implant, he developed an infective endocarditis of his mitral valve apparatus requiring replacement with mechanical valve prosthesis. His post-operative course was complicated by sternal wound dehiscence requiring extensive debridement of the sternum with a pectoral muscle flap reconstruction. Approximately 2 months after his mitral valve replacement, he developed fever and chills with blood cultures coming back positive. He was again diagnosed with a prosthetic valve infective endocarditis. A second mitral valve replacement was conducted using a porcine valve through a right thoracotomy with his post-operative course uneventful until 5 months after this most recent procedure. The patient was starting to complain of periodic episodes of chest discomfort. A chest X-ray revealed a mass on the ascending aorta suspicious for a pseudoaneurysm. A CT scan of the chest was performed which demonstrated a large pseudoaneurysm arising from the anterior aspect of the ascending aorta (Fig. 43.1).

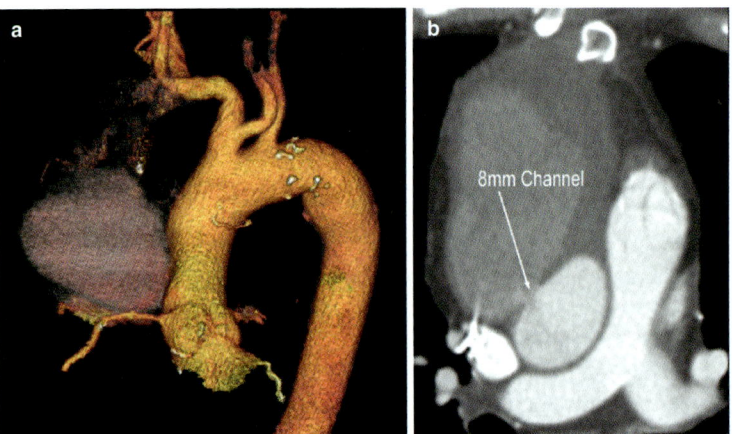

Fig. 43.1 (a, b) A 3D reconstruction depicting the location of the pseudoaneurysm in the ascending aorta. An oblique view of the same region shows the measurement of the defect

The pseudoaneurysm measured 7.6 cm × 8.0 cm and was thought to have originated from the cardioplegia site. Using reconstruction software, the specific defect
was identified with its width measuring 8 mm. He was felt to be at an extreme risk
for an open surgical repair and was consented for the use of an endovascular device
in an off-label fashion.

43.3 Endovascular Approach

The left common femoral artery was exposed and open retrograde cannulation using
an 18 G needle was done. The patient was heparinized and a sheath inserted to maintain wire access. Percutaneous retrograde cannulation of the right common femoral
artery was performed with an 18 G needle and similarly a 0.035 in. soft tip angled
glide wire was advanced into the thoracic aorta and a 5 Fr sheath exchanged. A
5 Fr pigtail angiographic catheter was advanced into the ascending aorta where
the anatomy was documented with an aortogram (Fig. 43.2a). The glide wire was
maneuvered so that it could transverse the defect and cannulate the pseudoaneurysm
sac. An aortogram of the sac was conducted to document all potential entry and exit
points (Fig. 43.2b). An intravascular ultrasound probe was loaded on the wire and
the probe advanced to the area of the defect. The width of the defect as measured by
IVUS was in agreement with measurements from the CT scan (Fig. 43.3), The defect
was 2 cm away from the right coronary artery and with the confirmed neck diameter of 8 mm, the patient was evaluated to be eligible to receive a septal occluder to
exclude the pseudoaneurysm sac. From the left groin, an Amplatzer septal occluder
(AGA Medical Corporation, Golden Valley, MN, USA) was advanced and deployed

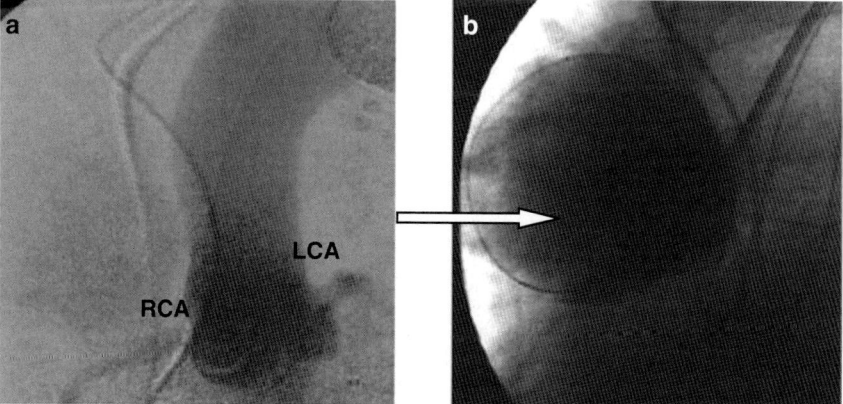

Fig. 43.2   (a, b) Dual angiograms demonstrating the ascending aorta pseudoaneurysm (*arrow*) as
well as the right (RCA) and left coronary (LCA) arteries

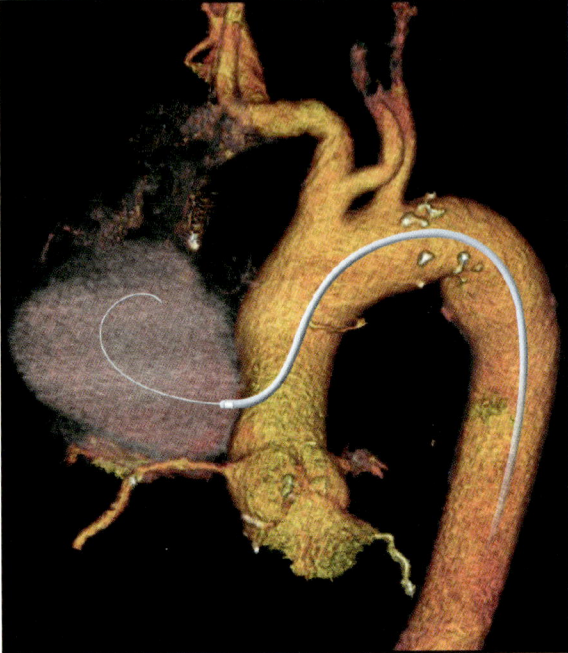

Fig. 43.3 An artist's illustration of the cannulation of the pseudoaneurysm

across the aortic pseudoaneurysm under fluoroscopic control (Fig. 43.4). The completion aortogram showed good position of the occluder device and minimal leak through the device (Fig. 43.5). The bilateral groins were closed in the usual fashion and the patient was transferred to the recovery room. His post-operative computed tomography scans revealed complete occlusion of the neck of the pseudoaneurysm (Fig. 43.6). He was discharged home in stable condition. Since the surgery, he has not had any complications or significant medical events. Surveillance imaging indicates that the pseudoaneurysm is starting to regress in size, with no evidence of arterial filling.

43.4 Discussion

Pseudoaneurysms of the ascending aorta can arise from cannulation sites from aortic perfusion catheters, cardioplegia cannulation sites, origin of saphenous vein grafts conduits, and aortotomy sites from aortic valve replacement during cardiopulmonary bypass. Pseudoaneurysms of the ascending aorta and aortic arch are difficult to treat with open surgical techniques associated with considerable morbidity and mortality due to the redo median sternotomy.

Total endovascular management of the ascending aorta while an attractive option is still in its infancy and requires an in-depth knowledge of the surgical anatomy. The

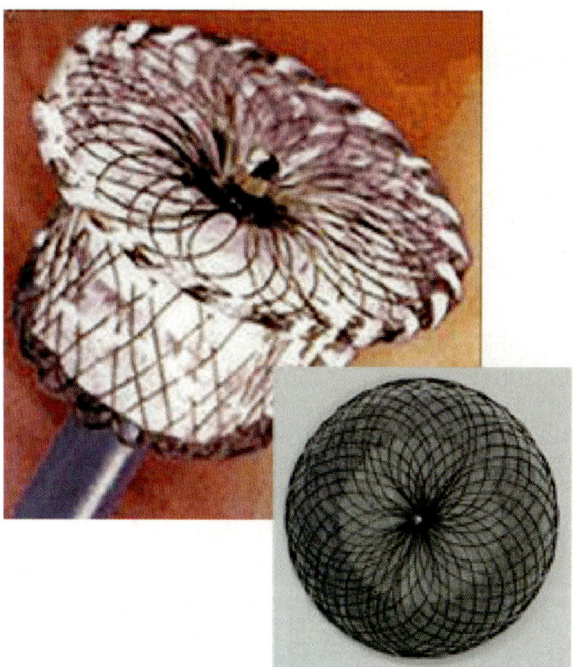

Fig. 43.4 An Amplatzer septal occluder (AGA Medical Corporation, Golden Valley, MN, USA) used to close the neck of the pseudoaneurysm

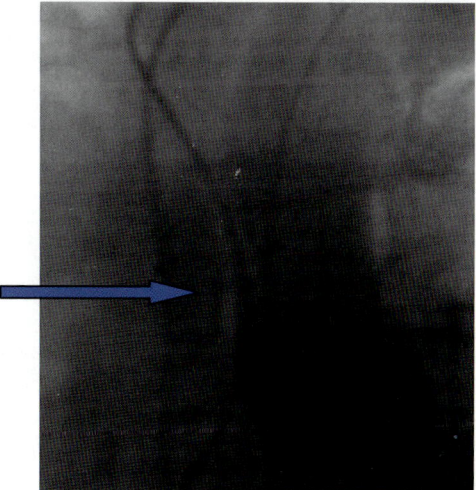

Fig. 43.5 A completion angiogram showing the postion of the Amplatzer with a slight blush of contrast in the pseudoaneurysm sac

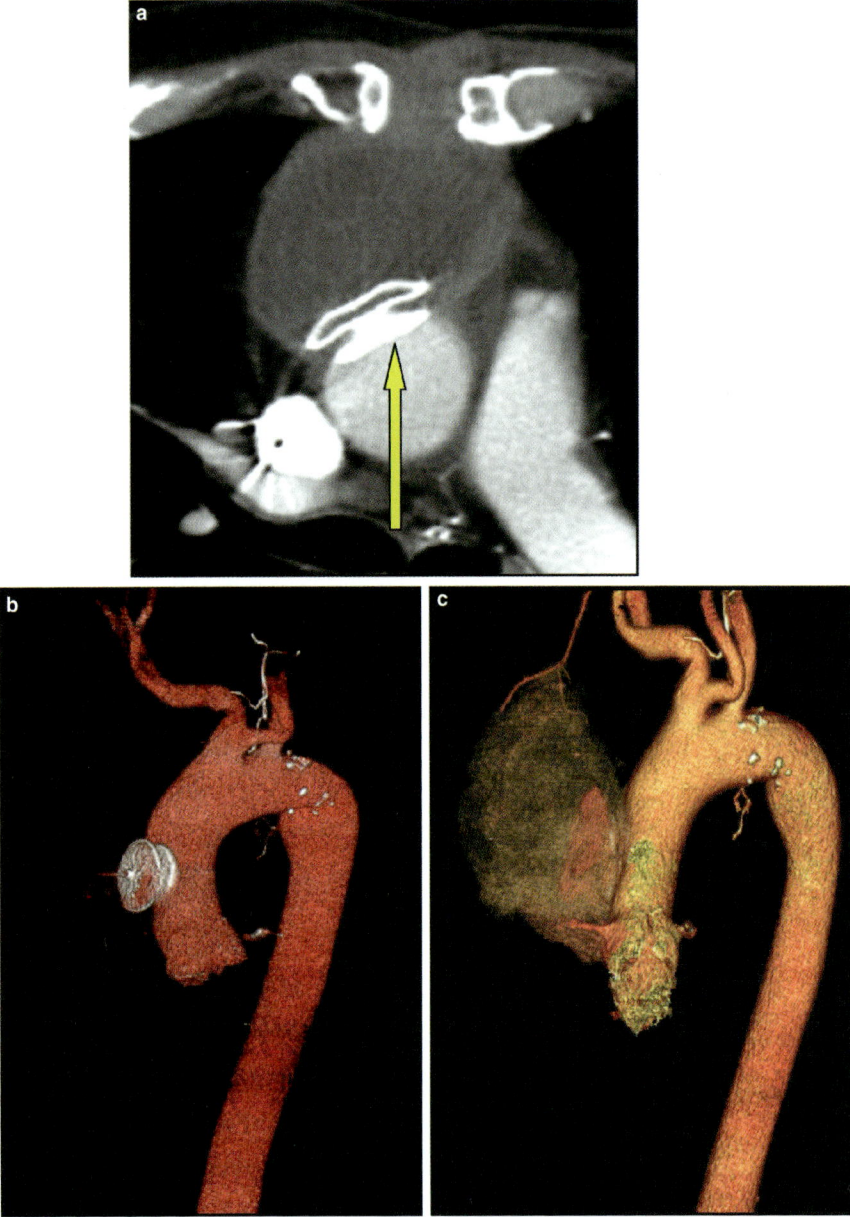

Fig. 43.6 (**a–c**) Sixty-four slice CT scan images demonstrating exclusion of the ascending aortic pseudoaneurysm with an Amplatzer occluder (*yellow arrow*). There are no signs of an endoleak

complex anatomy of the sinotubular junction, the variations in the aortic pathology, and the presentation of disease require a unique approach to each patient. The majority of ascending aortic aneurysms are atherosclerotic that will eventually require an elective replacement when the diameter is 6.0 cm or greater. There is no commercially available endoluminal graft for the management of ascending aortic pathology. Application of endoluminal graft technology to the ascending aorta has to take into account the short landing zones and the possibility of flow obstruction to both coronary artery circulation and the brachiocephalic vessels. In the past, customized grafts incorporating Gianturco Z stents and PTFE have been constructed to create grafts of varying diameters and lengths suitable for use in the ascending aorta.

Combination of endovascular techniques using coil embolization,[5] endoluminal grafts, and septa occluders[6] can be used to treat pseudoaneurysms of the ascending aorta. The application of the Amplatzer atrial septal occluder device to exclude a pseudoaneurysm of the ascending aorta is a novel technique which requires a discrete neck for deployment. Intravascular ultrasound approved to be a useful tool in determining or confirming the exact diameter of the neck for careful selection of the appropriately sized device.

In conclusion, the continued evolution of medical imaging and with improvements in device technology may make the ascending aorta more amenable to a total endovascular repair. Endograft design would need to address the challenges presented by the origin of the coronary arteries, the innominate artery, and the aortic valve. A concept device for the future would have components that would allow side branches for coronary artery perfusions and a method to affix the graft to the aortic wall, perhaps with the use of endostaples. For now, simple endovascular repair of the ascending aorta will remain a rare occurrence until the technological hurdles are beaten.

References

1. Sullivan KL, Steiner RM, Smullens SN, Griska L, Meister SG. Pesudoaneurysm of the ascending aorta following cardiac surgery. *Chest.* 1988;93:138–143.
2. Hatfield DR, Fried AM, Ellis GT, Mattingly Jr WT, Todd EP. Intraoperative control of an ascending aortic pseudo aneurysm by Fogarty balloon catheter: a combined radiologic and surgical approach. *Radiology.* 1980;135:515–517.
3. Kpodonu J, Wheatley GH 3rd, Ramaiah VG, Rodriguez-Lopez JA, Strumpf RK, Diethrich EB. Endovascular repair of an ascending aortic pseudoaneurysm with a septal occluder device: mid-term follow-up. *Ann Thorac Surg.* 2008;85(1):349–351.
4. Diethrich EB, Ramaiah VG, Kpodonu J, Rodriguez JA. *Endovascular and Hybrid Management of the Thoracic Aorta. A Case Based Approach.* 1st ed. West Sussex: Wiley-Blackwell; 2008.
5. Lin PH, Busch RL, Tong FC, Chaikof E, Martin LG, Lumsden AB. Intra-arterial thrombin injection of n ascending aortic pseudo aneurysm complicated by transient ischemic attack and rescued with systemic abciximab. *J Vasc Surg.* 2001;34:939–942.
6. Komanapalli CB, Burch G, Tripathy U, Slater MS, Song HK. Percutaneous repair of an ascending aortic pseudo aneurysm with a septal occluder device. *J Thorac Cardiovasc Surg.* 2005;130:603–604.

Chapter 44
Use of a Remote Wireless Pressure Sensor for Post-operative Surveillance of Thoracic Endoluminal Grafts

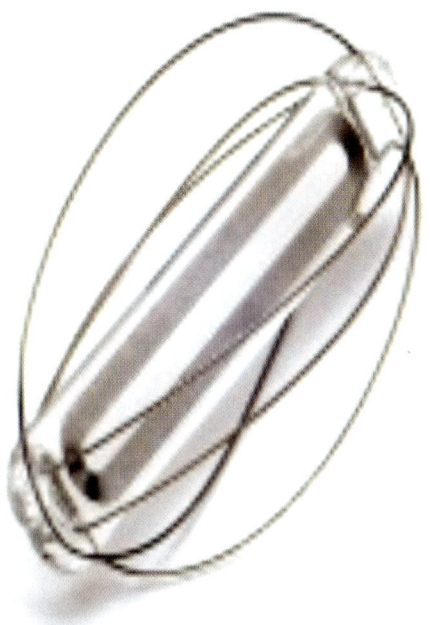

44.1 Introduction

Thoracic endografting for the treatment of thoracic aortic aneurysms requires life-long post-operative surveillance using various imaging techniques. Currently, the entirety of exclusion or absence of endoleaks is evaluated by intra-operative angiography and post-operative CT scans. Multiple contrast injections can lead to an increased risk of contrast-induced nephropathy as well as increased radiation to both patient and surgeon. Remote wireless pressure sensor monitoring is a new

J. Kpodonu, *Manual of Thoracic Endoaortic Surgery*,
DOI 10.1007/978-1-84996-296-4_44, © Springer-Verlag London Limited 2010

technology with potential benefit for post-operative surveillance of thoracic endo-grafts without the added risk of radiation exposure or contrast-induced nephropathy. Advantages of this new technology include frequent evaluations with multiple examinations performed on a given patient at any time within the year; systemic pressurization may be detected much earlier within a previously excluded aneurysm and lead to prompt evaluation and treatment. The microelectromechanical (MEMS) technology of the EndoSure sensor is currently being studied for use in the false lumen evaluation of treated type B dissections, blood pressure evaluation, and heart failure monitoring. The Acute Pressure Measurement to Confirm Aneurysm Sac Exclusion Trial (APEX) data demonstrated the efficacy of immediate exclusion of an abdominal aortic aneurysm sac using the pressure sensor with agreement between the sensor measurements and angiography regarding detection of type I and III endoleaks in 92.1% ($n = 70$) with a sensitivity of 94% and a specificity of 80%.[1-3] The data collected in this study led the Food and Drug Administration (FDA) to approve the device for the implantation in an abdominal aortic aneurysm prior to endoluminal graft exclusion.

44.2 Case Scenario

A 71-year-old woman with multiple co-morbidities including hypertension, severe COPD, and renal dysfunction underwent a CT scan of the chest for the assessment of pain that was radiating to her back. She was found to have a 6.5 cm × 5.1 cm saccular aneurysm (Fig. 44.1). She was not a suitable candidate for open surgical repair and was offered a less invasive approach using an endoluminal graft. In order to reduce her exposure to radiation and the risk of contrast-induced nephropathy associated with repeated CT scans, she was chosen to receive an EndoSure wireless pressure sensor (CardioMEMS, Inc., Atlanta, GA) for the surveillance of her tho-racic aneurysm. The sensor would be deployed during the same procedure used to insert and implant the endoluminal graft for her aneurysm (Fig. 44.2).

44.3 Technical Details

Under general anesthesia, open retrograde cannulation of the right common femoral artery was performed with an 18 G needle and a 0.035 in. soft tip angled glide wire was passed into the distal thoracic aorta and exchanged for a 9 Fr sheath under fluoroscopic visualization. Percutaneous access of the left common femoral artery was similarly performed and a 5 Fr sheath introduced. Five thousand units of heparin was given to keep the activated clotted time greater than 200 s. A 5 Fr angiographic pigtail catheter was advanced through the left groin sheath into the thoracic aorta. The fluoroscopic C-arm was positioned in a left anterior oblique angle and an oblique thoracic arch aortogram was performed to visualize the arch

Fig. 44.1 A 64-slice CT scan
of the chest demonstrating a
saccular aneurysm measuring
6.5 cm × 5.1 cm

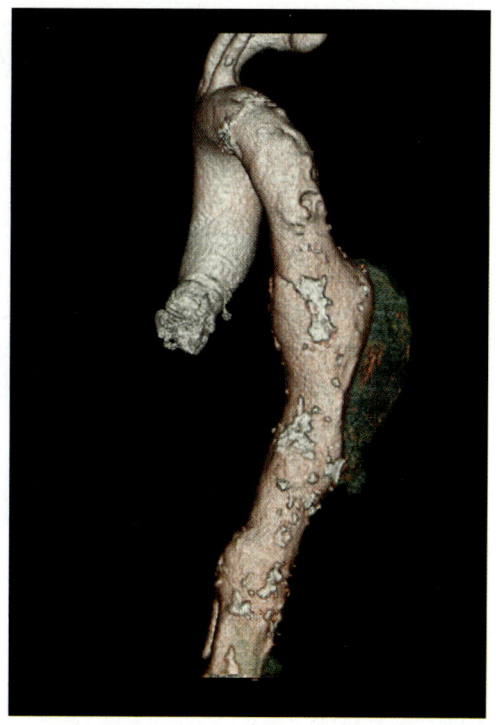

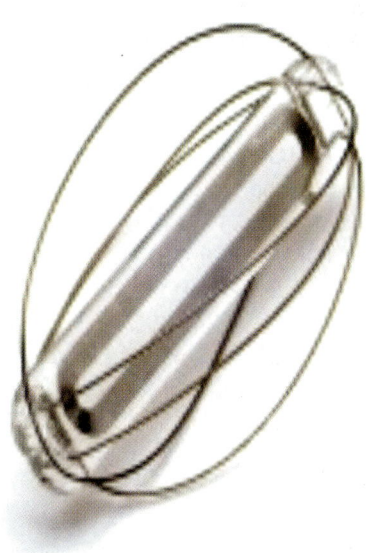

Fig. 44.2 An EndoSure
wireless pressure sensor
(CardioMEMS, Inc., Atlanta,
GA)

Fig. 44.3 A pre-deployment
angiogram demonstrating a
descending thoracic
aneurysm

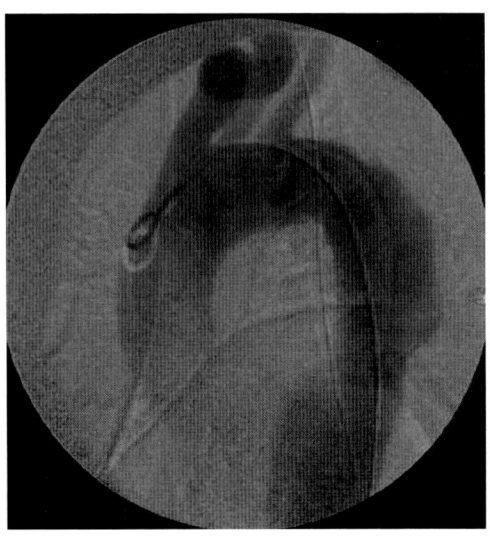

vessels and the descending thoracic aortic aneurysm (Fig. 44.3). Intravascular ultrasound (IVUS) using a 7 Fr probe (Volcano Therapeutics, Inc.) was performed. Based
on the measurements, a 34 mm × 15 cm Gore TAG (W.L. Gore, Flagstaff, AZ)
graft was chosen. The IVUS catheter was exchanged for an extra stiff 260 cm wire
Lunderquist (Cook, Bloomington, IN). An angiogram was performed to evaluate
the aneurysm sac with careful attention paid to the amount of free-flowing blood
contained within the sac. To properly deploy the sensor, a pocket free of thrombus
would be needed to ensure that the EndoSure sensor would not be crushed upon
deployment of the endoluminal graft. Crushing of the sensor can lead to erroneous
readings. Once eligibility was validated, a 30 mm × 15 mm EndoSure wireless
pressure sensor (Fig. 44.2) was loaded on a long delivery sheath through the left
groin and deployed into the aneurysm sac. The right 9 Fr sheath was exchanged for
a 22 Fr Gore sheath and a 34 mm × 15 cm TAG stent graft device was advanced
through the Gore sheath and subsequently deployed over an extra stiff wire. The
device was deployed within an area that had previously been identified for suitable
landing zones and marked on a "road map" angiogram. A Gore tri-lobe balloon was
used to perform post-deployment balloon angioplasty to the proximal and distal
segments of the graft to ensure proper apposition. Pressure readings taken from the
sensor before and post-exclusion of the aneurysm are shown in Fig. 44.4. An overall reduction in systolic, diastolic, and mean pressures can be seen with the pulse
pressure reduced to 0.54 mmHg immediately after endoluminal graft deployment.
A completion angiogram demonstrated exclusion of the aneurysm with no endoleak
(Fig. 44.5). All wires and sheaths were removed; the right common femoral artery
was closed in a transverse fashion with restoration of flow. A 6 Fr Angioseal closure

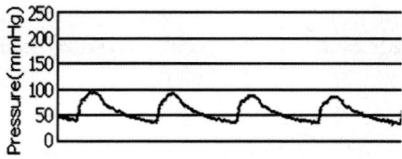
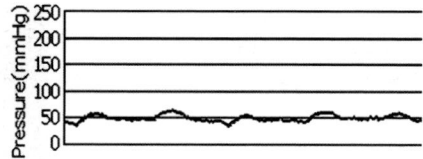

	Sensor	Art. Line	Ratio
Systolic	94	98	
Diastolic	30	38	
Mean	56	59	
Pulse	64	60	1.07

	Sensor	Cuff	Ratio
Systolic	62	107	
Diastolic	32	51	
Mean	47	70	
Pulse	30	56	0.54

Pre- Exclusion   **Post-Exclusion**

Fig. 44.4 Pre- and post-exclusion of pressure tracing readings from the EndoSure wireless pressure sensor (CardioMEMS, Inc., Atlanta, GA)

device was deployed to the left common femoral artery. Prior to leaving the OR, the patient was extubated and bilateral peripheral pulses were documented. A CT scan of the chest performed the following day showed exclusion of the descending thoracic aneurysm with no endoleak noted (Fig. 44.6). She was discharged home on the second post-operative day (POD #2) in satisfactory condition.

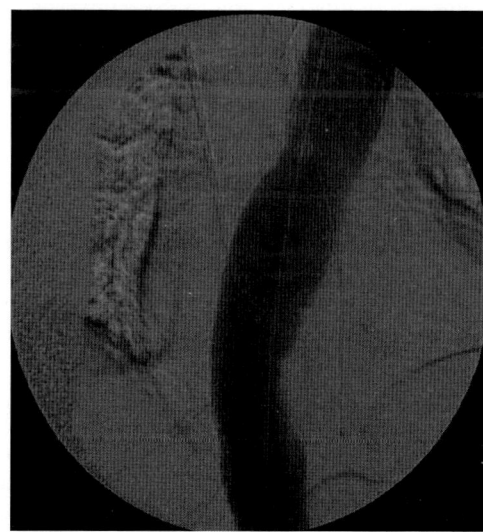

Fig. 44.5 A post-deployment angiogram showing exclusion of the aneurysm with no demonstrable endoleak

Fig. 44.6 Three-dimensional
reconstruction documents the
position of the wireless
pressure sensor within the
aneurysm sac

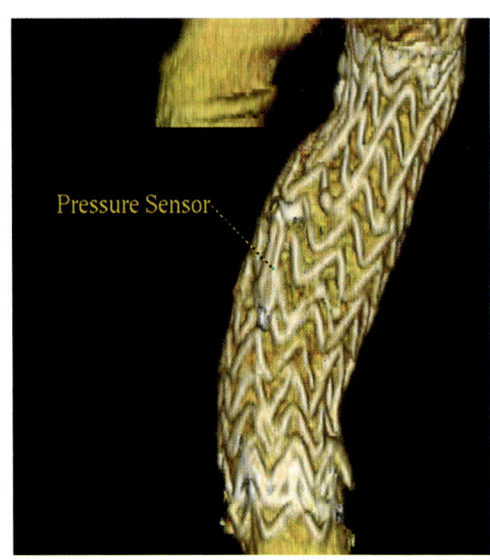

44.4 Discussion

The EndoSure wireless pressure sensor (CardioMEMS, Inc., Atlanta, GA) is primarily used for the surveillance of abdominal and lately thoracic aortic aneurysms. The sensor is deployed during the same procedure used to insert and implant the endoluminal graft for her aneurysm.[4,5] Advantages of this new technology include frequent evaluations with multiple examinations performed on a given patient at any time within the year; systemic pressurization may be detected much earlier within a previously excluded aneurysm and lead to prompt evaluation and treatment. The microelectromechanical (MEMS) technology of the EndoSure sensor is currently being studied for use in the false lumen evaluation of treated type B dissections, blood pressure evaluation, and heart failure monitoring. In conclusion, remote pressure sensing may, in the future, eliminate the need for serial contrast-enhanced CT scans as part of a post-operative surveillance program for thoracic aneurysms.

References

1. Baum RA, Carpenter JP, Cope C, et al. Aneurysm sac pressure measurements after endovascular repair of abdominal aortic aneurysms. *J Vasc Surg*. 2001;33:32–41.
2. Ohki T, Yadav J, Gargiulo N, et al. Preliminary results of an implantable wireless aneurysm pressure sensor in a canine model: will surveillance CT scan following endovascular AAA repair become obsolete? *J Endovasc Ther*. 2003;10(suppl. I):32.
3. Ohki T, Ouriel K, Silveira PG, et al. Initial results of wireless pressure sensing for endovascular aneurysm repair: the APEX Trial-Acute pressure measurement to confirm aneurysm sac exclusion. *J Vasc Surg*. 2007;45(2):236–242.

4. Kpodonu J, Ramaiah VG, Williams J, Shennib H, Diethrich EB. Novel way to confirm successful endovascular repair of a thoracic aortic aneurysm using a remote wireless pressure sensor. *Ann Thorac Surg*. 2007;84(1):272–274.
5. Diethrich EB, Ramaiah VG, Kpodonu J, Rodriguez JA. *Endovascular and Hybrid Management of the Thoracic Aorta. A Case Based Approach*. 1st ed. West Sussex: Wiley-Blackwell; 2008.

Index

J. Kpodonu, *Manual of Thoracic Endoaortic Surgery*,
DOI 10.1007/978-1-84996-296-4, © Springer-Verlag London Limited 2010